Mechanical Ventilation for Respiratory Failure

Demystifying the Box in the Corner of the Room

Mechanical Ventilation for Respiratory Failure

Demystifying the Box in the Corner of the Room

Editors

Richard M. Schwartzstein, MD

Ellen and Melvin Gordon Distinguished Professor of Medicine and
   Medical Education
Chief, Division of Pulmonary, Critical Care and Sleep Medicine
Department of Medicine
Harvard Medical School
Beth Israel Deaconess Medical Center
Boston, Massachusetts

Jeremy B. Richards, MD, MA

Chair of the Department of Medical Education
Department of Medical Education
Harvard Medical School
Mount Auburn Hospital
Cambridge, Massachusetts

Elias Baedorf Kassis, MD

Medical and Scientific Director of Respiratory Care
Assistant Professor of Medicine
Division of Pulmonary, Critical Care and Sleep Medicine
Department of Medicine
Harvard Medical School
Beth Israel Deaconess Medical Center
Boston, Massachusetts

 Wolters Kluwer

Philadelphia · Baltimore · New York · London
Buenos Aires · Hong Kong · Sydney · Tokyo

Senior Acquisitions Editor: Keith Donnellan
Senior Development Editor: Ashley Fischer
Editorial Coordinator: Vinodhini Varadharajalu
Marketing Manager: Kirsten Watrud
Production Project Manager: Matt West
Manager, Graphic Arts & Design: Stephen Druding
Manufacturing Coordinator: Bernard Tomboc
Prepress Vendor: S4Carlisle Publishing Services

Library of Congress Cataloging-in-Publication Data

ISBN-13: 978-1-975171-09-4

ISBN-10: 1-975171-09-8

Library of Congress Control Number: 2023908279

Contributors

Elias Baedorf Kassis, MD
Medical and Scientific Director of Respiratory Care
Assistant Professor of Medicine
Division of Pulmonary, Critical Care and Sleep
* Medicine*
Department of Medicine
Harvard Medical School
Beth Israel Deaconess Medical Center
Boston, Massachusetts

Diana Bouhassira, MD
Physician
Department of Pulmonary and Critical Care Medicine
The Johns Hopkins University School of Medicine
Baltimore, Maryland

Jakub Glowala, MD
Resident
Department of Medicine
McGaw Medical Center of Northwestern University
Chicago, Illinois

Sarah Ohnigian, MD
Instructor in Medicine
Harvard Medical School
Attending Physician
Beth Israel Deaconess Medical Center
Boston, Massachusetts

Jeremy B. Richards, MD, MA
Chair of the Department of Medical Education
Department of Medical Education
Harvard Medical School
Boston, Massachusetts
Mount Auburn Hospital
Cambridge, Massachusetts

Richard M. Schwartzstein, MD
Ellen and Melvin Gordon Distinguished Professor of
* Medicine and Medical Education*
Chief, Division of Pulmonary, Critical Care and
* Sleep Medicine*
Department of Medicine
Harvard Medical School
Beth Israel Deaconess Medical Center
Boston, Massachusetts

Kavitha C. Selvan, MD
Pulmonary and Critical Care Fellow
Department of Internal Medicine
The University of Chicago Pritzker School of Medicine
Chicago, Illinois

Ali Trainor, MD
Senior Fellow
Harvard Combined Fellowship in Pulmonary and
* Critical Care Medicine*
Massachusetts General Hospital and Beth Israel
* Deaconess Medical Center*
Boston, Massachusetts

Emmett A. Kistler, MD
Clinical Fellow
Division of Pulmonary and Critical Care
Department of Medicine
Beth Israel Deaconess Medical Center
Massachusetts General Hospital
Boston, Massachusetts

Jonah Rubin, MD
Instructor in Medicine
Harvard Medical School
Attending Physician
Division of Pulmonary and Critical Care Medicine
Corrigan Minehan Heart Center ICU
Massachusetts General Hospital
Boston, Massachusetts

Ryan Kronen, MD
Fellow in Global and Rural Health
Department of Medicine, Division of Allergy and
  Infectious Diseases
University of Washington School of Medicine
St. Louis, Missouri

Preface

Your patient is gasping for air, struggling to breathe. The monitor shows that the patient's oxygen saturation, obtained from the pulse oximeter on the patient's finger, is dropping into the 80s despite supplemental oxygen. You proceed with intubation and initiation of mechanical ventilation—now what do you do?

Patients with respiratory failure who require invasive mechanical ventilation are among the sickest in the hospital. Getting oxygen into the blood and carbon dioxide out of the body are among the most critical functions of the respiratory system, necessary to maintain aerobic metabolism and normal acid-base function. Positive pressure ventilators, at their core, are fairly simple pumps, but the multiple options for setting the parameters by which the pump functions, the sometimes-dizzying array of abbreviations to describe what the pump is doing, and the range of numbers and alarms on the machine can be daunting for healthcare providers, from nurses to respiratory therapists to medical students and residents and fellows in training. This book is designed to take the mystery out of mechanical ventilators and reduce the anxiety often associated with managing intubated and ventilated patients with acute respiratory failure.

The book is divided into four sections to guide you from the basic physiology of respiratory failure to some of the newest advances in ventilatory support. Providing care for acutely ill patients with respiratory failure requires not only that you know *what* to do but *why* you are doing it. For this reason, we start with Section 1, *Physiological Principles Underlying Respiratory Failure and Mechanical Ventilation*. Respiratory failure can be viewed as a malfunction of one or more components of the respiratory system, and mechanical ventilators provide the support missing from the broken component. The respiratory system can be conceptually and functionally divided into three parts—the respiratory system controller, the ventilatory pump, and the gas exchanger in the lungs. With this conceptual foundation, you will have the baseline knowledge and understanding to be ready to tackle the intricacies of the ventilator.

Section 2 provides the *Basics of Mechanical Ventilation*. These chapters address core principles underlying volume and pressure ventilation, pressure support ventilation, and positive end-expiratory pressure. You will be guided through initial settings of the ventilator and core elements of monitoring the status of the intubated and ventilated patient. This section also addresses the approach to liberating or "weaning" the patient from mechanical support and the uses of noninvasive forms of mechanical ventilation.

In Section 3, we address the *Application of Mechanical Ventilation to Common Disease States* from chronic obstructive pulmonary disease (COPD) to acute respiratory distress syndrome (ARDS) to interstitial lung disease (ILD), as well as complications associated with mechanical ventilation. Finally, in Section 4, we consider *Special Topics in Mechanical Ventilation*, which will provide you with a glimpse of contemporary issues gaining greater attention in the last few years including ventilator asynchrony and the use of esophageal balloons to guide decisions about acceptable pressures delivered during inspiration with the ventilator. We also address the growing concern about provoking dyspnea in our patients with the settings we select with mechanical ventilators; dyspnea and distress during mechanical ventilation can contribute to significant mental health issues in survivors.

At all times in this textbook, we emphasize *understanding*, not just knowing. Throughout the book, we frequently refer back to some of the early physiology chapters to remind you to review that material if it did not make sense on your first reading, and to emphasize how each concept or application builds upon core material. Each chapter also includes several case vignettes with multiple choice questions to highlight concrete clinical applications of the concepts covered and to enable you to assess your understanding of these principles and your ability to apply them clinically.

We hope you enjoy your exploration of mechanical ventilation and find the care of patients with respiratory failure as rewarding as we do.

Richard M. Schwartzstein, MD
Jeremy B. Richards, MD, MA
Elias Baedorf Kassis, MD

Contents

Physiologic Principles Underlying Respiratory Failure Mechanical Ventilation

Overview of Respiratory Failure

Richard M. Schwartzstein

LEARNING OBJECTIVES

- Describe the components of the respiratory system and why respiratory failure should be viewed as a "system" problem rather than a malfunction of the lungs alone.
- Explain how derangements of each component may lead to respiratory failure.
- Outline the ways in which the mechanical ventilator may "fix" or replace the malfunctioning part of the respiratory system.

INTRODUCTION

"The patient is going into respiratory failure! They need to be intubated, STAT!" The comments and cries for help can be heard almost daily in every hospital. Patients arrive with pneumonia or heart failure or get too much fluid during their admission or develop other complications of treatment and diseases that lead to a low oxygen level (Pa_{O_2}) or elevated carbon dioxide level (Pa_{CO_2}). Institution of mechanical ventilation can be lifesaving, and managing the patients with this intervention requires skills not often taught in medical school. This section of the book will provide you with a refresher on some of the basic physiologic principles of the respiratory system that are key to understanding the mechanical ventilator and the best ways to use it to support a patient in respiratory failure.

Although we often think of respiratory failure as the consequence of problems with the lungs, probably because of our focus on the blood gases (partial pressures of oxygen and carbon dioxide), the reality is that respiratory failure is really a "system" problem; the respiratory system no longer functions adequately to maintain life. For us to maintain life we need a functioning respiratory system thought of broadly as all the things necessary to get oxygen from the atmosphere to the blood and carbon dioxide back out. This perspective will help you understand how ventilators are constructed and how best to manipulate them in the care of your patients.

Let's start with a definition—what is respiratory failure? How do you decide a patient is in respiratory failure? Some will rely on a particular level of Pao_2 or $Paco_2$, but what level should we choose? Pao_2 less than 60 mm Hg? $Paco_2$ greater than 50? If you take care of patients with chronic lung disease, they often have blood gases that meet these criteria, but are nevertheless living relatively normal lives outside the hospital—are they in respiratory failure? Similar conundrums come up when we consider definitions for heart failure or renal failure. Does a specific level of ejection fraction or creatinine denote heart or renal failure and, if so, what does that mean for the patient?

The reality is that as humans we are blessed with a large "physiologic reserve." If one removes a lung, most people do quite well, assuming the remaining lung is normal. The same can be said of the renal system; a nephrectomy can be performed without causing major problems for the individual with one normal kidney remaining. When an individual experiences a myocardial infarction, damage is done to the heart, but in most instances, the patient does quite well after recovery from the acute incident.

So, how should we define "respiratory failure?" I think the simplest construct is that acute respiratory failure is a condition in which there is an abnormality of the respiratory system, which, if not corrected immediately, will lead to death if the patient is not treated with mechanical ventilation. Key to this definition is that we are looking at the entire respiratory system, not just the lungs.

This chapter provides an overview of respiratory failure as a failure of the respiratory system, which will serve as the basis for Chapters 2 to 4 and an understanding of how the mechanical ventilator replaces or supplements the broken parts of the system. This approach will assist in demystifying the ventilator and help you become comfortable with the basic function of the machine and the rationale for the changes you may need to make to optimize care for your patient.

THE RESPIRATORY SYSTEM

The goals of the respiratory system are to move, by bulk flow, gas from the outside world to the alveolus, where oxygen and carbon dioxide diffuse between the blood and alveolus, and then back to mouth by bulk flow. To achieve this function three components of the respiratory system are required: the respiratory controller, the ventilatory pump, and the gas exchanger (**Table 1-1**).

The Respiratory Controller

Why do we breathe? What determines the depth of our breaths? In the 5 seconds between breaths, how hypoxemic do we become? How hypercapnic? In fact, in the time between normal breaths, we cannot measure the changes in Pao_2 or $Paco_2$ because they are so small. Although major changes in blood levels of oxygen and carbon dioxide will stimulate the

TABLE 1-1	Components of the Respiratory System	
Element	**Function**	**Components**
Controller	To determine the rate and depth of breathing	Inspiratory neurons in the medulla Reticular activating system
Ventilatory pump	To create pressure to move gas from the mouth to the alveolus and back to the mouth	Bones of the chest wall (eg, ribs, sternum, clavicle, spine); pleural surfaces; airways; muscles of the chest wall
Gas exchanger	To diffuse oxygen into the blood and remove carbon dioxide from the blood	Pulmonary alveoli, pulmonary vasculature

peripheral and central chemoreceptors, thereby increasing the activity of the central controller, derangements in blood gases are not the stimulus for our regular breathing in the resting state.

When we sleep (or are unconscious), we have a central pattern generator in our brainstem that sets the rate and depth of breathing. Inspiratory neurons have a firing frequency, much like a pacemaker, that stimulates the inspiratory muscles to initiate a breath. When awake, however, other factors come into play. The reticular activating system, also located in the brainstem distinct from the inspiratory neurons, is a key component of the brain responsible for attention and sensation and appears to be a major element in "wakefulness." When awake, our breathing is not dependent on the activity of the brainstem. We know this because of an unusual group of people who are born with an abnormality in the region of the brainstem where the central pattern generator is located. These individuals, who are characterized as having congenital central hypoventilation syndrome (CCHS), stop breathing when they go to sleep but breathe relatively normally when awake; at night, they must be sustained with a mechanical ventilator, but when awake, they breathe quite normally. Thus, wakefulness or some element of the reticular activating system must be playing a role in our control of breathing when awake.

The cortex of the brain also has a key role to play in the control of breathing. Unlike many other vital functions of the body, for example, heart rate or peristalsis, we can speed up, slow down, or stop our breathing with conscious thought, at least to some degree. Given this additional level of control, our emotions and behaviors also affect our breathing.

There are multiple sources of information that feed into the controller that will modify the rate and depth of breathing, particularly during disease states (**Table 1-2**). Our peripheral chemoreceptors are stimulated by low Pao_2, high $Paco_2$, and low pH while the central chemoreceptors respond to high $Paco_2$ and low pH; messages are sent to the central controller from the chemoreceptors to change the rate and depth of breathing. Similarly, receptors from stretch and irritant receptors in the lungs, pulmonary vasculature, and right ventricle also play a role in the control of ventilation by sending signals to the central control regions of the brain (**Figure 1-1**). J-receptors in the lung respond to high pulmonary capillary pressures associated with heart failure, whereas irritant receptors in the airways are probably involved in the tachypnea associated with inhalation of noxious chemicals and the inflammation of respiratory infections. The lung contains slowly adapting receptors, some of which respond to stretch. Typically, expansion of the lung stimulates receptors that diminish the drive to breathe, whereas deflation (eg, atelectasis) increases the activity of the central controller. Part of the reason we "sigh" may be from stimuli from small regions of the lung that collapses because of repetitive small breaths (ie, when our tidal volume is low and relatively uniform).

TABLE 1-2 Examples of Pathologic Causes of Changes in Respiratory Control

Condition	Mechanism	Effect on Controller
Drug overdose	Depression of central controller	Decreased ventilation
Congestive heart failure	Stimulation of vascular receptor and J-receptors	Increased ventilation
Interstitial pneumonia	Stimulation of irritant receptors	Increased ventilation
Pulmonary embolism	Stimulation of vascular receptors	Increased ventilation
Pleural effusion	Stimulation of pulmonary stretch receptors	Increased ventilation
Acute asthma	Stimulation of irritant receptors in airways	Increased ventilation

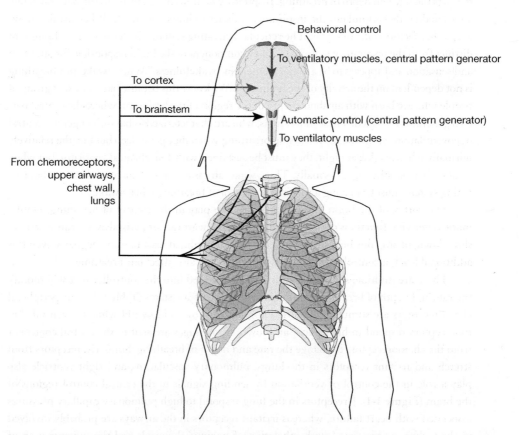

Figure 1-1: **The elements of ventilatory control.** Multiple factors contribute to the control of breathing. Conscious or volitional control arises from the cerebral cortex, and automatic control emanates from the brainstem. Information from mechanical and chemoreceptors throughout the respiratory system modulates the activity of the control centers. (From The Controller: Directing the Orchestra. In: Schwartzstein RM, Parker MJ. *Respiratory Physiology: A Clinical Approach.* Wolters Kluwer; 2006:126-148. Figure 6.1.)

The Ventilatory Pump

Bulk flow of gas from mouth to alveolus and back requires a pump, which is provided by the constituents and properties of the lungs and chest wall. The elements of the ventilatory pump include bones (ribs, vertebral bodies, sternum), muscles (intercostals, diaphragm, accessory muscles of ventilation such as the sternocleidomastoids and abdominal muscles), peripheral nerves that connect the controller to the muscles, pleura (which links motion of the chest wall to the lungs), the connective tissue of the chest wall and lungs, which provide elastic properties to these structures, and the airways that conduct the flow of gas from mouth to alveolus and back again (**Figure 1-2**). Failure of one of these elements may lead to respiratory failure as seen in a range of diseases (eg, neuromuscular disease such as polio or myasthenia gravis, abnormalities of the chest wall such as flail chest associated with trauma, and airways disease such as status asthmaticus) (**Table 1-3**).

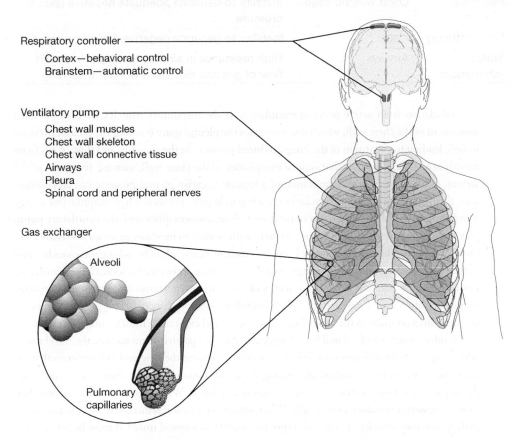

Respiratory controller
Cortex—behavioral control
Brainstem—automatic control

Ventilatory pump
Chest wall muscles
Chest wall skeleton
Chest wall connective tissue
Airways
Pleura
Spinal cord and peripheral nerves

Gas exchanger
Alveoli
Pulmonary capillaries

Figure 1-2: The components of the respiratory system. The respiratory system is composed of three key components: the controller, the ventilatory pump, and the gas exchanger. Each of these components has several elements. To achieve the functional goals of the respiratory system, each of these elements must be working effectively and in an integrated manner. To understand the way that diseases affect breathing and the ways that the body tries to compensate for these impairments and restore homeostasis, you must have a solid appreciation of the physiology of each of these parts. (From Getting Started: The Approach to Respiratory Physiology. In: Schwartzstein RM, Parker MJ. *Respiratory Physiology: A Clinical Approach*. Wolters Kluwer; 2006:1-8. Figure 1.1.)

TABLE 1-3 Examples of Pathologic Abnormalities in the Ventilatory Pump Leading to Respiratory Failure

Disease	Part of Ventilatory Pump Affected	Mechanism of Respiratory Failure
Poliomyelitis	Peripheral nerves	Inability to generate adequate negative pleural pressure
Myasthenia gravis	Peripheral nerves	Inability to generate adequate negative pleural pressure
Guillain-Barré	Peripheral nerves	Inability to generate negative pleural pressure
Kyphoscoliosis	Chest wall/rib cage	Decreased compliance of chest wall→ inadequate negative pleural pressure
Flail chest	Chest wall/rib cage	Inability to generate adequate negative pleural pressure
Pneumothorax	Pleura	Inability to generate negative pleural pressure
Status asthmaticus	Airways	High resistance in airways leading to reduced flow of gas and increased work of breathing

Inhalation is an active process; stimulation of the inspiratory muscles leads to outward movement of the chest wall, which decompresses the pleural space (causing the pleural pressure to fall), leading to expansion of the lungs, reduced pressure in the alveolus, and flow of gas from mouth to alveolus. Diseases that reduce compliance of the chest wall, increase resistance of the airway, or interfere with the generation of adequate negative pleural pressure can all compromise tidal volume and minute ventilation, leading to hypoxemia and/or hypercapnia. For a large number of the problems leading to respiratory failure, abnormalities with the ventilatory pump play a major or contributing role, particularly with respect to increases in airway resistance because of mucus/inflammation and/or bronchospasm. When work of breathing increases because of the reduced compliance of the lungs and/or chest wall or resistance is elevated, the ventilatory muscles may fatigue and accessory muscles of ventilation (eg, sternocleidomastoid, pectoralis major) are often called into action. When overall ventilation is increased, typically because of increases in dead space in the lungs, both inspiratory and expiratory muscles may be activated.

Under conditions of normal breathing, exhalation is a passive phenomenon; the recoil forces of the lung (both elastic forces related to the connective tissue in the lung and surface forces that are the consequence of the air-liquid layer lining the alveoli) lead to positive alveolar pressure when the inspiratory muscles are turned off at the end of inhalation. With alveolar pressure greater than mouth pressure, expiratory flow results. When minute ventilation is increased, however, as noted earlier, accessory muscles of exhalation (predominantly abdominal muscles) must be activated to increase expiratory flow and allow for increased respiratory rate and larger tidal volumes.

The Gas Exchanger

Gas exchange occurs at the level of the alveolus and pulmonary capillaries. Each alveolus is surrounded by a fine mesh of capillaries, which creates an enormous surface area across which diffusion of oxygen and carbon dioxide may occur. Although thickening of this membrane may rarely cause a diffusion impairment, many pathologies may lead to destruction of alveoli and/or capillaries, thereby reducing the total surface area for diffusion. As this surface area diminishes because of problems such as emphysema and pulmonary fibrosis, the number of pulmonary blood vessels through which the output of the right ventricle must travel diminishes. As one looks at the totality of the cross-sectional area of the thousands of pulmonary vessels in parallel, you see that this also diminishes. Assuming cardiac output remains constant, the velocity of the blood traveling through the pulmonary circulation must increase.

$$\text{Velocity of a fluid through a tube} = \frac{\text{Flow through the tube}}{\text{Cross - sectional area of the tube}}$$

This increase in velocity does not affect gas exchange to any significant degree at rest because of the rapidity with which oxygen and carbon dioxide diffuse; in other words, it takes so little time for diffusion to occur and for equilibrium to be achieved between the alveolus and the blood that even though the red blood cell spends less time in contact with the alveolus, Pa_{O_2} and Pa_{CO_2} are maintained (**Figure 1-3**). With increases in cardiac output, however, as

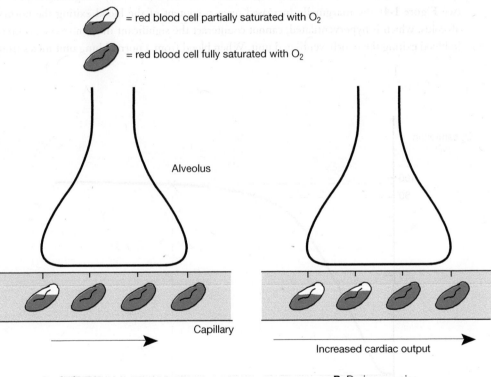

Figure 1-3: **Diffusion of oxygen. A,** At rest, equilibration between the alveolus and the blood occurs quickly. By the time a red blood cell (RBC) is one-third of the way through the alveolar capillary, the hemoglobin has picked up all the oxygen with which it is going to bind. **B,** During exercise, however, cardiac output increases, resulting in more rapid transit of RBCs through the capillary. In the diagram, equilibration between alveolus and blood is now shown as occurring farther along the capillary. If a pathologic process is present in the lung that prolongs diffusion time, equilibration may not occur between the alveolus and the blood. The result is a decrease in Pa_{O_2} during exercise. (From The Gas Exchanger: Matching Ventilation and Perfusion. In: Schwartzstein RM, Parker MJ. *Respiratory Physiology: A Clinical Approach.* Wolters Kluwer; 2006:95-125. Figure 5.10.)

occurs during exercise and at times with sepsis or vascular shunts, one might see the effects of a diffusion abnormality as a fall in oxygen saturation.

As noted earlier, diffusion problems are an unusual cause of gas exchange problems at rest. Much more important are disturbances in the relationship between ventilation and perfusion of alveoli. For gas exchange to occur, there needs to be an alignment within the lung of where gas is going and where blood flow is distributed. When there is a perfect match, we say the ventilation ($\dot{V}$) to perfusion ($\dot{Q}$) ratio ($\dot{V}/\dot{Q}$) is 1. When ventilation is reduced relative to perfusion because of disease process affecting the airways, oxygen is taken up by the blood faster than the gas is being replenished in the alveolus; this reduces the alveolar partial pressure of oxygen (P_{AO_2}). With a lower P_{AO_2}, blood flowing through that lung unit will obtain less oxygen and the arterial oxygen partial pressure (P_{aO_2}) and oxygen content of the blood will go down. Increasing ventilation to normal units to raise the P_{AO_2} will not compensate for this problem because the O_2 saturation and O_2 content of the blood exiting the hyperventilated unit are already near maximum; the oxygen content of the blood is only marginally improved (see **Figure 1-4**); the marginally increased oxygen content of the blood exiting the normal alveolus, which is hyperventilated, cannot counteract the significant drop in oxygen content in blood exiting the poorly ventilated unit. When blood from a normal lung unit mixes from

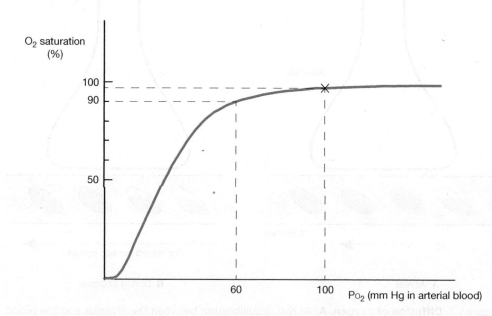

Figure 1-4: An example of the oxygen-hemoglobin saturation curve. A normal alveolus receiving normal ventilation will have a P_{O_2} of approximately 100. The blood perfusing that unit will be approximately 97% saturated with oxygen (point X). If you hyperventilate the unit maximally, you may be able to raise the P_{O_2} in the alveolus to about 130-140 mm Hg; this will raise the O_2 saturation of the hemoglobin in the blood to 100%, but this is only a marginal increase in oxygen content. (From The Gas Exchanger: Matching Ventilation and Perfusion. In: Schwartzstein RM, Parker MJ. *Respiratory Physiology: A Clinical Approach.* Wolters Kluwer; 2006:95-125. Figure 5.8.)

blood coming from a poorly ventilated unit, the resulting Pao_2 is determined by the average O_2 content of the two streams of blood.

Many of the common respiratory diseases you encounter from asthma and chronic obstructive pulmonary disease (COPD) to pneumonia to congestive heart failure are characterized by mismatch between ventilation and perfusion sufficient to lead to acute respiratory failure. They all respond reasonably well to supplemental oxygen, although the patient may require intubation because of failure of the ventilatory pump to facilitate clearance of secretions and inflammatory material or to our inability to reliably administer the supplementary oxygen necessary to maintain an adequate oxygen saturation of the blood.

In some severe cases of $\dot{V}/\dot{Q}$ mismatch, when $\dot{V} = 0$, supplemental oxygen may not raise the Pao_2 significantly. We consider this scenario to be evidence of pulmonary shunt. Because of problems with normal hypoxic pulmonary vasoconstriction, an adaptive process that causes vasoconstriction of pulmonary vessels perfusing a hypoxic alveolus thereby redirecting blood flow to better ventilated (and oxygenated) alveoli, blood continues to go to units that are not receiving any ventilation. Although supplemental oxygen will raise the partial pressure of poorly ventilated alveolus, it cannot raise the Pao_2 in an alveolus that is receiving no ventilation (more on this in Chapter 3). For most of these patients, who typically are suffering from acute respiratory distress syndrome (ARDS), institution of mechanical ventilation is essential to preserve life.

Linking the Different Parts of the Respiratory System to Hypoxemia and Hypercapnia

Although there is a tendency to think that all patients with a low Pao_2 or a high $Paco_2$ have a problem with the gas exchanger, the reality is that abnormalities of the respiratory controller and the ventilatory pump can also lead to abnormal blood gases. Consider the patient presenting to the emergency department with an opiate overdose; the respiratory rate is low and the tidal volume, the size of the breath, is small. There is nothing wrong with the lungs or the chest wall, but the Pao_2 will be low and the $Paco_2$ elevated. Similarly, imagine a patient with severe episode of myasthenia gravis and severe muscle weakness. The respiratory rate is very rapid, but the tidal volumes are very small. There is nothing wrong with the lungs or controller, yet the Pao_2 is low and the $Paco_2$ is high. How can we be sure that a pneumonia isn't also present in these patients? We could obtain a chest radiograph, but early in the course of pneumonia, you may not always see an infiltrate. We could listen to the breath sounds with our stethoscope for abnormal findings suggestive of pneumonia, but these are not always present either. The best way to assess whether there is an abnormality in the gas exchanger is to determine the alveolar-to-arterial oxygen difference or A-aDo_2 (which will be discussed in more detail in Chapter 3). An abnormal A-aDo_2 tells us that there is a problem with the gas exchanger. If the A-aDo_2 is normal, the patient's hypoxemia is due to a problem with the controller or ventilatory pump (or the patient is in an environment in which the air being breathed has a low PO_2, eg, high altitude).

THE MECHANICAL VENTILATOR: REPLACING THE BROKEN PART OF THE RESPIRATORY SYSTEM

If you were to design a ventilator, you would start by saying, "what are the problems I have to fix?" With our overview in this chapter, you would surmise that to correct all forms of respiratory failure, I need a machine that will address potential problems with the controller, the ventilatory pump, and the gas exchanger.

The Controller

All positive pressure ventilators enable you to set the number of breaths to be delivered to the patient each minute (the respiratory rate). Not all patients require this, of course, but the ventilator must be able to determine the rate and size of the breath, the latter of which requires integration of the controller and the ventilatory pump in the healthy patient. With the ventilator, we think of the controller as discretely separate from the pump function of the respiratory system. Of course, the controller in the brain also determines several things in addition to the rate of breathing; the ratio of inspiration to expiration, the inspiratory flow, and the changes in flow throughout the inspiration are not things you think about consciously, but your respiratory control centers determine these things for you. For the patient with a damaged or suppressed controller (eg, from sedation), the medical team must determine these settings on the ventilator; you must adjust the "control" function that is not performing properly.

The Ventilatory Pump

If the respiratory system is not able to generate a negative alveolar pressure sufficient to overcome high resistance of the airways or low compliance of the lungs and chest wall, respiratory failure will follow. The mechanical ventilator replaces or supplements this "damaged" part of the respiratory system by "pushing" air into the lungs; the positive pressure ventilator produces a pressure at the upper airway that is greater than in the alveolus, resulting in flow of gas into the lungs.

The Gas Exchanger

For a patient with hypoxemia because of a problem with the gas exchanger (diffusion abnormality or ventilation/perfusion mismatch), we can supply higher concentrations of oxygen in the inspired gas via the mechanical ventilator. If the hypoxemia is due to hypoventilation (a consequence of a problem with the respiratory controller leading to a low rate or tidal volume or a problem with the ventilatory pump contributing to a low tidal volume), the mechanical ventilator can be used to set the rate and the tidal volume.

KEY POINTS

Respiratory failure results when one or more elements of the respiratory system malfunction—the respiratory controller, the ventilatory pump, or the gas exchanger. Mechanical ventilators are designed to supplement or replace the "broken" part of the system, thereby restoring the patient's homeostasis with respect to the respiratory system. As you begin your study and use of mechanical ventilators, many of the seeming complexities of the various settings you must implement will make more sense if you remind yourself of the link between that aspect of the mechanical ventilator and the part of the respiratory system it is designed to replace.

STUDY QUESTIONS AND ANSWERS

Questions

1. Which of the following is not a component of the ventilatory pump?
   A. Airways
   B. Brainstem
   C. Phrenic nerve
   D. Intercostal muscles

2. A 30-year-old previously healthy patient with bilateral infiltrates and evidence of bacterial pneumonia has a Pao_2 of 55 mm Hg with supplemental oxygen delivering 60% oxygen. The decision is made to intubate the patient and place him on mechanical ventilation. You would characterize his respiratory failure as being due to:
   A. a controller problem.
   B. dysfunction of the ventilatory pump.
   C. abnormality of the gas exchanger.
   D. All of the above

3. A 20-year-old woman with a history of asthma develops acute shortness of breath. When you examine her you find normal breath sounds on the left with reduced breath sounds, but not wheezes, on the right. Oxygen saturation without supplemental oxygen is 97%. A chest radiograph shows a large right pneumothorax. You characterize her respiratory problem as being due to dysfunction of:
   A. the controller.
   B. the ventilatory pump.
   C. the gas exchanger.
   D. All of the above

4. A 75-year-old patient has been mechanically ventilated for 1 week because of respiratory failure. Her Pao_2 is now 75 mm Hg with Fio_2 0.3. Each time you disconnect her from the ventilator, her oxygen saturation drops, and the patient's respiratory rate is noted to be 2-3 breaths/min. You decide the problem that is keeping her from being extubated resides with the:
   A. controller.
   B. ventilatory pump.
   C. gas exchanger.
   D. All of the above

Answers

1. **Answer B. Brainstem**
   Rationale: The brainstem is essential for the control functions of the respiratory system but is not part of the ventilatory pump. The airways allow bulk transfer of gas from the mouth to the alveoli and back. The phrenic nerve is essential for connecting the controller to the diaphragm. The intercostal muscles are used to help move the rib cage to facilitate breathing.

2. **Answer C. Abnormality of the gas exchanger**
   Rationale: The patient has a very low oxygen level because of his pneumonia and disruption of the gas exchanger (alveoli and pulmonary vessels). There is no history to suggest problems with the controller or ventilatory pump.

(continued)

3. **Answer B. The ventilatory pump**

   Rationale: Motion of the chest wall and lung is linked via the pleural space. Movement of the chest wall decompresses or compresses the pleural space, which changes intrathoracic pressure and consequently alveolar pressure. By disrupting the "connection" of the chest wall to the lung, a pneumothorax disrupts the ventilatory pump.

4. **Answer A. Controller**

   Rationale: The patient's endogenous respiratory rate is abnormally low; hypoventilation is leading to the fall in her oxygen saturation when disconnected from the ventilator. This may be due to sedation or a new pathology in her brain. Because the oxygenation is adequate when she is receiving mechanical support, the gas exchanger appears to be performing well. If the ventilatory pump was the concern, the respiratory rate would be elevated, an indication that the brain is trying to compensate for a weakened "pump" function.

SUGGESTED READINGS

Getting Started: The Approach to Respiratory Physiology. In: Schwartzstein RM, Parker MJ. *Respiratory Physiology: A Clinical Approach*. Wolters Kluwer; 2006:1-8.

The Controller: Directing the Orchestra. In: Schwartzstein RM, Parker MJ. *Respiratory Physiology: A Clinical Approach*. Wolters Kluwer; 2006:126-148.

The Gas Exchanger: Matching Ventilation and Perfusion. In: Schwartzstein RM, Parker MJ. *Respiratory Physiology: A Clinical Approach*. Wolters Kluwer; 2006:95-125.

Principles of Respiratory Mechanics: Applications to Mechanical Ventilation

Richard M. Schwartzstein

LEARNING OBJECTIVES

- Describe the determinants of flow through tubes.
- Identify the factors that alter resistance in mechanically ventilated patients.
- Explain how changes in resistance lead to a fall in pressure along a tube.
- Describe the determinants of compliance of the respiratory system and their implications for managing mechanically ventilated patients.
- Describe the factors that contribute to the stability of the alveolus and the physiologic abnormalities that predispose to alveolar collapse.
- Explain how one can monitor changes in resistance and compliance in mechanically ventilated patients.

INTRODUCTION

In Chapter 1, we described the elements of the respiratory system, one of which is the ventilatory pump, which is responsible for creating a negative pressure in the alveolus during inhalation, which results in the flow of air from mouth to alveolus, and a positive pressure during exhalation, which drives the air back in the opposite direction. As you recall, inspiration requires muscle force, whereas exhalation at normal levels of ventilation is largely passive, depending on the recoil forces of the lungs. With positive pressure ventilation, the pressure differential that leads to a flow of gas into the lungs is generated by the ventilator rather than the inspiratory muscles. Nevertheless, the principles of flow through tubes, including resistance and compliance (a measure of the "stiffness" of the system), remain in force and must be applied to the patient receiving mechanical ventilation to understand how to manage the ventilator. Patients with asthma and chronic obstructive lung disease (COPD), for example, typically have increased airway resistance; those with interstitial lung disease, diffuse pneumonia, acute respiratory distress syndrome (ARDS), and a variety of chest wall problems are characterized by reduced compliance.

FLOW THROUGH TUBES

Driving Pressure

Consider a tube through which there is a fluid flowing (**Figure 2-1**). There is a pressure on each end of the tube (P_1 and P_2) and a resistance (R) within the tube itself. According to Ohm's law, the pressure differential, or *driving pressure,* between the ends of the tubes determines the flow, for any given resistance (**Figure 2-1**).

Most commonly, the ΔP between the ends of the tube is taken as pressure at the mouth (P_{mouth}) and pressure at the alveolus (P_{alv}). The pressure at the mouth is determined by the settings of the ventilator, and the pressure at the alveolus can be measured under static conditions with a maneuver called the plateau pressure (P_{plat}), described later. For any given flow through the tube, the rate at which pressure falls is determined by the resistance of the tube.

Resistance

The resistance of a tube is determined by a number of factors. The first consideration is the diameter of the tube. According to Poiseuille's law, resistance is proportional to $1/r^4$. Consequently, very small changes in radius of the tube will result in large differences in resistance. If you have a plug of mucus reducing the effective radius of the tube, you will need to set the ventilator to deliver a much greater pressure to deliver the same flow of gas.

As soon as the trachea divides into the mainstem bronchi, and they divide into lobar bronchi, segmental bronchi, etc., the relationship between radius and resistance becomes a bit more complicated. Each time a tube subdivides into two smaller tubes, one creates tubes in parallel; although the radius of each individual tube is smaller after the division, the cross-sectional area of the tubes in parallel is greater than the cross-sectional area of the tube from which they originated. Consequently, the resistance of the tubes in parallel is less than the tube from which they originated. As gas flows from the mouth to the periphery of the

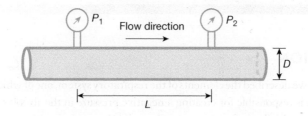

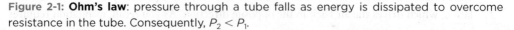

Figure 2-1: Ohm's law: pressure through a tube falls as energy is dissipated to overcome resistance in the tube. Consequently, $P_2 < P_1$.

lung, we move from a single large tube (the trachea) to thousands of very small tubes in parallel (respiratory bronchioles) with a very large cross-sectional area (**Figure 2-2**). Consequently, resistance is higher in central airways than in the periphery of the lungs.

The radius of a flexible tube is determined by the pressure difference between the inside (P_i) and outside (P_o) of the tube. This difference is called the transmural pressure (P_{tm}). Thus,

$$P_{tm} = P_i - P_o$$

The pressure outside the tube can be considered the same as intrathoracic pressure, which is best represented as the pleural pressure. When a patient is receiving positive pressure ventilation, the pressure inside the airways will be positive and usually greater than the intrathoracic pressure. However, if the patient is making forceful expiratory efforts, P_{tm} may become negative, which will compress and, in some cases in smaller airways with thin walls, may collapse the airway entirely. This is particularly a consideration in patients with emphysema in whom the destruction of lung parenchyma reduces many of the supporting structures that help to keep small airways open.

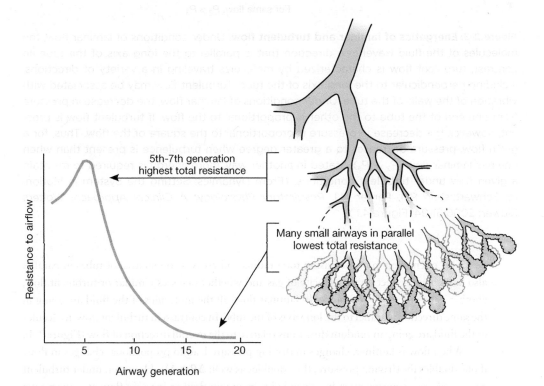

Figure 2-2: Distribution of resistance in the lung. Although the smallest airways, as individual tubes, have the highest resistance, they are arranged in parallel. This arrangement means that the resistances of the small bronchi add as reciprocals, thereby leading to extremely low resistance to airflow in the periphery of the lung. The highest areas of resistance are found in the more central airways, with the peak airway resistance occurring in the fifth to seventh generation of airways. (From Dynamics: Setting the System in Motion. In: Schwartzstein RM, Parker MJ. *Respiratory Physiology: A Clinical Approach*. Wolters Kluwer; 2006:61-94. Figure 4.2.)

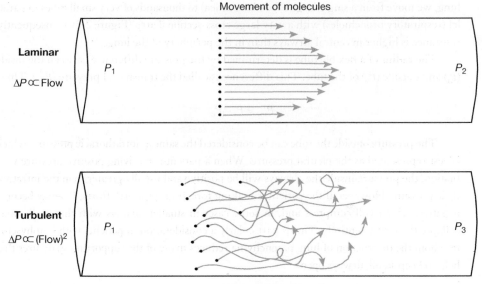

Movement of molecules

Laminar

$\Delta P \propto$ Flow

P_1 P_2

Turbulent

$\Delta P \propto$ (Flow)^2

P_1 P_3

For same flow, $P_2 > P_3$

Figure 2-3: Energetics of laminar and turbulent flow. Under conditions of laminar flow, the molecules of the fluid travel in a direction that is parallel to the long axis of the tube. In contrast, turbulent flow is characterized by molecules traveling in a variety of directions, including perpendicular to the long axis of the tube. Turbulent flow may be associated with vibration of the walls of the tube. Under conditions of laminar flow, the decrease in pressure from one end of the tube to the other is proportional to the flow. If turbulent flow is present, however, the decrease in pressure is proportional to the square of the flow. Thus, for a given flow, pressure decreases to a greater degree when turbulence is present than when one has laminar flow ($P_2 > P_3$). Stated in another way, more energy is required to maintain a given flow under turbulent conditions. (From Dynamics: Setting the System in Motion. In: Schwartzstein RM, Parker MJ. *Respiratory Physiology: A Clinical Approach*. Wolters Kluwer; 2006:61-94. Figure 4.1.)

This phenomenon of increasing total radius and cross-sectional area of tubes in parallel also has a major effect on the velocity of gas and whether one sees laminar or turbulent flow, another determinant of resistance. In laminar flow, all the molecules of the fluid are going in the same direction, parallel to the long axis of the tube. In contrast, in turbulent flow, molecules of the fluid are going in random directions relative to the overall direction of flow (**Figure** 2-3).

When flow is laminar, changes in driving pressure lead to proportional changes in flow; if one doubles the driving pressure, flow doubles as well: $\Delta P \propto \Delta \dot{V}$. However, under turbulent conditions, more energy must be expended to maintain flow or increase flow at a given rate: $\Delta P \propto \Delta (\dot{V})^2$. To double the flow, one must increase the driving pressure (the pressure difference between the two ends of the tube) by a factor of 4. In essence, the resistance under turbulent conditions is higher than under laminar conditions.

What determines whether flow is laminar or turbulent? The answer to this lies in fluid mechanics, but for the biology of the lung, we can reduce it to a few simple variables that relate to something called Reynolds number (RN). If RN is greater than 2000, one is likely to have turbulent conditions.

$$RN \propto \frac{(\text{Density})(\text{Velocity})}{\text{Viscosity}}$$

Because the viscosity of the gas we breathe does not change significantly, RN largely depends on the density and velocity. The next question is: how do we think about the velocity of the gas as it travels in the lung? Velocity is determined by the following relationship:

$$\text{Velocity} = \text{Flow/Cross-sectional area of the tube}$$

For a given flow, the greater the radius of the tube, the lower the velocity and the less likely one will have turbulent flow with the resulting increase in resistance. In the periphery of the lung, with thousands of airways in parallel, the cross-sectional area of the tubes is high and velocity is low; in contrast, as one moves toward the central airways, cross-sectional area goes down and velocity increases. Consequently, turbulent flow and the highest resistance is found in the more central airways. Imagine a patient with asthma with very narrowed airways because of inflammation, increased mucus production, and bronchoconstriction. Airway radius is significantly reduced, velocity increases, and we get turbulent flow, which produces vibrations of the airways that we hear as "wheezes."

The density of a gas does come into play with upper airway obstruction. A patient with laryngospasm or laryngeal edema, for example, has a severe narrowing of the airway, leading to high velocity of the gas moving across it, which produces turbulent flow and leads to increased work of breathing. One intervention to buy time for primary treatment of the problem to work is to have the patient breathe heliox, a mixture of helium and oxygen (in contrast to the nitrogen/oxygen mixture in the atmosphere that we normally breathe). Per the equation for RN, this reduces the density of the gas (helium is less dense than nitrogen), which may forestall turbulent flow, reduce resistance, and minimize the work of breathing. There are some data suggesting that severe asthma patients with acute respiratory failure who are receiving mechanical ventilation may benefit from heliox as well.

Pressure Within a Tube

We noted earlier in this chapter that the radius of an airway is related to the transmural pressure across the wall of the airway. The same is true for the alveolus into which the airway empties on inspiration. High pressure in the alveolus will lead to large alveolar volume, which may cause lung damage, particularly in patients with ARDS (see Chapter 14). The relationship between the pressure at the mouth being delivered by the ventilator and the pressure in the alveolus is determined by the flow and resistance, per Ohm's law.

The pressure we measure in an airway may be viewed as the "potential energy" of the molecules in the gas; if the gas is moving (ie, there is flow in the tube), the molecules also have kinetic energy. The potential energy is manifest as the hydrostatic pressure we measure when we say the pressure in the airway or alveolus is X cm H_2O. As the gas moves down the airway to the alveolus, potential energy is transformed into heat because of the work to overcome resistance; consequently, the hydrostatic pressure goes down as gas flows from mouth to alveolus on inhalation, and from alveolus to mouth on exhalation. If resistance is high (as one might expect in a patient with bronchospasm or significant airway inflammation), the ventilator may be delivering gas at a high pressure at the mouth, but by the time the gas reaches the alveolus, a large proportion of that pressure has been dissipated and the alveolar pressure may not be dangerously high or at risk of overdistension. The challenge in managing patients with lung disease leading to respiratory failure is that the effect of the disease on the lung is often heterogeneous; some regions of lung may be very diseased while other regions of the lung remain relatively normal. This will lead to a larger volume of gas going into some regions than other. In a healthy individual, the highest resistance in the lungs is at the level of the fourth or fifth generation of airways (each time an airway divides into two airways is called a "generation"); this location reflects the velocity of the gas, which is an important determinant of laminar versus turbulent flow via Reynold's number, and because of the branching pattern of the airways, which also contributes to turbulent flow.

In a patient receiving mechanical ventilation, resistance of the airways may be elevated because of narrowing of the airway. The most common causes of narrowing are (1) airway inflammation, (2) mucus in the airways, (3) bronchospasm, (4) fluid/edema of the airways, and (5) aspirated material.

Because we cannot measure the resistance in each airway and the flow into individual alveoli, we must still be cautious when delivering gas at high pressures, and the plateau pressure (explained later) provides us with the best sense of the pressure in the alveolus. Similarly on exhalation, areas of high resistance will empty more slowly than regions of lung with low resistance; consequently, at the end of exhalation, some parts of the lung will be at higher lung volume than others and are prone to hyperinflation.

COMPLIANCE

Compliance is defined as the change in volume achieved by a change in pressure within a flexible structure. Imagine a balloon that is inflated to a certain volume and has a particular pressure within it. You now blow more air into the balloon, increasing the pressure within it. The volume increases further. The change in volume divided by the change in pressure equals the compliance of the balloon:

$$\text{Compliance} = \Delta V/\Delta P$$

Compliance is determined largely by the physical characteristics of the structure that lead to a recoil force, which will move the volume of the structure back to its "resting volume," that is, the volume that it would assume if there were no forces being exerted on the structure. Compliance may change as the structure varies in the range of absolute volume; for example, the lung becomes less compliant the more it is inflated.

The lung and chest wall are both flexible structures that have a resting position. A force *must be exerted on them to move them from their resting position.* If that force is removed, they will recoil back to their respective resting positions. Remember that the chest wall consists of the bones and cartilage of the rib cage and vertebral column and the muscles and connective tissue that hold them all together. The resting position of the chest wall is about two-thirds to three-fourths of the way between residual volume (RV) and total lung capacity (TLC).

The determination of the three key lung volumes (TLC, functional residual capacity [FRC], and RV) is based upon the balance of forces between the ventilatory muscles, the lung recoil (the lungs always exert a force to a lower volume), and the chest wall, which may exert a force inward or outward depending on the volume of the chest wall relative to its resting position (if the chest wall is above its resting volume, it will exert a force inward; if the chest wall is below its resting volume, it will exert a force outward; see **Table 2-1**). The RV also depends in some individuals, particularly patients with increased expiratory airway resistance, on the time it takes during a forced exhalation to reach the equilibrium between the balance of forces.

For the purpose of mechanical ventilation, the most relevant volume for us to consider is FRC, also called "relaxation volume." This is the volume of the respiratory system at the end of a passive exhalation, and it is primarily determined by the balance of forces of the lung inward (to a lower volume) and the chest wall outward (to a higher volume)—see **Table 2-1** in cases of increased airway resistance or very short expiratory time; the end-expiratory volume may be higher than FRC because there is not adequate time for the system to exhale gas to reach the relaxation volume.

FRC is important because the lower the FRC, the more likely that alveoli will collapse, in keeping with the Law of Laplace:

$$P = 2T/r$$

where P is pressure generated in the alveolus by the recoil forces; T the tension in the wall of the alveolus leading to an inward force that creates the pressure; and r the radius of the alveolus. The smaller the radius of the alveoli, the lower the lung volume, and the greater the chance of alveolar collapse. If alveoli collapse on exhalation and do not reopen on inhalation, the result is a pulmonary shunt, which leads to hypoxemia that may not respond well to supplemental oxygen. Such conditions require us to use positive end-expiratory pressure to increase the end-expiratory lung volume (and prevent the lung from reaching FRC) and avoid alveolar collapse (more on this in Chapter 14).

The recoil forces of the lung include both elastic forces (because of the collagen in the lung tissue) and surface forces (because of the air-liquid interface in the alveoli). Diseases that increase the elastic properties and/or weight of the lung (eg, pulmonary inflammation and fibrosis; pulmonary edema—either cardiogenic or non-cardiogenic) will reduce the compliance of the lung and lead to a lower FRC. In addition, processes that disrupt the nature or quantity of surfactant (a detergent substance produced by type II pneumocytes to reduce surface forces in the liquid lining the lung) in the alveoli will increase surface tension and recoil forces and lead to reduced compliance and lower FRC, thereby predisposing to alveolar collapse (see **Figure 2-4**). Diseases that destroy lung tissue, for example, emphysema, reduce

TABLE 2-1 Balance of Forces Determining Lung Volumes[a]			
	Lungs	**Chest Wall**	**Muscles**
Total lung capacity (TLC)	↓	↓	↑
Functional residual capacity (FRC)	↓	↑	Muscles are relaxed
Residual volume (RV)	↓	↑	↓

[a]Each of the major lung volumes we consider in respiratory mechanics is determined by a balance of forces between the lungs, chest wall, and ventilatory muscles to cause the respiratory system to get bigger or larger. The direction of the arrows (up or down) reflects the direction of the force exerted by the chest wall, lungs, and respiratory muscles to make the volume of the respiratory system larger or smaller.

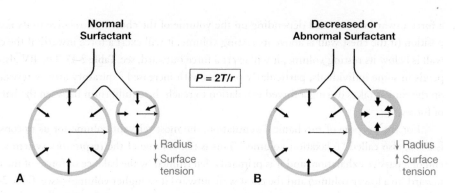

Figure 2-4: **Effect of surfactant on alveolar size.** Surfactant is a detergent that reduces surface tension in the liquid lining the alveolus; this reduces the recoil force of the alveolus and helps to stabilize alveoli during exhalation when lung volume and alveolar radius decline. **A,** Normal lung: In the normal lung, as alveolar volume diminishes, the density of surfactant in the surface layer increases, leading to a fall in surface tension, which prevents the pressure in the alveolus from rising and pushing the air into the larger alveolus. **B,** Absent or minimal surfactant: Per the Law of Laplace, if there were diminished surfactant, the increased surface tension will increase pressure in the alveolus and predispose to air moving from the smaller alveoli to larger alveoli, leading to alveolar collapse and shunt.

the inward recoil force of the lung, thereby changing the balance of forces and leading to an increase in FRC.

Abnormalities of the chest wall can also alter FRC. The most common abnormality is increased weight of the chest wall because of obesity or severe edema. This weight diminishes the normal outward recoil force of the rib cage, impairs the downward movement of the diaphragm, and reduces FRC. Similarly, when the abdomen is distended with an increase in the intra-abdominal pressure, as occurs in conditions such as pancreatitis or cirrhosis with significant ascites, the force of the abdomen pressing on the diaphragm also leads to a decrease in FRC and predisposes to alveolar collapse.

MONITORING COMPLIANCE AND RESISTANCE WITH POSITIVE PRESSURE VENTILATION

The concepts we have been discussing are relevant to the daily management of patients receiving mechanical ventilation. We can determine whether a patient has abnormal respiratory system compliance or airway resistance with simple techniques involving the assessment of the pressure needed to inflate the lung. These techniques are best done with the patient being passive, that is, not making any respiratory efforts.

Beginning at the end of exhalation, you note the pressure at the airway opening (Pao) as indicated by the ventilator. Ideally this is done with an "expiratory hold," which means that you close the valves in the ventilator so that no air is going into or out of the lungs; under these conditions, the pressure at the airway opening equals the pressure in the alveolus (in a tube with no flow, the pressure at each end of the tube must be the same). Next, you deliver a known volume of gas (usually 400-450 mL) into the patient with the ventilator and note the highest or "peak" pressure required to push the air into the lung. The peak pressure reflects the energy that must be applied to overcome both the resistance of the airways and the recoil

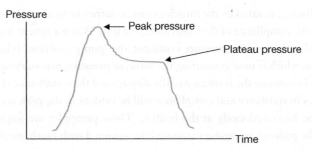

Figure 2-5: Peak and plateau pressure. This figure shows a single breath with positive pressure ventilation. The peak pressure occurs when air is being pushed into the lung. The peak pressure reflects *both* resistive and recoil (elastic and surface tension) forces. The plateau pressure occurs when you create an "inspiratory hold," that is, the inspiratory and expiratory valves are closed and static conditions have been created. NOTE: these pressures assume that the patient is not making any respiratory efforts during the measurements.

forces of the lung and chest wall. If this pressure is elevated above normal (in a patient with a completely normal airway resistance and respiratory system compliance, the peak pressure should be less than 20 cm H_2O), either airway resistance or respiratory system compliance is abnormal.

To determine the source of the abnormality, one performs an "inspiratory hold"—the valves of the ventilator are closed after the gas has been completely pushed into the lungs. The pressure at the airway opening will again reflect the pressure in the alveolus because there is no gas moving into or out of the lung. The pressure during the inspiratory hold is called the "plateau pressure." Because there is no gas flow at this time, the pressure reflects only the recoil forces of the lung and chest wall; airway resistance is not relevant when there is no flow. The maneuver to produce the peak and plateaus pressures is shown in **Figure 2-5**.

You can calculate the compliance of the respiratory system by the formula noted earlier in the chapter: compliance $= \Delta V/\Delta P$. If the difference between the peak and plateau pressure is greater than 10 cm H_2O, it is likely that airway resistance in the patient's lungs is elevated (see **Figure 2-5**). Remember, if the compliance of the lungs is reduced, the cause may be the lungs (increased elastic or surface forces) or the chest wall (eg, rib cage abnormality, obesity, increased intra-abdominal pressure).

If the peak and plateau pressures change over several minutes by the same amount (ie, each goes up by 15 cm H_2O), and the difference between the two stays the same, something has changed in the compliance of the system. One can make this conclusion because changes in resistance would affect the difference between peak and plateau pressures; with no change in that difference, resistance must be constant. A change in the recoil forces, on the other hand, would affect both the peak and plateau pressure; changes in recoil forces lead to a change in compliance. It now takes more pressure to expand the respiratory system.

CONCLUSION

The chest wall, lung parenchyma, and airways function like a pump during spontaneous breathing to move gas from the atmosphere down to the alveoli and then back out to the atmosphere. The inspiratory muscles move the chest wall to generate a negative pressure within the alveoli, thereby creating a pressure gradient from mouth to alveolus that produces a flow of gas. The force generated by the muscles must be sufficient to overcome the resistance of the airways and the compliance of the lungs and chest wall. When a patient has respiratory failure and is treated with a positive pressure ventilator, the "pump function" is largely transferred to the ventilator, which is now generating the force, or pressure, necessary to make gas flow into the lungs and overcome the resistance of the airways and the compliance of the respiratory system. Changes in resistance and compliance will be evident in the peak and plateau pressures, which can be measured easily at the bedside. These principles are important for assessing changes in the patient's respiratory status while sustained with mechanical ventilation.

KEY POINTS

- Flow through tubes reflects principles embodied in Ohm's law ($\Delta P =$ Flow $\times$ Resistance). One must also consider conditions of flow, that is, laminar or turbulent.
- The highest resistance in the lungs tends to be in the more central airways.
- The compliance of the lung and chest wall (compliance $= \Delta V/\Delta P$) tells us about the stiffness of the respiratory system and must be considered when providing positive pressure ventilation. Various lung diseases may increase or decrease lung compliance.
- Recoil forces of the lung (which affect lung compliance) include elastic forces as well as forces arising from the surface tension of the liquid/air interface in the alveolus; the surface tension is affected by surfactant. Conditions in which surfactant is depleted or not functioning normally will have increased recoil forces, lower FRC, and greater propensity to collapse in accord with the Law of Laplace.
- The resistance of the airways and the compliance of the respiratory system can be estimated and monitored by assessing the peak and plateau pressures when a breath is delivered by positive pressure ventilation.

STUDY QUESTIONS AND ANSWERS

Questions

1. A patient with respiratory failure because of pneumonia is being treated with positive pressure ventilation (with a set tidal volume and inspiratory time). On examination, you hear wheezes throughout both lungs. You predict the following:
    A. Peak pressure will be elevated.
    B. Plateau pressure will be elevated.
    C. Laminar flow is present.
    D. Compliance of the respiratory system is reduced.

2. You are caring for a patient with a history of heart failure who is admitted to the intensive care unit (ICU) with respiratory failure because of pneumonia and hypoxemia. She is given intravenous fluids to treat her hypotension. Several hours later she appears to be in more respiratory distress. What do you predict?
    A. Airway resistance is decreased.
    B. Respiratory system compliance is increased.
    C. The peak pressure is down while the plateau pressure is up.
    D. The peak and plateau pressures are up the same amount.

3. You are called to see a patient who was admitted to the ICU with smoke inhalation because of a house fire. He remains hypoxemic despite administration of 100% oxygen by mask. He is going into respiratory failure and is intubated. Following intubation, he requires 100% oxygen from the ventilator to maintain an O_2 sat of 90%. His peak and plateau pressures are both very high on the ventilator. You suspect the underlying issue is:

   A. increased airway resistance.
   B. a problem with surfactant in the lung.
   C. increased lung compliance.
   D. a partial airway obstruction from an aspiration.

Answers

1. **Answer A. Peak pressure will be elevated**
   Rationale: The wheezes are evidence of increased airway resistance and turbulent flow (because of increased velocity through a narrowing of the airway, which increases Reynolds Number and predisposes to turbulent flow). The peak pressure will be elevated to maintain a given flow to achieve the desired tidal volume. The plateau pressure, which is determined during an inspiratory hold at the end of the breath at time when there is no flow, will not be changed by change in airway resistance.

2. **Answer D. The peak and plateau pressures are up the same amount**
   Rationale: The patient likely has developed acute heart failure with pulmonary edema. The excess water in the lungs reduces the lung compliance, which leads to an increase in the plateau pressure. Although airway resistance might be up a small amount with pulmonary edema if there is also edema of the airways or fluid in the airways (which might cause peak pressure to be up more than plateau pressure), most often in this scenario peak and plateau pressures will be elevated to the same degree because of the fall in lung compliance.

3. **Answer C. Increased lung compliance**
   Rationale: The patient has likely developed ARDS, which leads to deficiency in and abnormal function of surfactant, which leads to increased surface tension in the air-liquid interface in the alveoli, increased recoil forces, and collapse of alveoli that do not fully reopen on inspiration. Compliance of the lungs is reduced leading to increased peak and plateau pressure. The collapse of alveoli will lead to severe hypoxemia because of shunt. In contrast, increased airway resistance, because of partial airway obstruction, would lead to an increase in peak pressure, but would not alter plateau pressure significantly.

Principles of Gas Exchange and Acid-Base Physiology: Application to Mechanical Ventilation

Richard M. Schwartzstein

LEARNING OBJECTIVES

- Describe the five physiologic causes of hypoxemia.
- Distinguish ventilation/perfusion mismatch from pulmonary shunt.
- Explain the concept of dead space and its impact on minute ventilation and carbon dioxide elimination.
- Demonstrate the use of the alveolar gas equation for analyzing causes of hypoxemia.
- Link the concepts of gas exchange to the management of the ventilator.
- Describe the basic principles of the physiology of acid-base disturbances.
- Explain the use of the ventilator to manage acid-base considerations in patients with acid-base disorders.

INTRODUCTION

One of the cardinal features of a large proportion of cases of acute respiratory failure is a problem with the gas exchanger. As we discussed briefly in Chapter 1, the gas exchanger is one of the three major components of the respiratory system, along with the controller and the ventilatory pump. In Chapter 2, we examined a number of features of the pump function of the respiratory system and the mechanics of how the ventilatory pump works and the importance of these concepts for the management of the ventilator. In this chapter, we review the basics of gas exchange and their implications for oxygenation and the elimination of carbon dioxide. Although we can usually overcome hypoxemia by increasing supplemental oxygen, high concentrations of inhaled oxygen (fraction of inspired gas that is oxygen, ie, F_{IO_2}), particularly above 0.6, can be toxic to the lung, and high levels of Pa_{O_2} have, in some studies, also been associated with adverse outcomes; consequently, one of our goals is to employ ventilator strategies to minimize the F_{IO_2}. Carbon dioxide levels can usually be normalized by increasing ventilation with the ventilator, but in some patients with chronic respiratory conditions preceding the acute respiratory failure, a "normal" Pa_{CO_2} may inhibit their ability to be liberated from the ventilator and breathe on their own.

In addition, the lung is the major organ for maintenance of normal acid-base balance. Respiratory acids account for a far greater fraction of the acid produced by the body each day than do metabolic acids. Cessation of breathing will lead to life-threatening acidemia in a matter of minutes—compare that to the relatively slow buildup of metabolic acid over days associated with acute renal failure. Thus, an understanding of these key principles will help you design the best strategies for caring for the patient with acute respiratory failure.

GAS EXCHANGE AND VENTILATION/PERFUSION RELATIONSHIPS

The gas exchange "unit" in the lung is the alveolus with its associated capillaries. Diffusion of oxygen occurs across the very thin alveolar and capillary walls, taking oxygen from high concentration in the alveolus to the lower concentration in the pulmonary arterial blood returning to the lungs from the body. In the other direction, a high content of carbon dioxide in the pulmonary arterial blood diffuses into the alveolus and is then eliminated from the body on the next exhalation.

For this system to work well, the blood must flow to regions of lung that are also being ventilated well, that is, there must be good matching of ventilation ($\dot{V}E$) and perfusion ($\dot{Q}$). Under normal circumstances, because of branching patterns of the airways and blood vessels and the effects of gravity on blood flow, there is typically more perfusion and ventilation in the dependent compared to nondependent portions of the lung. This effect, however, is seen to a greater extent with perfusion than ventilation. Consequently, there is typically more perfusion relative to ventilation in the bases of the lung (upright person), and relatively more ventilation than perfusion in the apices.

If ventilation and perfusion are matched perfectly, we say there is a $\dot{V}/\dot{Q}$ of 1. If there is ventilation with no perfusion, as sometimes occurs in the most nondependent regions of lung, or if the alveolar pressure is greater than capillary pressure (more on this later in the chapter), we call that region of the lung "dead space." The gas or ventilation going to that unit is not participating in gas exchange because there is no capillary blood into and out of the alveolus within which gas transfer can occur; the ventilation is, in a sense, "wasted."

The opposite extreme is seen if there is perfusion to a region of lung but no ventilation, either because an airway is completely obstructed or because the alveoli are collapsed or completely filled with fluid or inflammatory material. We call this situation a "pulmonary shunt"; no gas transfer is occurring and the blood leaves the alveolar capillary with the same Po_2 and Pco_2 as it had when it entered the capillary.

If there is high resistance in airways leading to alveolus or high compliance (reduced elastic recoil) of the lung region, the flow of gas into and out of the alveolus will be reduced; if perfusion is relatively normal, there will be reduced ventilation relative to perfusion, that is, $\dot{V}/\dot{Q}$ less than 1 (see **Figure 3-1**), that is, there is "wasted perfusion" of the alveolus. If ventilation is reduced compared to perfusion, the amount of oxygen in the alveolus will go down; oxygen is being taken out of the alveolus by the blood in the capillary but it is not being replaced normally because ventilation (gas flow into the alveolus) is reduced. This will contribute to hypoxemia. This effect, in normal lungs, is minimized by the vasoconstrictor response of the pulmonary arterioles to low alveolar oxygen (low Pao_2), an evolutionary adaptation to redirect blood flow to better ventilated units. In diseased lungs, however, this vasoconstriction does not occur as well as in a normal lung, resulting in $\dot{V}/\dot{Q}$ mismatch.

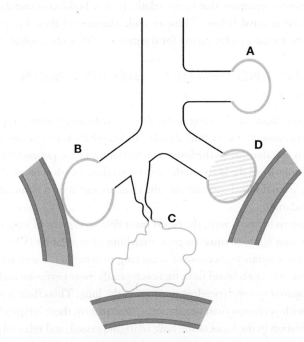

Figure 3-1: Ventilation/perfusion relationships within the lung. Alveolus "A" represents dead space; the alveolus is being ventilated but not perfused (no blood flow). Alveolus "B" is a normal alveolus; it is receiving both ventilation and perfusion in normal amounts. Alveolus "C" represents an alveolus that has poor elastic recoil and high resistance in the airway leading to the alveolus. Ventilation is reduced in this alveolus because of the high airway resistance and the high compliance of the lung, which reduces the recoil of the lung unit so it does not empty well. Ventilation is reduced whereas perfusion may be relatively normal, which leads to $\dot{V}/\dot{Q}$ mismatch. Alveolus "D" is collapsed and filled with fluid; there is no ventilation but the unit is still being perfused. This represents a pulmonary shunt where $\dot{V} = 0$.

MINUTE VENTILATION, DEAD SPACE, AND CARBON DIOXIDE ELIMINATION

Minute ventilation ($\dot{V}E$) is the number of liters per minute that goes into (or comes out of) the lungs. The air that enters the lung may go to regions with no perfusion (dead space) or to alveoli that are being perfused. The number of liters per minute going to dead space is noted as $\dot{V}D$, and ventilation going to perfused alveoli is noted as $\dot{V}A$; consequently, $\dot{V}E = \dot{V}A + \dot{V}D$. The elimination of carbon dioxide is directly related to alveolar ventilation. $Paco_2$ is represented by the following relationship:

$$Paco_2 \; \alpha \; \dot{V}co_2/\dot{V}A$$

The higher the amount of CO_2 produced by the body ($\dot{V}co_2$), the greater the $Paco_2$ for a given level of alveolar ventilation; the higher the alveolar ventilation, the lower the $Paco_2$ for any given amount of CO_2 being produced by the body.

There are two forms of dead space in the lung: anatomic dead space and alveolar dead space. Anatomic dead space is the volume of gas that is inhaled but never reaches the alveoli. Remember, the last gas inhaled stays in the upper airways and never reaches the alveoli where gas exchange might take place. This volume is typically estimated based on the patients' size—1 mL/lb ideal body weight; in the average individual, anatomic dead space is 150 to 170 mL. Alveolar dead space, depicted in **Figure 3-1**, is quite small in a healthy individual but may be substantial in disease states. Consequently, the fraction of dead space in a resting breath (tidal volume of 400-450 mL) is about 0.3; this fraction is called the V_d/V_t ratio (dead space to tidal volume ratio).

Minute ventilation is the product of tidal volume multiplied by the respiratory rate. For the same $\dot{V}E$, one might have very different $\dot{V}A$ depending on the tidal volume; the more shallow the tidal volume for a given $\dot{V}E$, the greater the proportion of the breath that will go to dead space and not participate in gas exchange. If you wish to reduce the $Paco_2$ in your patient with acute respiratory failure who is mechanically ventilated, you could consider raising the tidal volume or the respiratory rate; the former will be more "efficient" in lowering the $Paco_2$ (results in a decrease in V_d/V_t), but other considerations (eg, low tidal volume strategy to minimize volutrauma as discussed in Chapters 13 and 15) may preclude relying solely on changes in tidal volume to adjust the $Paco_2$.

Implications for Management of the Ventilator

Minute ventilation in a healthy adult is approximately 5 to 6 L/min. If dead space is increased because of the underlying illness, minute ventilation will need to be increased to maintain a normal $Paco_2$. Alternatively, if the patient has active inflammation and increased metabolic activity, often evidenced by fever, carbon dioxide production will likely be increased, again warranting increased ventilation to maintain a normal $Paco_2$.

As noted earlier, alveolar dead space results when an alveolus is receiving ventilation but is not being perfused. In healthy individuals in the upright position, this may occur in the apices of the lung, which receive ventilation but may not be perfused because the pulmonary artery pressure is not sufficient to result in blood flow to the upper lung regions or is so minimal as to result in compression of the capillary by alveolar pressure (see **Figure 3-2**). When a patient is receiving positive pressure ventilation, increases in pressure in the alveolus (P_{alv}), which is best assessed by measuring the plateau pressure with an inspiratory hold at the end of an inspiration (see Chapter 2), may rise to a point such that the P_{alv} is greater than the blood pressure in the capillary. Under these conditions, the capillary may be compressed by

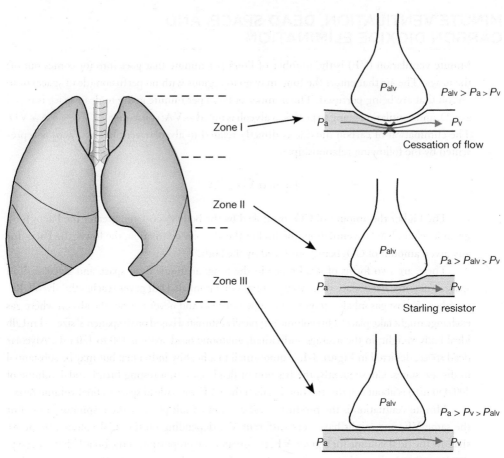

Figure 3-2: Zones of the lung. The lung is depicted as it would appear in a person standing upright. The most apical zone, zone I, of the lung receives the least blood flow because of gravity. $P_a < P_{alv}$ and the pulmonary vessel is compressed by the alveolus. In zone II, a gradual increase in flow occurs as one moves from the top to the bottom of the zone. P_a becomes increasingly large as one travels down the zone. Throughout the zone, however, $P_a > P_{alv} > P_v$. In zone III, the pressure in the alveolus has little impact on blood flow because $P_a > P_v > P_{alv}$. (From The Gas Exchanger: Matching Ventilation and Perfusion. In: Schwartzstein RM, Parker MJ. *Respiratory Physiology: A Clinical Approach.* Wolters Kluwer; 2006:95-125. Figure 5.5.)

the pressure in the alveolus, thereby preventing perfusion of the alveolus; the result is that one has now created alveolar dead space with a consequent reduction in $\dot{V}A$—one has effectively created "zone I" lung (see **Figure 3-2**). Under these conditions, $Paco_2$ may rise.

In patients with heterogeneous lung disease, with some relatively normal regions and some with significant $\dot{V}/\dot{Q}$ mismatch, which reduces alveolar ventilation, normal levels of $Paco_2$ may be achieved by increasing total ventilation, which increases ventilation primarily of the normal units. The normal units (with $\dot{V}/\dot{Q}$ near 1) are able to compensate for the diseased units with low $\dot{V}/\dot{Q}$ because of the way in which carbon dioxide binds to hemoglobin (see **Figure 3-3**). If the disease in the lung is quite extensive, there may not be sufficient normal lung units to allow for "compensation" of the poorly ventilated units to achieve a normal $Paco_2$.

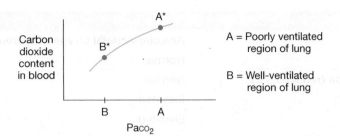

$A =$ Poorly ventilated region of lung

$B =$ Well-ventilated region of lung

Figure 3-3: Carbon dioxide binding to hemoglobin. Carbon dioxide is carried in the blood on hemoglobin and is also dissolved in the liquid portion of the blood, which determines the $Paco_2$. The content of carbon dioxide in the blood is the combination of the "bound" and "dissolved" CO_2. The relationship between $Paco_2$ and CO_2 content in the blood is linear, as shown. A poorly ventilated unit (A^*) will not eliminate much CO_2 resulting in a high $Paco_2$ content (A^*) and high $Paco_2$ (A). A well-ventilated unit, on the other hand, may have a low $Paco_2$ (B) and low CO_2 content (B^*). When the blood from the two regions of the lung mixes, the resulting CO_2 content and $Paco_2$ may be normal.

For patients with chronic lung disease leading to chronic hypercapnia, the elevated levels of $Paco_2$ can be viewed as an adaptive response to minimize the work of breathing. If $Paco_2$ is elevated, every alveolus receiving ventilation and perfusion will contain high levels of carbon dioxide when equilibrium is established between the blood and the alveolus. Consequently, fewer liters of alveolar gas will be needed to eliminate whatever CO_2 is being produced metabolically each minute; $\dot{V}A$ will be lower. For patients with disorders of the ventilatory pump, this may reduce dyspnea. In patients with diseases such as emphysema associated with chronic hypercapnia who develop acute respiratory failure, it is important to target the $Paco_2$ with mechanical ventilation to the patient's baseline level or even allow it to be slightly higher to allow $\dot{V}E$ to be as low as possible, which reduces the work of breathing and facilitates weaning from the ventilator and ultimate extubation (more on this issue in Chapter 11).

OXYGENATION, THE ALVEOLAR GAS EQUATION, AND THE CAUSES OF HYPOXEMIA

Oxygen delivery to the tissue is essential for life because we are largely dependent on aerobic metabolism for the function of our major organs. These organs are dependent on adequate oxygen delivery to their respective tissues. As noted earlier for carbon dioxide, the content of oxygen in the blood is a combination of oxygen bound to hemoglobin and oxygen dissolved in the liquid portion of the blood. The delivery of oxygen to the tissue is dependent on the oxygen content of the blood and the cardiac output generated by the cardiovascular system.

$$O_2 \text{ delivery} = O_2 \text{ content} \times \text{Cardiac output}$$

There are five physiologic causes of hypoxemia, and these can be distinguished in part by the calculation of the alveolar-arterial oxygen difference (A-aDo_2) (see Table 3-1).

The A-aDo_2 tells us about the functioning of the alveoli and associated capillaries. We calculate the Po_2 in the alveolus (Pao_2) using the alveolar gas equation:

$$Pao_2 = Fio_2 (P_{atm} - P_{H_2O}) - Paco_2/R$$

TABLE 3-1 Physiologic Causes of Hypoxemia	
Mechanism	**Alveolar-Arterial Oxygen Difference**
Altitude	Normal
Hypoventilation (reduced V̇E)	Normal
V̇/Q̇ mismatch	Elevated
Shunt	Elevated
Diffusion abnormality	Elevated

The first part of the equation tells us about the P_{O_2} of the inhaled gas (remember the partial pressure of a gas $[P_g]$ in the atmosphere is the fraction of that gas in the total gas volume multiplied by the P_{atm} or barometric pressure, which will vary with altitude, P_{H_2O} is the vapor pressure in the gas in the alveolus because the air we breathe is fully saturated by the upper airway or by the mechanical ventilator for the intubated patient; P_{H_2O} is 47 mm Hg and must be subtracted from the total gas pressure). The second part of the equation tells us about the alveolar ventilation (as we discussed earlier in the chapter, P_{aCO_2} is inversely related to alveolar ventilation) and the exchange rate between oxygen consumed and CO_2 produced in metabolism (the respiratory quotient, or R), which determines the P_{aCO_2}. For the average American diet, the mix of carbohydrates, protein, and fat utilized for metabolism leads to a respiratory quotient (R) of 0.8.

The first part of the equation is affected by supplemental oxygen, which increases the F_{IO_2}, and altitude; the higher you are, the lower the barometric pressure is (the fraction of oxygen in the air is 0.21 at sea level and on the top of Mt. Everest; the P_{O_2} is lower at altitude because the barometric pressure is lower). Alveolar ventilation also affects the P_{O_2} in the alveolus because the greater the V̇A, the more rapidly oxygen is replenished in the alveolus as gas diffuses across the alveolar wall into the capillary blood. The greater the V̇A, the lower the P_{aCO_2} (which is roughly the same as in P_{ACO_2}) and the higher the P_{AO_2} (see **Figure 3-4**).

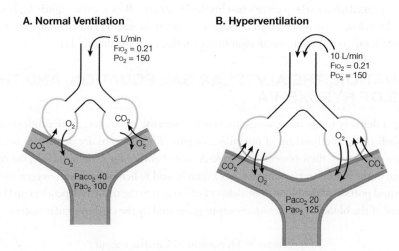

Figure 3-4: Hyperventilation, alveolar P_{O_2} and P_{CO_2}. A, normal ventilation of 5 L/min. At the level of the alveolus, CO_2 and O_2 equilibrate with the blood perfusing the alveoli, leading to an alveolar P_{CO_2} of 40 mm Hg and P_{O_2} of 100 mm Hg. By doubling the ventilation (and holding CO_2 production the same), air is removed more quickly from the alveolus with fresh air (no carbon dioxide and a large amount of oxygen) replenishing it. More CO_2 is removed; more oxygen is available for diffusion into the blood. The new steady state is a lower P_{CO_2} and a higher P_{O_2} (B).

Having calculated the alveolar P_{O_2}, we now compare it to the arterial P_{O_2}. Because there is a small amount of $\dot{V}/\dot{Q}$ mismatch even in normal lungs, and because some of the veins in the heart empty into the left atrium, the Pa_{O_2} is slightly lower than the PA_{O_2}. The difference between the two increases with age because of increases in $\dot{V}/\dot{Q}$ mismatch over the age of 30 (normal A-aD_{O_2} usually is less than the age multiplied by 0.3). If the A-aD_{O_2} is larger than that number, one knows that there is a problem with the gas exchanger.

Physiologic Causes of Hypoxemia

As outlined in **Table 3-1**, there are five physiologic causes of hypoxemia (note: we are describing physiologic/pathophysiologic mechanisms, not disease states per se). With hypoventilation, gas in the alveolus is not replenished as quickly as normal and CO_2 accumulates in the alveolus, whereas O_2 continues to be removed from the alveolus and taken up by blood in the capillaries. The result ultimately is that the equilibrium between alveolus and capillary blood is shifted to a higher P_{CO_2} and a lower P_{O_2}; both the alveolar and arterial oxygen levels are reduced and A-aD_{O_2} remains normal.

At high altitude, the barometric pressure is reduced, which lowers the partial pressure of oxygen that is inhaled leading to a lower PA_{O_2}. When the gas in the alveolus comes into equilibrium with the blood perfusing the alveolus, the arterial O_2 will be lower than normal but the A-aD_{O_2} will be normal.

The remaining three physiologic causes of hypoxemia are associated with diseases that affect the gas exchanger (alveoli and associated pulmonary capillaries). With diseases that affect ventilation of alveoli in some regions of lung, usually because of increased airway resistance, the alveolar O_2 in those regions of the lung is diminished, whereas normal regions of lung remain unaffected. Together, this leads to hypoxemia with a widened A-aD_{O_2}. Shunt is an extreme form of $\dot{V}/\dot{Q}$ mismatch in which alveoli receive no ventilation in some regions of lung (either because of alveolar collapse or alveoli being fully filled with fluid and/or inflammatory material); blood perfusing these alveoli cannot pick up oxygen or offload carbon dioxide. Hypoxemia results with a widened A-aD_{O_2}.

Unlike focal lung diseases for which the normal regions of lung can compensate for CO_2 elimination via hyperventilation (see **Figure 3-3**), oxygenation is not corrected by increases in alveolar ventilation in the normal lung units. This is because of the different binding relationship of oxygen to hemoglobin compared to carbon dioxide and oxygen. Rather than the linear curve seen for the relationship between Pa_{CO_2} and $\dot{V}E$, the relationship between Pa_{O_2} and oxygen content of the blood is sigmoid shaped (see **Figure 3-5**). Consequently, hyperventilating a normal unit and raising the alveolar and arterial P_{O_2} does not significantly increase O_2 *content* of the blood, and there is no meaningful compensation for the diseased unit that fails to provide adequate oxygenation for blood perfusing it.

Although shunt is one end of the spectrum of $\dot{V}/\dot{Q}$ mismatch, it behaves differently with respect to its response to supplemental oxygen than other forms of $\dot{V}/\dot{Q}$ mismatch; this difference can be used to distinguish between the two conditions clinically. Patients who are hypoxemic because of $\dot{V}/\dot{Q}$ mismatch will have a significant response in Pa_{O_2} with administration of supplemental oxygen. In patients who have regions of lungs with reduced ventilation, the alveolar O_2 falls, leading to hypoxemia. With administration of supplemental oxygen, however, the PA_{O_2} will rise in these units because they are receiving some ventilation and Pa_{O_2} will rise. In contrast, in patients with significant regions of lung demonstrating shunt physiology, supplemental oxygen will not have a significant effect on Pa_{O_2} because

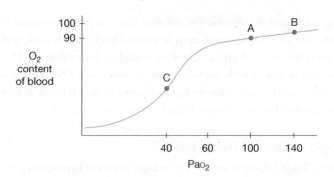

Figure 3-5: Relationship between Pao$_2$ and O$_2$ content. Because of the sigmoid shape of the oxygen-hemoglobin binding relationship, the O$_2$ content of blood is near maximum in normal lung units with a Pao$_2$ of 100 (A). By hyperventilating these units and raising the Pao$_2$ to 140 mm Hg (B), one does not increase the oxygen content of the blood significantly and cannot compensate for a disease unit with a Pao$_2$ of 40 and low oxygen content (C).

the lung units exhibiting shunt receive no ventilation; the Pao$_2$ does not rise in the lung units demonstrating shunt. In the normal units that do see the supplemental oxygen and experience an increase in alveolar Po$_2$, the capillary blood is already nearly fully saturated, and the supplemental oxygen does not result in a significant increase in oxygen content of the blood (see **Figure 3-5**).

Finally, diffusion abnormalities, which are most commonly because of disease processes that reduce the surface area for diffusion between alveoli and capillaries (eg, emphysema, interstitial lung diseases), usually do not lead to hypoxemia at rest because there is significant reserve capacity for diffusion, that is, equilibrium between the gas in the alveolus and capillary is achieved well before the red blood cell (RBC) exits the alveolar capillary. Consequently, delays because of thickening of the diffusion interface do not become clinically apparent until the velocity of the RBC through the capillary increases two- to threefold as occurs during exercise (see **Figure 3-6**).

Implications for Management of the Ventilator

Acute hypoxemic respiratory failure is common because of derangements in any of the three components of the respiratory system. For controller problems leading to hypoventilation, elevated levels of Paco$_2$, and hypoxemia with a normal A-aDo$_2$, establishing normal levels of V̇A is usually adequate to sustain the patient. If the patient has hypoxemia with an elevated A-aDo$_2$ but responds well to supplemental oxygen with a significant rise in Pao$_2$, one can conclude that V̇/Q̇ mismatch is the underlying mechanism or process causing the hypoxemia. If supplemental oxygen fails to increase the Pao$_2$ significantly, then one is likely dealing with significant shunt physiology. Additional measures, such as utilizing positive end expiratory pressure (PEEP), should be considered (more on this in Chapters 7 and 13).

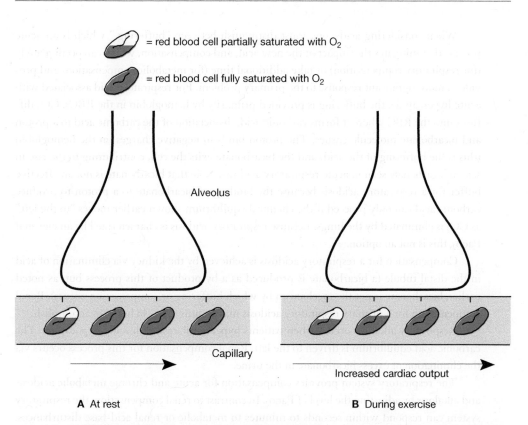

Figure 3-6: **Diffusion of oxygen. A,** At rest, equilibration between the alveolus and the blood occurs quickly. By the time a red blood cell (RBC) is one-third of the way through the alveolar capillary, the hemoglobin has picked up all the oxygen with which it is going to bind. **B,** During exercise, however, cardiac output increases, resulting in more rapid transit of RBCs through the capillary. In the diagram, equilibration between alveolus and blood is now shown as occurring farther along the capillary. If a pathologic process is present in the lung that prolongs diffusion time, equilibration may not occur between the alveolus and the blood. The result is a decrease in Pao₂ during exercise. (From The Gas Exchanger: Matching Ventilation and Perfusion. In: Schwartzstein RM, Parker MJ. *Respiratory Physiology: A Clinical Approach*. Wolters Kluwer; 2006:95-125. Figure 5.10.)

ACID-BASE BALANCE AND THE RESPIRATORY SYSTEM

Acids are produced in the body primarily because of the process of generating energy from carbohydrates (CHO), protein and fat. When burning CHO, we produce carbonic acid, which can dissociate to a proton and bicarbonate. Alternatively, carbonic acid dissociates to a molecule of water and carbon dioxide.

$$H_2O + CO_2 \longleftrightarrow H_2CO_3 \longleftrightarrow H^+ + HCO_3^-$$

The respiratory system removes large amounts of "respiratory" acid via elimination of carbon dioxide, which keeps this reaction moving to the left. The metabolism of proteins leads to additional "metabolic" acids, which are removed via the kidneys. Finally, metabolism of fats leads to ketoacids, which are further metabolized.

When considering acids, one must distinguish between "buffering," which is an acute process that mitigates the impact of the new acid, and compensation, which can occur acutely (for respiratory compensation) or take additional time (for metabolic compensation) and provides a more significant response to the primary problem. For respiratory acid associated with acute hypercapnia, the buffering is provided primarily by hemoglobin in the RBCs. CO_2 diffuses into the RBC where it forms carbonic acid; dissociation of the carbonic acid to a proton and bicarbonate molecule ensues. The proton binds to negative charges on the hemoglobin (this is the buffering of the acid) and the bicarbonate exits the cell, contributing to the rise in serum bicarbonate seen in acute respiratory acidosis. Note that bicarbonate is not an effective buffer for a respiratory acidosis because the binding of bicarbonate to a proton to produce carbonic acid can only proceed if the chemical equilibrium shown earlier moves "to the left" as CO_2 is eliminated by the lungs. Because respiratory acidosis is characterized by an elevated $Paco_2$, this is not an option.

Compensation for a respiratory acidosis is achieved by the kidney via elimination of acid in the distal tubule (a bicarbonate is produced as a by-product of this process but, as noted earlier, bicarbonate is not the mechanism by which buffering or compensation occurs). Renal compensation for a primary respiratory acidosis may require 24 to 48 hours to accomplish.

Respiratory alkalosis occurs when patients hyperventilate and develop hypocapnia. The carbonic acid equilibrium is driven to the left. Renal compensation for this process occurs via the elimination of excess bicarbonate in the urine.

The respiratory system provides compensation for acute and chronic metabolic acidosis and alkalosis by adjusting the level of $Paco_2$. In contrast to renal compensation, the respiratory system can respond within seconds to minutes to metabolic or renal acid-base disturbances. Metabolic (renal) compensation may take up to 48 hours to complete.

Implications for Management of the Ventilator

Much of what is described regarding respiratory acidosis and alkalosis and respiratory compensation for metabolic processes occurs because of the activity of various control mechanisms in the body that respond to changes in pH, receptors in the pulmonary interstitium, airways, and vasculature, along with behavioral factors, such as anxiety or fear. For patients with acute respiratory failure managed with mechanical ventilation and receiving sedative medications, the healthcare team may need to adjust the ventilator, effectively taking over for the controller. When regulating the minute ventilation for an acute respiratory acidosis or to compensate for a metabolic acidosis, you must consider whether you wish to increase the respiratory rate, the tidal volume, or both. Increasing the respiratory rate, which will decrease expiratory time, could be a problem in patients with high expiratory airway resistance and flow limitation (more on this in Chapter 11). Alternatively, increasing the tidal volume may be problematic if it results in a volume and/or plateau pressure that places the patient at risk for volutrauma. Clinical judgment must be used in these situations.

When choosing to adjust ventilation to achieve a target $Paco_2$ via alterations in respiratory rate, there is a simple calculation one can make to get a rough estimate of the change needed. Recall the relationship between $Paco_2$ and alveolar ventilation:

$$Paco_2 \, \alpha \, \dot{V}co_2/\dot{V}A$$

Assuming CO_2 production is constant while you are making your changes, $Paco_2$ is inversely related to alveolar ventilation. If you want to reduce $Paco_2$ to 4/5 of its present value, you increase ventilation by 5/4. You are adjusting total ventilation, not alveolar ventilation, per se, but because tidal volume is being held constant, you are not altering the ratio of dead space to tidal volume in each breath. This allows total ventilation to be a reasonably good proxy for alveolar ventilation.

If you choose to increase tidal volume to reduce the $Paco_2$ but find that $Paco_2$ rises rather than falls, beware of the possibility that you have inadvertently created more alveolar dead space by increasing alveolar pressure (assessed with plateau pressure). If P_{alv} rises to the point that it exceeds capillary pressure in the alveolus, perfusion to the alveolus will cease and dead space will result (see discussion of Zone 1 Lung in Figure 3-2).

SUMMARY

Acute respiratory failure is commonly associated with disturbances in oxygenation and elimination of carbon dioxide. An understanding of the five physiologic causes of hypoxemia enables you to analyze your patient's situation and focus in on changes in the ventilator that will be most effective in addressing the problem and minimizing the F_{IO_2} of supplemental oxygen required, thereby avoiding potential toxicity associated with hyperoxia in the lungs and other tissues. Similarly, a solid understanding of the principles underlying the elimination of carbon dioxide from the body allows you to regulate the ventilator in a manner that optimizes $Paco_2$.

Patients with acute respiratory failure often have multisystem disease that can lead to metabolic disturbances and acid-base disorders. When these are superimposed on hypoxemia and/or hypercapnia, a range of acid-base disturbances may result. For patients receiving significant sedation, the control mechanisms of the respiratory system may be suppressed, making it necessary for the healthcare provider to understand core principles of these interactions to facilitate optimal management of the mechanical ventilator.

KEY POINTS

- There are five core physiologic mechanisms underlying hypoxemia. Those that are associated with derangements of the gas exchanger have an abnormal alveolar to arterial oxygen difference ($A\text{-}aDo_2$).
- Excessive "doses" of supplemental oxygen, that is, high F_{IO_2}, may lead to oxygen toxicity of the lung; efforts should be made to reduce F_{IO_2} to less than 0.6.
- Ventilation-perfusion mismatch can be distinguished from pulmonary shunt by the response to supplemental oxygen. Pao_2 rises significantly with supplement oxygen in cases of $\dot{V}/\dot{Q}$ mismatch; shunt does not.
- Minute ventilation comprises alveolar ventilation and dead space ventilation; only alveolar ventilation contributes to gas exchange.
- Dead space can be subdivided into anatomic and alveolar dead space.
- Changes in the size of the breath will change the dead space to tidal volume ratio because anatomic dead space in the upper and central airways is the major component of dead space in most patients.
- Alveolar dead space typically rises in primary diseases of the lungs.
- $Paco_2$ is directly proportional to CO_2 production by the body and inversely related to alveolar ventilation.
- Increased alveolar pressure may lead to compression of alveolar capillaries, which can create alveolar dead space.

STUDY QUESTIONS AND ANSWERS

Questions

1. A 60-year-old man is intubated for hypoxemic respiratory failure because of pneumonia. His initial arterial blood gas showed Pao_2 50 mm Hg, $Paco_2$ 35 mm Hg, and pH 7.44. Supplemental oxygen is administered. With Fio_2 0.6, the Pao_2 rises to 58 mm Hg. The most likely mechanism responsible for his hypoxemia is:
   A. high altitude.
   B. hypoventilation.
   C. $\dot{V}/\dot{Q}$ mismatch.
   D. shunt.
   E. diffusion abnormality.

2. A patient with acute respiratory failure has a $Paco_2$ of 55 mm Hg with a pH of 7.29. You decide to reduce the tidal volume and increase the respiratory rate to increase the minute ventilation and reduce the $Paco_2$. When the arterial blood gas is checked, the $Paco_2$ is now 60 mm Hg. Oxygenation has not changed significantly.
   What is the best explanation for this result?
   A. The patient's carbon dioxide production must have increased.
   B. The patient's carbon dioxide production must have decreased.
   C. The dead space to tidal volume ratio increased with the reduction in tidal volume and alveolar ventilation fell.
   D. The change in the ventilator settings led to increased pulmonary shunt.
   E. None of the above

3. A patient with acute respiratory distress syndrome (ARDS) is being intubated and mechanically ventilated. Plateau pressures have been relatively high. In an effort to enhance oxygenation, the team increases the tidal volume and minute ventilation. The next blood gas shows an unexpected increase in the $Paco_2$. The most likely explanation for this change is:
   A. creation of dead space with high intra-alveolar pressure.
   B. increased respiratory system compliance.
   C. increased carbon dioxide production.
   D. a decrease in the intrapulmonary shunt.

Answers

1. **Answer D. Shunt**
   Rationale: The A-aDo_2 is 58 mm Hg, which exceeds the upper limit of normal for a 60-year-old man (age $\times$ 0.3 = 18). With an abnormal A-aDo_2, the hypoxemia is due to $\dot{V}/\dot{Q}$ mismatch, shunt, or a diffusion abnormality. Diffusion problems typically do not cause hypoxemia at rest. The minimal response to supplemental oxygen is more consistent with shunt than $\dot{V}/\dot{Q}$ mismatch.

2. **Answer C. The dead space to tidal volume ratio increased with the reduction in tidal volume and alveolar ventilation fell**
   Rationale: $Paco_2$ is inversely proportional to alveolar ventilation. Increasing total ventilation does not guarantee that alveolar ventilation goes up. By decreasing the tidal volume, the portion of each breath made up by dead space likely increased, which then leads to a decrease

in alveolar ventilation despite the increase in total ventilation. The change in tidal volume should not increase pulmonary shunt and Pa_{CO_2} is less likely to be affected by shunt than oxygenation, which did not change significantly.

3. **Answer A. Creation of dead space with high intra-alveolar pressure**

   Rationale: A patient with ARDS typically has low pulmonary compliance because of surfactant dysfunction. An increase in tidal volume will lead to an increase in alveolar pressure, which may be accentuated because of the low compliance. The high alveolar pressure may compress alveolar capillaries impairing perfusion and leading to creation of alveolar dead space. The change in ventilator settings should not affect CO_2 production nor alter intrapulmonary shunt.

Effects of Mechanical Ventilation on Cardiovascular Function

Richard M. Schwartzstein

LEARNING OBJECTIVES

- Describe the cardiovascular system response to increased work of breathing.
- Explain the effect of changes in intrathoracic pressure on cardiac function, contrasting spontaneous breathing with positive pressure ventilation.
- Define preload and afterload in the context of changing intrathoracic pressure.
- Explain the relationship between lung volume and pulmonary vascular resistance.
- Describe the impact of intra-alveolar pressure on pulmonary vascular resistance.

INTRODUCTION

A major feature of positive pressure ventilation is an increase in intrathoracic pressure during inspiration. Positive pressure may be present only during inspiration or may be present throughout the respiratory cycle if one applies positive end-expiratory pressure (PEEP) with the ventilator. The heart and great veins sit within the chest; consequently, as flexible structures, they are affected by these changes in pressure.

The right ventricle (RV) pumps blood through the pulmonary arterial system. Although this system has a much lower resistance than the systemic circulation, changes in lung volume and alveolar pressure may alter resistance and have an impact on right ventricular function and cardiac output. Although the focus of healthcare providers tends to be on gas exchange and lung mechanics for patients in the intensive care unit with acute respiratory failure, it is important that you understand the multiple interactions between the respiratory and cardiovascular systems and how mechanical ventilation can alter the hemodynamics of your patient.

WORK OF BREATHING AND CARDIOVASCULAR FUNCTION

Patients with acute respiratory failure often appear to be in "respiratory distress." Although the patient may or may not be able to describe if they are having breathing discomfort, or dyspnea, the physical exam, including observation of the patient's breathing, may tell you about the work of breathing. When we state the patient is in respiratory distress, we are describing physical findings or signs on exam. This is distinct from saying the patient has dyspnea, which is a symptom. Although we may suspect patient experiences of pain and breathing discomfort, by definition, only the patient can tell you if they are having a symptom. In Chapter 19, we will address the issue of dyspnea during mechanical ventilation.

The signs of respiratory distress are usually correlated with evidence of increased muscular efforts to generate a negative inspiratory pressure and aid in generating a high inspiratory flow and large tidal volume. These efforts are typically a reflection of increased respiratory drive (stimulation of the respiratory controller) and mechanical derangements of the ventilatory pump (eg, increased airway resistance or decreased lung or chest wall compliance), which necessitate greater driving pressure to produce the desired flow. Accessory muscles of ventilation are muscles whose primary function is something other than generating gas flow into or out of the lungs. Accessory muscles of **inhalation** include the external intercostal muscles, the pectoralis, the sternocleidomastoid, and the scalene muscles; these are called into action to assist the diaphragm to move the chest wall outward and generate a negative intrathoracic pressure for inspiration. Accessory muscles of **exhalation** include the internal intercostals and the abdominal muscles; remember, under normal conditions, exhalation during resting breathing is passive; the recoil force of the lungs is sufficient to exhale and muscle activity is not required.

With a normal respiratory system, the ventilatory muscles receive less than 20% of cardiac output, even during exercise. During a severe asthma attack, however, oxygen demand goes up significantly in these muscles as they must work to overcome airway resistance and the reduced compliance of the lungs and chest wall, most commonly seen if there is dynamic hyperinflation associated with flow limitation. With an increased end-expiratory lung volume associated with dynamic hyperinflation, the inspiratory muscles are shortened and become less effective in generating force. Cardiac output increases with contributions from both greater stroke volume and faster heart rate. In some cases, lactic acidosis develops because the increased work of breathing exceeds aerobic capacity of the inspiratory muscles. Patients with exacerbations of chronic obstructive lung disease (COPD) may demonstrate similar consequences of increased work of breathing.

Oxygen delivery to tissues depends on both cardiac output and oxygen content of the blood.

$$O_2 \text{ delivery} = \text{Cardiac output} \times \text{Oxygen content}$$

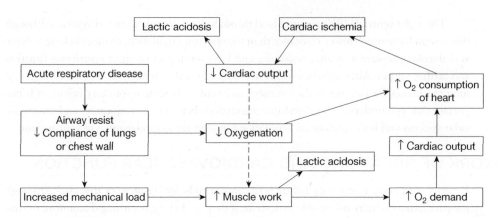

Figure 4-1: Effect of work of breathing on cardiac function. Acute respiratory failure is often the consequence of increased airway resistance and/or decreased lung and chest wall compliance, both of which will increase the work performed by the inspiratory muscles to generate a negative intrathoracic pressure. The increased oxygen demands of the muscles place an increased burden on the heart to generate greater cardiac output. To the extent that Pao_2 may be low and the energy demands of the ventilatory muscles may not be fully met by aerobic metabolism, lactic acid production will increase, which could compromise cardiac function. One can get into a downward spiral of compromised ventilatory muscle and cardiac function.

If the patient is hypoxemic with reduced oxygen saturation or is significantly anemic, oxygen delivery will fall, further placing the patient at risk for metabolic acidosis. If the patient has underlying systolic dysfunction of the heart in addition to their acute respiratory disease, stroke volume may be impaired, which will compromise cardiac output and O_2 delivery. For a patient with significant coronary artery disease, the increased demand placed on the heart by the work of breathing may provoke cardiac ischemia, which risks further systolic dysfunction, reduced O_2 delivery to the respiratory muscles, decreased inspiratory capacity, worse oxygenation, and a vicious cycle that can lead to death (**Figure 4-1**).

Intubation and initiation of positive pressure breathing is often undertaken as a means of interrupting this cycle. By reducing or removing the work of breathing and improving oxygenation, mechanical ventilation reduces the excess demand placed on the cardiovascular system by acute respiratory illness. Additional hemodynamic consequences, however, may follow.

HEMODYNAMIC EFFECTS OF BREATHING

With the swings in intrathoracic pressure associated with breathing, blood flow into the thorax will vary with the phase of the respiratory cycle. Because spontaneous breathing is characterized by negative pressure within the thorax during inspiration, whereas positive pressure ventilation is associated with positive intrathoracic inspiratory pressure, the effects on hemodynamics will differ between the two conditions. We will compare and contrast these effects during inspiration and expiration with spontaneous and assisted ventilation.

Preload

Preload is the length of a myocyte just prior to ventricular contraction. The overlap of actin and myosin within the cardiac sarcomere, which is set by the length of the myocyte at the end of diastole, determines the force of contraction when the fiber is electrically stimulated to contract. Because we cannot measure the length of the myocyte directly, we use the volume of the RV or left ventricle (LV) as a surrogate measure of the length of individual sarcomere. A plot of the relationship between ventricular end-diastolic volume and the resulting stroke volume on the next contraction is the Starling relationship (**Figure 4-2**).

The end-diastolic volume of the RV is determined by the amount of blood returning to the right atrium (RA) from the vena cava. Both the inferior and superior vena cava originate outside of the thorax and the pressure within them is positive. The portion of the vena cava within the thorax and the RA is subject to the changing intrathoracic pressure during the respiratory cycle; in the healthy individual, the pressure in the thorax is always negative during quiet breathing but becomes more negative during inspiration. This fall in pressure in the RA and intrathoracic vena cava increases the pressure gradient for blood to flow from the extrathoracic to the intrathoracic vascular structures and increase "venous return" to the right heart, thereby moving the patient's position on the Starling curve (**Figure 4-2**) to the right, which results in a greater stroke volume and cardiac output. During exhalation, intrathoracic pressure increases and the venous return falls. For an individual in acute respiratory distress with increased work of breathing, the swings in intrathoracic pressure are accentuated as are the hemodynamic consequences.

Although the output from the RV goes to the lungs and ultimately becomes the return of pulmonary venous blood from the lungs to the LV, the impact of the respiratory cycle is different for each ventricle. During inspiration, as the lung expands, the volume of the pulmonary veins, which are tethered open by the surrounding lung tissue, increases. The veins then act like a reservoir, collecting blood from the lungs but not passing it along to the left atrium and LV. Thus, there is movement to the left on the Starling curve for the LV during inspiration with reduced stroke volume and cardiac output. In addition, the size of the LV during inspiration may be reduced because of the enhanced RV filling, which shifts the interventricular septum (which separates the RV and LV) to the left. The reduced preload of the LV during inspiration is responsible for the fall in blood pressure associated with inspiration, which we call pulsus paradoxus. The size of the pulsus paradoxus is determined by the variation in intrathoracic pressure during the respiratory cycle.

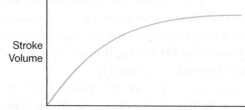

Figure 4.2: Starling curve. Stoke volume is dependent on actin-myosin overlap in the myocyte, which is determined by the end-diastolic ventricular volume (preload). Factors that reduce preload result in a movement along the curve to the left, with resulting decrease in stroke volume.

During positive pressure breathing, the sequence of events just described changes. Now intrathoracic pressure increases during inspiration and, if PEEP is present, during expiration as well. Consequently, the driving pressure for blood moving from the extrathoracic vena cava to the intrathoracic vena cava diminishes; venous return to the RV falls and shifts to the left on the Starling curve with reduced output to the LV and a fall in cardiac output to the systemic circulation. For a patient with marginal blood pressure, this reduction in venous return to the heart throughout the respiratory cycle may lead to frank hypotension and a hemodynamic emergency. Consequently, in patients with marginal intravascular volume who are about to be treated with positive pressure ventilation, be prepared to provide supplementary fluids.

During positive pressure ventilation, particularly if tidal volumes are large, there is some evidence that the lungs may exert a compressive force on the heart, further reducing cardiac filling and stroke volume. Again, blood pressure may be compromised.

Afterload

To fully understand the impact of positive pressure ventilation on afterload, we must first address the definition of the term; afterload is the wall stress within the myocardium as it generates a force in the ventricular chamber, which we measure as the intraventricular pressure during systole (assuming a normal aortic valve, the intraventricular pressure during systole equals systolic blood pressure). Although pressure in the ventricle and aorta during systole is commonly the same, this does not mean that afterload equals systolic blood pressure, a common misconception, because the wall stress experienced by individual contractile units in the process of generating that pressure varies with the radius of the chamber and the number of contractile units available to generate the pressure. Afterload is defined by the Law of Laplace:

$$\text{Wall stress} = Pr/\text{Wall thickness}$$

P, or pressure, is the pressure generated by the force of contraction; the higher the pressure, the greater the wall stress to achieve the pressure. The "r" represents the radius of the ventricular chamber at the onset of contraction. The ventricle generates a pressure within the chamber by a contraction of myocytes around the circumference of the chamber; in the process of making the circumference smaller, a vector force is generated inward to produce the intraventricular pressure. The greater the radius, the smaller the inward vector factor force and the greater the wall stress to achieve a given intraventricular pressure (see **Figure 4-3**). This is why a patient with chronic mitral regurgitation and a large, dilated ventricle may have greater afterload with a blood pressure of 100 mm Hg than a healthy individual with a normal size ventricle and systolic blood pressure of 120 mm Hg.

The "thickness" component of the Law of Laplace refers to the number of contractile units available to generate the force. In a patient with chronic hypertension (and high wall stress), the body adapts by generating new contractile units, a process that we call "hypertrophy." The stress is now dispersed across more contractile units, thereby reducing the "afterload" for any given unit.

The effect of positive pressure breathing on afterload is related to the changing intrathoracic pressure during the respiratory cycle. Under conditions of spontaneous breathing, the intrathoracic pressure is generally negative and moves from smaller to larger negative values

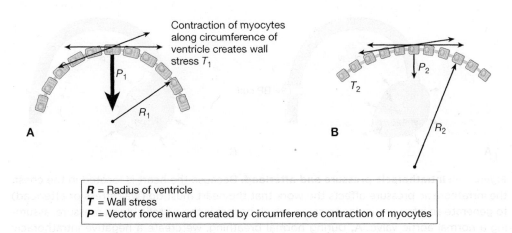

Contraction of myocytes along circumference of ventricle creates wall stress T_1

R = Radius of ventricle
T = Wall stress
P = Vector force inward created by circumference contraction of myocytes

Figure 4-3: Afterload and the Law of Laplace. The Law of Laplace defines cardiac afterload, which is equivalent to wall stress.

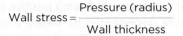

$$\text{Wall stress} = \frac{\text{Pressure (radius)}}{\text{Wall thickness}}$$

As myocytes contract along the circumference of the ventricle, they act to shorten or decrease the circumference. This has the effect of generating a vector force inward toward the center of the ventricle, which we measure as pressure. **A,** a ventricle with a relatively small radius at the onset of contraction. **B,** a ventricle with a larger radius at the onset of contraction. For a given wall stress, the pressure generated with a small radius is greater than the pressure generated with a large radius.

during inspiration and back down during exhalation. The negative intrathoracic pressure around the heart exerts a force that tends to expand the heart, which causes the intraventricular pressure to fall. If the desired intraventricular pressure during systole is +120 mm Hg and the intrathoracic pressure is –10 mm Hg, the heart must contract more forcefully to overcome the intrathoracic pressure and reach a pressure of 120 mm Hg (see **Figure 4-4**, panel A); wall stress (or afterload) is increased. In contrast, the institution of positive pressure breathing makes the intrathoracic pressure positive throughout the respiratory cycle, with the least positive values at the end of exhalation and the most positive values at the end of inspiration; wall stress (or afterload) is decreased when the positive pressure in the thorax is "assisting" the myocardium in producing the desired intraventricular systolic pressure (see **Figure 4-4**, panel B).

For patients with acute myocardial ischemia and resultant pulmonary edema, the institution of positive pressure ventilation reduces wall stress and may reduce myocardial oxygen demand, thereby potentially alleviating the ischemia. In addition, the impact of positive pressure in the thorax on venous return to the right heart (reduced preload) also reduces afterload by virtue of reducing the volume (and radius) of the ventricle (yes, reducing preload reduces afterload—take another look at the Law of Laplace if this is confusing).

Patients with asthma or COPD and acute respiratory distress and work of breathing typically have very large negative pressure in the thorax during inspiration. This has the effect of increasing afterload, which is relieved by institution of positive pressure ventilation.

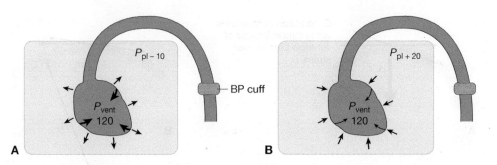

Figure 4-4: Intrathoracic pressure and afterload. Because the heart is located in the chest, the intrathoracic pressure affects the work that the heart must do (wall stress or afterload) to generate an intraventricular pressure, which becomes the systolic blood pressure, assuming a normal aortic valve. **A,** During normal breathing, we create a negative intrathoracic pressure (represented by pleural pressure [Ppl], P_{pl} –10 mm Hg in this example), which tends to expand the heart. Thus, to generate an intraventricular pressure of 120 mm Hg, the heart must contract with a force that would generate a total of 130 mm Hg of pressure to overcome the negative intrathoracic pressure. **B,** During positive pressure breathing, we create a positive intrathoracic pressure (represented by pleural pressure, P_{pl} +20 mm Hg in this example), which tends to compress the heart. Thus, to generate an intraventricular pressure of 120 mm Hg, the heart must contract with a force that would generate a total of only 100 mm Hg of pressure to supplement the positive intrathoracic pressure and achieve the desired blood pressure.

EFFECT OF POSITIVE PRESSURE VENTILATION ON PULMONARY VASCULAR RESISTANCE

There are two types of blood vessels in the lungs: large vessels and small vessels. The large vessels travel in the lung parenchyma and vary in diameter with lung volume; thus, at low lung volume, the radius is small and resistance is high in these vessels. The small vessels are surrounding the alveoli. As the distending pressure increases in the alveoli, that is, as they get larger, these small vessels are compressed and resistance goes up. Consequently, the effect of lung volume is opposite for the two types of vessels leading to a U-shaped curve when we look at the total pulmonary vascular resistance (PVR; **Figure 4-5**).

Generally, patients with acute respiratory failure tend to have an end-expiratory lung volume that is near functional residual capacity (FRC; the normal end-expiratory volume at which the force of chest wall recoil outward is equal and opposite to the inward recoil force of the lungs). There are two conditions, however, associated with end-expiratory lung volume that may vary considerably from FRC and consequently, vascular resistance will increase; this increase in resistance may affect cardiac output and blood pressure.

In patients with severe obstructive lung disease and tachypnea, expiratory time is reduced; in the setting of flow limitation, this will lead to dynamic hyperinflation. With shortened expiratory time (whether with spontaneous breathing or in a patient treated with mechanical ventilation), the inhaled volume cannot be exhaled fully, and the subsequent breath starts at a higher lung volume. This process continues until the lung has reached a new equilibrium at which the volume of gas inhaled equals the volume exhaled (see **Figure 4-6**). The new equilibrium is achieved because the elastic recoil force of the lung is greater at higher lung volume (greater driving force for exhalation) and because the diameter of airways increases at

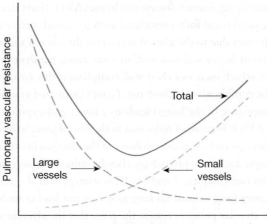

Figure 4-5: Effect of lung volume on pulmonary vascular resistance. The large blood vessels in the lung are distended by the surrounding lung tissues as the lung expands. In contrast, the smaller alveolar vessels have increased resistance as the lung increases in size because of the distending pressure of the alveolus compressing these small, thin-walled vessels.

higher volumes, thereby reducing resistance to expiratory flow. At these higher lung volumes, however, PVR increases because of compression of small pulmonary vessels as a result of the high transpulmonary pressure (**Figure 4-5**). The higher PVR may impair right ventricular function, leading to increased right ventricular pressure and volume, with a shift of the interventricular septum to the left, which compromises left ventricular compliance and filling. The institution of treatment with intubation and initiation of mechanical ventilation must take these findings into account to avoid further compromise of hemodynamics. Particular attention must be given to allowing sufficient expiratory time to reduce dynamic hyperinflation.

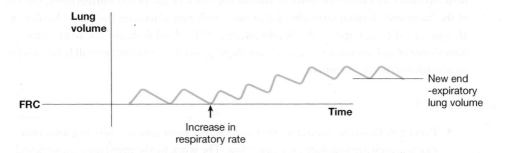

Figure 4-6: Dynamic hyperinflation. For a patient with expiratory flow limitation, exhalation may consume all of the time allotted for exhalation (T_i, inspiratory time; T_e, expiratory time); this is in contrast to a healthy individual in whom expiratory flow takes up only a portion of expiratory time. In the graphic shown, the patient (who has significant expiratory resistance and flow limitation) is initially coming down to functional residual capacity (FRC) at the end of the exhalation. With an increase in respiratory rate from 12 to 20 breaths/min, however, expiratory time is shortened and the expiratory time is no longer sufficient to allow all the air inhaled to come out in the allotted time for exhalation; end-expiratory volume begins to rise. This process continues on successive breaths until the patient establishes a new equilibrium (same amount of gas inspired and expired) at a higher end-expiratory lung volume. See Chapter 11, COPD, for additional information on dynamic hyperinflation.

Patients with acute respiratory distress syndrome (ARDS) have decreased lung compliance because of the enhanced recoil forces associated with increased surface tension in the air-liquid interface of the alveolus due to the altered surfactant the altered surfactant in this condition. In addition, the use of heavy sedation and, in some cases, paralytics may reduce the tone of chest wall muscles, which increases chest wall compliance; this reduces the outward recoil of the chest wall. The combination of these two factors (increased compliance of the chest wall and decreased compliance of the lungs) leads to a lower end-expiratory lung volume, which can cause increased PVR because of reduction in the size of extra-alveolar vessels (**Figure 4-5**). PEEP is used to increase end-expiratory volume of the alveolus in order to reduce the possibility of alveolar collapse and shunt physiology, thereby enhancing oxygenation and reducing the risk of atelectrauma (see Chapters 3 and 13). This strategy will also improve PVR by increasing the end-expiratory lung volume (as long as it does not lead to such high pressures during inhalation that the alveolar pressure rises to the point that the alveolar vessels are compressed).

The reduced compliance of the lungs in ARDS also predisposes to higher alveolar pressure with mechanical ventilation to achieve the desired tidal volume. Although efforts are made to avoid pressures above 20 to 25 cm H_2O to avoid volutrauma, higher pressures are sometimes required. Higher alveolar pressure may compress alveolar arterioles and capillaries, leading to higher PVR, greater work for the RV, and the creation of zone I lung and pulmonary dead space (see Figure 3-2, Chapter 3).

SUMMARY

Although the natural focus of the healthcare provider caring for a patient with acute respiratory failure is centered on the respiratory system, the heart and lungs are intimately connected by the pulmonary vasculature and experience a common intrathoracic environment with varying pressure throughout the respiratory cycle. Variations in intrathoracic pressure may have significant effect on both preload and afterload of the RV and LV, which may alter hemodynamics and blood pressure as well as the work of the heart. Furthermore, the size of the lungs and elevated intra-alveolar pressure will have effects on the extra-alveolar and alveolar vasculature, respectively, thereby altering PVR, blood flow, and the work of the RV. Knowledge of and attention to these relationships between the two organs will help you optimize cardiopulmonary function.

KEY POINTS

- Patients with severe inspiratory airway resistance must generate very negative intrathoracic pressure to achieve adequate flow. The work by the inspiratory muscles and demand for a greater portion of cardiac output will increase the work of the heart. Initiation of positive pressure ventilation in such a patient will reduce the need for a high cardiac output and will reduce myocardial oxygen demand.
- During inspiration with positive pressure ventilation, venous return to the RV (preload) is reduced.
- The use of PEEP reduces venous return to and preload of the RV.
- During inspiration with positive pressure ventilation, afterload or wall stress of the ventricle is reduced.
- PVR is affected by lung volume; both very high and very low lung volumes are associated with elevated PVR.
- PVR may increase with high intra-alveolar pressure.

STUDY QUESTIONS AND ANSWERS

Questions

1. A is admitted after three days of high fever, nausea, and a multilobar pneumonia. Because of progressive hypoxemia, the patient is intubated and started on positive pressure ventilation. Blood pressure is low after initiation of mechanical ventilation and you are considering starting vasopressors. At this point, you should:

   A. diurese the patient.

   B. give crystalloid fluids to the patient.

   C. raise the PEEP.

   D. increase the respiratory rate.

2. You are caring for a patient with severe emphysema who is in acute respiratory failure and receiving positive pressure ventilation with PEEP set at 5 cm H_2O. The $Paco_2$ is elevated, and you decide to increase minute ventilation by increasing the respiratory rates. You re-check the arterial blood gas and find that the $Paco_2$ is even higher than before. What is the best explanation for this finding?

   A. The patient has developed heart failure.

   B. Right ventricular preload has increased.

   C. Alveolar pressure has increased.

   D. PEEP is too low.

3. A patient with acute myocardial ischemia and pulmonary edema is in respiratory failure and is intubated and treated with positive pressure ventilation. The major benefit of initiating positive pressure ventilation in this setting is:

   A. decreased afterload.

   B. decreased stroke volume.

   C. reduced PVR.

   D. increased intra-alveolar pressure.

Answers

1. **Answer B. give crystalloid fluids to the patient**

   Rationale: With fever and nausea for several days, the patient probably has intravascular volume depletion and is to the far left on the Starling curve. This will reduce stroke volume, cardiac output, and blood pressure. When positive pressure ventilation is started, intrathoracic pressure is increased and venous return goes down farther and blood pressure is further compromised. The patient should be given crystalloid fluids to enhance preload and cardiac output.

   Diuresis would exacerbate the problem by further reducing preload. Elevating PEEP, by further increasing intrathoracic pressure, will decrease venous return and exacerbate the problem. Increasing the respiratory rate will either not have an effect on hemodynamics or may worsen them if there is significant expiratory airway resistance and dynamic hyperinflation, which will elevate intrathoracic pressure.

2. **Answer C. Alveolar pressure has increased**

   Rationale: In a patient with COPD and severe expiratory airflow obstruction, it is important that you provide adequate expiratory time; failure to do so will lead to dynamic hyperinflation, increased lung volume, and increased intra-alveolar pressure, which will compress and

(continued)

may occlude the pulmonary capillaries leading to the creation of dead space. Consequently, even though total ventilation may be increased by raising the respiratory rate, the alveolar ventilation, which determines $Paco_2$, will be reduced because of the creation of alveolar dead space (the alveolus is receiving ventilation but no perfusion). Changing the respiratory rate is unlikely to precipitate heart failure and may reduce right ventricular preload because of the higher intrathoracic pressure as described earlier. Further elevations in PEEP will exacerbate the high intra-alveolar pressure and worsen the problem of increased dead space.

3. **Answer is A. Decreased afterload**

   Rationale: Afterload, or wall stress, is exemplified by the Law of Laplace for the heart. By increasing intrathoracic pressure, the LV has to do less work (generate less wall tension) to achieve a desired intraventricular pressure, which leads to the blood pressure needed by the body. In addition, the impact of positive pressure in the thorax on the preload (reduces intraventricular filling) will reduce the radius of the ventricle, further reducing afterload, myocardial oxygen consumption, and ischemia, which may enhance the contractile force generated by the ventricle leading to improved stroke volume and cardiac output. PVR may actually increase with positive pressure ventilation because of increased intra-alveolar pressure.

Basics of Mechanical Ventilation

Basics of Mechanical Ventilation

Pressure and Volume Control Ventilation

Jeremy B. Richards • Diana Bouhassira

LEARNING OBJECTIVES

- Describe ventilator settings for pressure and volume control ventilation.
- Identify appropriate clinical circumstances for initiating a controlled mode of mechanical ventilation.
- Discuss the differences between volume control and pressure control ventilation.
- Delineate the physiologic effects of volume and pressure control ventilation.
- Determine when to adjust ventilator settings for patients on pressure or volume control ventilation.

INTRODUCTION

Controlled mechanical ventilation is a broad clinical term describing ventilatory modes in which a patient's respiratory cycle is completely controlled by the ventilator. Controlled mechanical ventilation is subdivided into either pressure control ventilation or volume control ventilation, with either pressure or volume, respectively, being set by the ventilator. Controlled modes of mechanical ventilation are indicated for patients with severe, advanced respiratory failure, and understanding the intricacies of volume and pressure control ventilation is essential for healthcare providers caring for intubated and mechanically ventilated patients. In this chapter, we review the indications for using controlled modes of ventilation, as well as the ventilator settings and clinical management approaches to using volume or pressure control ventilation.

PHYSIOLOGIC CONTEXT

Pressure and volume are two important clinical and physiologic concepts in mechanical ventilation. Pressure is the force exerted by a gas on a surface and is measured in either Pascals or, much more commonly in clinical practice, in millimeters of mercury (mm Hg) with respect to the cardiovascular system and centimeters of water (cm H_2O) for the respiratory system. Volume is the amount of space that a gas occupies and is measured in either milliliters (mL) or liters (L). The relationship between pressure and volume is known as Boyle's law, which states that when the volume of a gas increases, the pressure decreases. In addition, the concept of compliance is critical in understanding the relationship between volume and pressure in respiratory physiology. Compliance is defined as the "change in volume" divided by the "change in pressure" (see **Figure 5-1**), and compliance may be affected by either lung physiology or chest wall processes (the respiratory system comprises *both* the lungs *and* the chest wall). The implications of Boyle's law and the concept of respiratory system compliance are discussed in more detail later; understanding the relationships between pressure and volume is critically important when determining initial ventilator settings and for monitoring the effects of either pressure control or volume control ventilation on a patient's respiratory system.

In order to maintain a patient's respiratory status, it is important to control both the pressure and volume of their ventilation. There are a variety of different types of mechanical ventilators, with the two major modes being positive pressure ventilators and negative pressure ventilators. Positive pressure ventilators provide positive pressure to the lungs, whereas negative pressure ventilators generate negative pressure external to the thoracic cavity, resulting in expansion of the rib cage and chest wall, which results in a negative pressure in the thorax and flow of air into the respiratory system. Negative pressure ventilation is rarely used in contemporary clinical practice (it was a mainstay for the treatment of respiratory failure because of neuromuscular disease, particularly polio, in the 1950s) and will not be discussed further in this chapter.

Pressure and volume can also be controlled manually using an Ambu bag or similar device. An Ambu bag is a hand-held device which, when squeezed manually, delivers positive

Boyle's law	Compliance
$P_1V_1 = P_2V_2$	$C = \dfrac{\Delta V}{\Delta P}$

Figure 5-1: **Boyle's law and compliance are critical physiologic concepts for understanding the mechanics of mechanical ventilation**.

pressure ventilation to the lungs. It can be used for both rescue breathing and regular ventilation depending on a patient's clinical circumstances and the clinical settings. Pressure and volume cannot be precisely regulated through standard manual bagging techniques, as neither the volume delivered through an Ambu bag nor the pressure generated by manually bagging a patient are measured.

In this context, this chapter focuses on positive pressure ventilation in general and controlled mechanical ventilation specifically. With controlled mechanical ventilation, either volume or pressure can be set by a healthcare provider and precisely delivered by the ventilator. Furthermore, the effects of setting a given volume or pressure (via Boyle's law and the patient's respiratory system compliance) can be accurately measured by the ventilator, allowing the healthcare provider to adjust ventilator settings to achieve optimal physiologic outcomes from controlled modes of mechanical ventilation.

INDICATIONS FOR CONTROLLED MECHANICAL VENTILATION

In general, the foundational indications for the initiation of mechanical ventilation are either inadequate ventilation (eg, the elimination of carbon dioxide from the body) or impaired gas exchange (eg, the update of oxygen across the alveolar-capillary basement membrane). Issues with ventilation and/or gas exchange can manifest as several specific indications for choosing to initiate controlled mechanical ventilation, including:

1. **Acute or chronic respiratory failure:** Respiratory failure is broadly defined as a clinical circumstance in which a patient is unable to maintain adequate oxygenation and/or ventilation on their own, requiring initiation of supplemental oxygen and/or mechanical ventilation. As described in Chapter 1, respiratory failure may be the consequence of abnormalities in any of the three elements of the respiratory system: the controller, the ventilatory pump, or the gas exchanger. Respiratory failure can be acute, chronic, or acute on chronic in onset. Acute respiratory failure generally refers to a deterioration in a patient's respiratory status over seconds, minutes, hours, or days, with the additional implication that the cause of the patient's respiratory failure may be reversible. Chronic respiratory failure describes long-standing impairment in either gas exchange or ventilation, with the implication that the patient's respiratory dysfunction is not reversible. Acute on chronic respiratory failure refers to an acute worsening of a patient's baseline compromised oxygenation and/or ventilation, with the anticipation that with treatment and supportive care, the acute component of the patient's respiratory deterioration will be reversible.

2. **Cardiac arrest:** Cardiac arrest is broadly defined as a condition in which the heart stops pumping blood and the patient requires resuscitation, including chest compressions and exogenous ventilation, in order to survive. Intubation and initiation of mechanical ventilation is a component of advanced cardiac life support for select patients who suffer cardiac arrest, and it is typically a component of postarrest care for patients who remain comatose after return of spontaneous circulation.

3. **Anesthesia:** When patients receive deep sedation or are put under general anesthesia in order to have surgery or other medical procedures performed, mechanical

ventilation is necessary because of suppression of the respiratory controller by the anesthetic agents. A state of anesthesia and/or altered mental status can also occur from ingestion or overdose of respiratory depressants such as opiates, benzodiazepines, alcohol, and other such substances. Because of impairment of the patient's respiratory controller from anesthetic effects, initiation of ventilation, typically with intubation and positive pressure ventilation, is necessary to maintain oxygenation and to achieve elimination of carbon dioxide.

4. **Airway protection:** This is when an endotracheal tube is inserted into the patient's airway in order to maintain airway patency and to allow for initiation of mechanical ventilation. A patient may require intubation for airway protection in the setting of altered mental status (eg, because of opiates, anesthesia, or other causes of depressed respiratory controller function) or from airway compromises (eg, because of mucus plugging, external airway compression, or other causes of decreased airway patency). One determines the need for airway protection by assessing the patient's gag reflex and ability to cough.

VOLUME CONTROL OR PRESSURE CONTROL?

There are no major studies demonstrating a significant difference in patient-centered outcomes between volume control versus pressure control ventilation, and the decision to use volume control or pressure control frequently is based on institutional preference and local practice patterns. In general, volume control ventilation tends to be more commonly used than pressure control ventilation, although this varies significantly based on local and regional practice patterns. As noted earlier, pressure and volume are linked by the concept of compliance: $\Delta V/\Delta P$ = compliance. With volume ventilation, if one sets the ventilator to provide a given volume, the resulting pressure is the dependent variable; if one utilizes pressure ventilation and delivers gas until a predetermined pressure is achieved, the resulting volume becomes the dependent variable.

In general, there are no disease-specific indications for choosing volume control versus pressure control ventilation, although the seminal ARDSNet study of patients with acute respiratory distress syndrome (ARDS) demonstrated decreased mortality for patients randomized to receive lower tidal volumes delivered via volume control ventilation. As such, in general, it may be preferable to employ volume control ventilation for patients with ARDS (see Chapter 13 for more extensive discussion of ventilator use to treat ARDS).

There are limited data indicating that pressure control ventilation may result in improved gas exchange and oxygenation in select populations (eg, obese patients, patients undergoing surgery). There are, however, no studies demonstrating significant differences between volume control and pressure control ventilation within heterogeneous populations of critically ill patients. As such, the decision to initiate volume control versus pressure control ventilation will primarily depend on local practice patterns and a patient's specific clinical circumstances. In general, volume control ventilation is a reasonable initial choice for patients requiring initiation of controlled mechanical ventilation. For patients with very high inspiratory drive to breathe, pressure control ventilation may be preferred because it typically provides a higher inspiratory flow than does volume ventilation; by meeting the patient's demand for high flow, dyspnea on the ventilator may be minimized.

RESPIRATORY RATE

Terminology

For either volume control or pressure control ventilation, the respiratory rate (RR) delivered by the ventilator is set by the healthcare provider. The set RR is the minimum obligatory number of breaths per minute that the patient will receive while they are maintained on controlled mechanical ventilation. If the patient initiates additional breaths above the set RR, the ventilator will support those additional breaths by providing either the set tidal volume (for volume control ventilation) or the set inspiratory pressure (for pressure control ventilation). To acknowledge that additional, patient-triggered breaths are supported (or "assisted") by the ventilator, volume- or pressure-controlled ventilation is sometimes referred to as "volume assist control" or "pressure assist control" ventilation. Given that all contemporary ventilators support or "assist" additional, patient-triggered breaths, however, "volume control ventilation" and "volume assist control ventilation" are practically and functionally synonymous. Consequently, we use the terms "volume control ventilation" and "pressure control ventilation" in this chapter (as is common in clinical practice) rather than "volume assist control" or "pressure assist control" ventilation.

Set Versus Actual Respiratory Rate

For both volume and pressure control modes of ventilation, the RR delivered by the ventilator must be set by the healthcare provider. As noted earlier, the patient may trigger extra breaths on top of the set RR, resulting in an actual RR that is higher than the set RR.

How does the ventilator determine that a patient is triggering extra, additional breaths above the set RR? There are two different methods by which the mechanical ventilator can detect a patient's inspiratory effort: pressure-triggered or flow-triggered breaths. In a pressure-triggered mode, the ventilator will initiate an inspiratory cycle (either delivering a set tidal volume for volume control ventilation or a set airway pressure for pressure control ventilation) when a patient generates a specific amount of negative intrathoracic pressure. By contracting the diaphragm, a patient can generate negative intrathoracic pressure, which is detected by a pressure monitor within the ventilator tubing. Typical pressure trigger thresholds are –0.5 to –1 cm H_2O. After detecting the threshold decrease in intrathoracic pressure, the ventilator will either deliver a set tidal volume (for volume control ventilation) or a set inspiratory airway pressure (for pressure control ventilation). Very low or very high trigger thresholds may result in patient-ventilator dyssynchrony (see Chapter 15).

VOLUME CONTROL VENTILATION

Regardless of the specific indication for initiation of controlled mechanical ventilation, healthcare providers must understand how to properly control the volume and pressure of the ventilator in order to ensure that patients who are intubated receive adequate ventilation. There are two types of volume control ventilation: constant pressure and constant flow.

In constant flow volume control, the ventilator delivers a set number of breaths per minute at a set flow. V_t is determined by the healthcare provider, and the flow can either be set by the ventilator or be adjusted by the provider. The flow rate and the inspiratory time together result in the preset V_t being delivered during each inspiratory cycle. In certain circumstances, the inspiratory flow can be increased or decreased, resulting respectively in a shorter or longer inspiratory phase of the respiratory cycle.

VOLUME CONTROL VENTILATION: INITIAL SETTINGS

Several settings on the ventilator must be configured prior to initiating volume control ventilation. The first setting is the type of ventilation—when initiating controlled mechanical ventilation, either volume-controlled or pressure-controlled ventilation must be selected. The second setting is the backup RR, which can be fixed at either a high or low number depending on the patient's needs. The third setting is the amount of air that is pushed into the lungs with each breath (the tidal volume or V_t), which is dictated by a number of both patient-level and clinical factors. The fourth setting is the level of positive end-expiratory pressure (PEEP), which helps to keep the lungs inflated during exhalation and reduces the likelihood of atelectasis. Finally, the fraction of inspired oxygen (FIo_2) must be set, informed by the patient's oxygenation status and clinical circumstances. Chapter 8, Section "Setting the Ventilator," provides an in-depth consideration of setting the PEEP and FIo_2.

In addition to these initial settings, as noted earlier, inspiratory flow can be used as a signal to the ventilator that a patient is attempting to initiate a breath. When a patient contracts their diaphragm and generates negative intrathoracic pressure, air starts flowing into the lungs, and the increase in inspiratory flow can be detected by the ventilator and used as a signal for the ventilator to deliver the set tidal volume (for volume control ventilation) or set inspiratory pressure (for pressure control ventilation). The differences between pressure- and flow-triggered breaths are depicted in **Figure 5-2**.

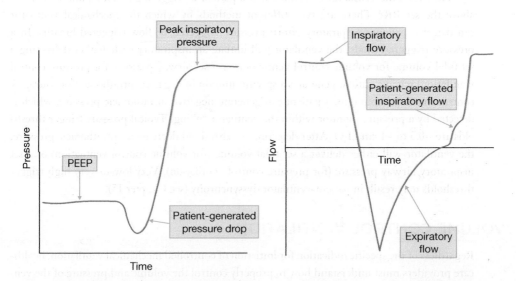

Figure 5-2: Pressure-time and flow-time tracings depicting different triggers for inspiration for mechanically ventilated patients. **A,** a pressure-mediated trigger, in which the patient generates negative intrathoracic pressure, which results in a downward deviation in the pressure tracing. In response to this downward deviation in pressure, the ventilator cycles from exhalation (providing PEEP) to inhalation (delivering a preset tidal volume or inspiratory pressure). **B,** a flow-mediated trigger, in which an upper deviation in flow, generated by a patient's inspiratory effort, results in the ventilator cycling from providing PEEP to delivering a preset inspiratory tidal volume or pressure. PEEP, positive end-expiratory pressure.

VOLUME CONTROL VENTILATION: CLINICAL MONITORING

For all patients who are intubated and initiated on mechanical ventilation, it is critical to monitor the vital signs and overall clinical status. Basic vital sign monitoring includes assessment of the patient's heart rate, blood pressure, RR, and oxygenation via pulse oximetry. In addition, given that controlled mechanical ventilation is characterized by setting a minimum obligatory RR and a set tidal volume, assessing for synchrony of the patient with the ventilator settings is critical.

Rate or Volume Dyssynchrony

A patient may be dyssynchronous with regard to either RR or tidal volume. A patient who is breathing above the RR set on the mechanical ventilator is dyssynchronous with regard to rate. Of note, it is extremely rare for a patient to have a lower RR than what is set by the ventilator as a backup rate (ie, the rate that will be provided in the absence of patient-initiated breaths)—if a patient's observed RR is lower than the ventilator's set rate, one should ensure that the patient has not somehow become disconnected from the ventilator (eg, the ventilator tubing has been dislodged or obstructed).

If a patient's exhaled tidal volume is significantly different than the V_t that the ventilator is set to deliver, then the patient is dyssynchronous with regard to volume. Although there is no universally accepted definition of volume dyssynchrony, a practical guideline is that if a patient's exhaled tidal volume is consistently more than 10% different than the set V_t, then the patient is dyssynchronous.

When a patient is dyssynchronous with regard to rate or volume, the healthcare provider must determine the cause(s) of dyssynchrony. One of the most common causes of rate or volume dyssynchrony is inadequate sedation. Natural, spontaneous breathing is characterized by variation in patients' RRs and tidal volumes—it is not normal or comfortable to breathe at a set rate and a homogeneous tidal volume breath over breath, minute over minute, hour over hour. Consequently, patients who are treated with mechanical ventilation frequently require adequate sedation to obligate ventilator synchrony. Other potential causes of dyssynchrony include inadequate respiratory flow, as dyspneic patients may prefer higher inspiratory flow, as the sensation of inspiratory flow can help mitigate the symptoms of dyspnea. Impaired ventilation and/or oxygenation can also stimulate an augmented respiratory drive and can contribute to rate or volume dyssynchrony.

Monitoring Pressure

For patients initiated on volume control ventilation, the ventilator delivers a set tidal volume during every inspiratory cycle. This set volume, based on the principle of Boyle's law and the patient's respiratory system compliance, will generate a positive pressure within the thorax. Specifically, delivering a set tidal volume during inhalation will result in a peak inspiratory pressure (PIP) as gas is flowing into the lung and a plateau pressure, which is determined by creating an "inspiratory hold" at the end of inspiration during which no gas is allowed into or out of the lungs (see Chapter 2), both of which need to be monitored as high PIPs and/or plateau pressures are associated with increased morbidity and mortality.

PIPs are generated by the movement of air through the patient's respiratory system during inhalation. The PIP is directly proportional to the resistance of a patient's respiratory system, with processes such as mucus plugging, obstructive airways disease, narrow endotracheal tube, and/or external airway compression resulting in elevated PIPs.

The plateau pressure can be characterized as the distending pressure required to inflate the lung and chest wall to the desired V_t. The set V_t and the patient's respiratory system compliance (again, defined as the change in volume divided by the change in pressure) directly determine the plateau pressure—patients with low respiratory system compliance will have higher plateau pressures (more pressure is required to stretch stiff, poorly compliant lungs or chest wall), whereas patients with high respiratory system compliance will have lower plateau pressures (less pressure is required to stretch loose, highly compliant lungs/chest wall).

As discussed in Chapter 8, Section "Setting the Ventilator," elevated plateau pressures have been strongly and repeatedly associated with increased mortality for patients with ARDS. Specifically, a plateau pressure of ≥30 cm H_2O has been shown to significantly increase mortality in mechanically ventilated patients. If a patient is found to have a high PIP and/or high plateau pressure, the first step is to reduce the set V_t, as a lower V_t will result in lower airway pressures. When decreasing the set V_t, the healthcare provider should continue to follow the PIP and plateau pressures, as well as the patient's minute ventilation, exhaled CO_2, and $Paco_2$ to ensure that ventilation is not prohibitively compromised by decreasing the set V_t.

PRESSURE CONTROL VENTILATION

In pressure control ventilation, the ventilator provides a flow of gas until a preset pressure is achieved; the volume of air flowing into the lungs varies based on the compliance of the respiratory system and patient effort to inhale. In constant pressure volume control, the ventilator delivers a set number of breaths per minute at a set pressure. The V_t generated by a set inspiratory pressure is directly dependent on the patient's respiratory system compliance. Specifically, a patient with low respiratory system compliance will have lower tidal volumes in response to a given set inspiratory pressure as compared to a patient with higher respiratory system compliance. In addition, if the patient is actively inspiring, that is, using their inspiratory muscles to expand the chest wall and reduce intrathoracic pressure, inspiratory flow and volume will increase.

PRESSURE CONTROL VENTILATION: CLINICAL MONITORING

Clinical monitoring for patients receiving pressure control ventilation is similar to what one provides for patients receiving volume control ventilation; one must follow the patient's vital signs and overall clinical status. Additionally, specifically for pressure control ventilation, the delivered tidal volume much be closely followed. Because the V_t is not set with pressure control ventilation, the inspiratory pressure must be increased if the V_t is too low or decreased if the V_t is too high. Changes in V_t should be coupled with close monitoring of the patient's ventilatory status, including minute ventilation, exhaled CO_2, and $Paco_2$.

COMPLICATIONS OF CONTROLLED MECHANICAL VENTILATION

Controlled mechanical ventilation, either volume or pressure control ventilation, is the most common mode of ventilation used in the intensive care unit (ICU). Although mechanical ventilation is a lifesaving intervention for many patients, it is not without its complications.

The most common complication of continuous mandatory ventilation (CMV) is ventilator-associated pneumonia (VAP), which occurs in 5% to 10% of patients on mechanical ventilation. Other complications include airway trauma, mucus plugging, and atelectasis.

The development of VAP is a multifactorial process, but the use of mechanical ventilation is the primary risk factor; the presence of the endotracheal tube, which bypasses the protective mechanisms of the larynx and may serve as a conduit for bacteria to enter the lung, and the inability to cough effectively with sedation contribute to the risk of developing VAP. The risk of VAP increases with the duration of time a patient is on mechanical ventilation, as well as with the number of days spent in the ICU. Patients who are immobile or have comorbidities such as chronic obstructive pulmonary disease (COPD) or diabetes are also at increased risk for developing VAP. The best way to prevent VAP is through diligent hand hygiene and oral care by both healthcare providers and family members. In addition, patients should be turned at least every 2 hours to prevent pooling of secretions and to promote drainage. Finally, keeping the head of the bed elevated 30 degrees or more, which may reduce gastroesophageal reflux, will also help reduce the risk of VAP.

In addition, mode-specific complications of controlled mechanical ventilation include volutrauma and/or barotrauma. Volutrauma is defined as structural lung injury because of overdistension of the lungs during mechanical ventilation; it is a direct consequence of delivering a tidal volume that is too large for a given patient's respiratory physiology or pathophysiology. Barotrauma is defined as structural lung injury because of administration of excessive pressure during mechanical ventilation. Of note, volutrauma can occur during either volume control *or* pressure control ventilation—monitoring the airway pressure generated by volume control ventilation and adjusting the set V_t as needed can decrease the risk of barotrauma, and monitoring the delivered tidal volume generated by pressure control ventilation and adjusting the set airway pressure as needed to avoid excessive tidal volume can decrease the risk of volutrauma.

Volu- or barotrauma can manifest as macroscopic lung injury, such as a pneumothorax, or microscopic injury, such as diffuse alveolar damage and acute lung injury. Once volu- or barotrauma occurs, the therapeutic focus is to minimize further ventilator-associated damage by minimizing airway pressures (for patients receiving volume control ventilation) or lung volumes (for patients receiving pressure control ventilation).

SUMMARY

There are two types of controlled mechanical ventilation: pressure control and volume control. In volume control ventilation, the machine is set to deliver a specific amount of air (the set V_t) to the lungs with each breath, and airway pressures (PIP and plateau pressures) are generated in response to the set V_t. In pressure control ventilation, the amount of air that is delivered to the lungs during inhalation is determined by the inspiratory pressure set on the ventilator. The ventilator maintains a constant rate of inspiratory flow (assuming the patient is passive; inspiratory flow increases if the patient is assisting inspiration), regardless of the V_t delivered during the inspiratory cycle. Understanding the basics of respiratory physiology, including Boyle's law and the concept of respiratory system compliance, is critical for understanding and responding to the effects of either volume or pressure control ventilation and for taking optimal care of mechanically ventilated, critically ill patients.

KEY POINTS

- Controlled mechanical ventilation is a clinical term describing ventilatory modes where a patient's respiratory cycle is completely controlled by the ventilator.
- Volume control ventilation and pressure control ventilation are two types of controlled mechanical ventilation, in which either volume or pressure is set by the ventilator.
- Understanding the relationships between pressure and volume is crucial for healthcare providers managing intubated and mechanically ventilated patients.
- Indications for controlled mechanical ventilation include acute or chronic respiratory failure, cardiac arrest, anesthesia, and airway protection, among other medical issues.
- The choice between volume control and pressure control ventilation is often based on institutional preference, with no significant difference in patient outcomes based on the available.
- Volume control ventilation delivers a set volume, whereas pressure control ventilation delivers inspiratory flow until a predetermined pressure is achieved.
- Basic settings for volume control ventilation include type of ventilation, backup respiratory rate, tidal volume, PEEP, and Fio_2.
- Monitoring for patient-ventilator synchrony and assessing for rate or volume dyssynchrony is important in volume control ventilation.

STUDY QUESTIONS AND ANSWERS

Questions

1. A 23-year-old woman is admitted to the ICU with acute respiratory failure because of an opiate overdose and aspiration pneumonia. On admission to the ICU, she is sedated and not meaningfully responsive. She is treated with volume control ventilation, with the following settings: tidal volume is 320 mL (7 mL/kg of predicted body weight), RR is 12 breaths/min, PEEP is 8 cm H_2O, and Fio_2 is 60%. Her PIP is 34 cm H_2O and plateau pressure is 32 cm H_2O. Which of the following is the most appropriate next step in her management?

   A. Increase the RR to 18 breaths/min.
   B. Decrease the tidal volume to 280 mL (6 mL/kg of predicted body weight).
   C. Place the patient in prone position.
   D. Decrease the PEEP to 5 cm H_2O.
   E. Administer a bronchodilator.

2. The respiratory therapist pages you to ask you to review a patient's arterial blood gas. The patient is a morbidly obese 60-year-old man who was intubated yesterday for acute hypoxic and hypercapnic respiratory failure because of a submassive pulmonary embolism. He has been maintained on pressure control ventilation over the course of his hospitalization, and his current ventilator settings are: inspiratory pressure 25 cm H_2O (peak pressure 25 cm H_2O), RR 24 breaths/min, PEEP 12 cm H_2O, and Fio_2 50%. His tidal volumes on these settings are 280 to 300 mL. His most recent arterial blood gas results demonstrate a pH of 7.29, $Paco_2$ 61 mm Hg, and Pao_2 70 mm Hg.

   Which of the following is the most appropriate next step in his care?

   A. Change from pressure control to volume control ventilation.
   B. Increase the PEEP to 16 cm H_2O.
   C. Increase the inspiratory pressure to 28 cm H_2O.
   D. Decrease the RR to 20 breaths/min.
   E. Decrease the Fio_2 to 40%.

3. A 23-year-old woman was intubated 2 days ago for acute hypoxic and hypercapnic respiratory failure because of a severe asthma exacerbation. She was initially paralyzed because of ventilator dyssynchrony, as she was overbreathing the ventilator and had wildly vacillating tidal volumes despite increasing doses of sedative medications. This morning, paralytics were stopped, and you are now called to assess her because of recurrent ventilator dyssynchrony. She is currently on volume control ventilation with the following settings: tidal volume 340 mL (7 mL/kg of predicted body weight), set RR 24 breaths/min, PEEP 5 cm H_2O, and F_{IO_2} 50%. Her actual RR is 36 breaths/min, and her actual tidal volumes range from 100 to 800 mL with significant vacillation from one breath to the next. She is currently receiving propofol 60 µg/kg/min for sedation and analgesia. An arterial blood gas has been ordered and is pending. Which of the following is the next most appropriate step in her care?

   A. Increase her tidal volume to 400 mL (8 mL/kg of ideal body weight).

   B. Make no changes until the arterial blood gas results are available.

   C. Change from volume control to pressure control ventilation.

   D. Increase her set RR to 36 breaths/min.

   E. Add fentanyl boluses and an infusion to her medication regimen.

Answers

1. **Answer B. Decrease the tidal volume to 280 mL (6 mL/kg of predicted body weight)**

   Rationale: This patient's plateau pressure is above 30 cm H_2O, which is the upper limit of acceptable plateau pressures for patients receiving volume control ventilation. Based on the compliance relationship between volume and pressure, reducing the set tidal volume will result in decreased airway and plateau pressures (thereby decreasing the resultant morbidity and mortality associated with increased plateau pressures). There are no data indicating that the patient's RR needs to be increased—without either the exhaled CO_2 or $Paco_2$, one cannot determine if the patient's minute ventilation is adequate or not. As such, given that the patient's plateau pressure is demonstrably above the upper acceptable limit, decreasing the patient's tidal volume is the management priority. The observation that the peak and plateau pressures are within 10 cm H_2O is consistent with normal resistance in the airways; consequently, a bronchodilator is not indicated. There is insufficient information to justify placing the patient in a prone position or decreasing the PEEP—the Pao_2 and Pao_2/F_{IO_2} ratio could inform the indication for such interventions, but based on the available information, decreasing the tidal volume is the most important next step in the patient's care.

2. **Answer C. Increase the inspiratory pressure to 28 cm H_2O**

   Rationale: His arterial blood gas results demonstrate an acute on chronic respiratory acidosis, with an estimated baseline $Paco_2$ of ~50 mm Hg and an acute decrease in ventilation resulting in an increase in his $Paco_2$ to 60 mm Hg. In this setting, increasing his minute ventilation to endeavor to optimize elimination of carbon dioxide is the primary therapeutic mandate. Minute ventilation may be increased by either increasing the RR or increasing the tidal volume, and for patients receiving pressure control ventilation, the tidal volume is modulated by changing the inspiratory pressure. Specifically, increasing the set inspiratory pressure would be expected to increase the tidal volume, such that answer option C is the most correct answer of the available choices. To be clear, increasing the RR would also be a reasonable choice, but this was not one of the answer options for this question (and decreasing the RR, as offered in answer option D, is incorrect). The patient's oxygenation is adequate, as

(continued)

STUDY QUESTIONS AND ANSWERS (*continued*)

demonstrated by a Pao_2 of 70 mm Hg and a Pao_2/Fio_2 ratio of 140, such that changing the patient's PEEP and/or Fio_2 is not indicated at this time (answer options B and E are not correct). Finally, there is no immediate indication to change ventilatory modes from pressure control to volume control ventilation (although volume control ventilation might provide you with greater control of tidal volume, e.g., if airway resistance increases, tidal volume will go down with pressure ventilation because more of the pressure will be used to overcome resistance rather than to distend the lung); rather, adjusting the patient's inspiratory pressure to augment his minute ventilation and to address his acute on chronic respiratory acidosis is the most important next step in his care.

3. **Answer E. Add fentanyl boluses and an infusion to her medication regimen**
   Rationale: In this scenario, the patient is prohibitively dyssynchronous with regard to both rate and volume, and increased analgesia (to reduce pain and dyspnea associated with the underlying asthma and mechanical ventilation) in an effort to achieve more optimal ventilator synchrony is indicated. Ventilator dyssynchrony is frequently because of inadequate sedation and an overactive respiratory controller, such that increasing sedation (if a patient is not yet ready to be liberated from mechanical ventilation) is needed to align the set and actual RR and tidal volume. One does not need to wait for the results of the arterial blood gas to make changes to address dyssynchrony—even if the blood gas results were reassuring, the patient is still dyssynchronous and this needs to be addressed. Changing the patient's tidal volume and/or RR (answer options A and D) will not be sufficient to adequately address this degree of dyssynchrony—sedation and, possibly, reinitiation of paralytics (if the patient is adequately sedated) are more appropriate interventions.

Suggested Readings

Chatburn R. Classification of mechanical ventilators. *Respir Care*. 1992;37:1009-1025.

Naik BI, Lynch C 3rd, Durbin CG Jr. Variability in mechanical ventilation: what's all the noise about? *Respir Care*. 2015;60(8):1203-1210.

Nichols D, Haranath S. Pressure control ventilation. *Crit Care Clin*. 2007;23(2):183-199, viii-ix.

Pavone M, Verrillo E, Onofri A, Caggiano S, Cutrera R. Ventilators and ventilatory modalities. *Front Pediatr*. 2020;8:500.

Pierson DJ. Indications for mechanical ventilation in adults with acute respiratory failure. *Respir Care*. 2002;47(3):249-262.

Sassoon C. Mechanical ventilator design and function: the trigger variable. *Respir Care*. 1992;37:1056-1069.

Sassoon C, Gruer S. Characteristics of the ventilator pressure and flow-trigger variables. *Intensive Care Med*. 1995;21:159-168.

Singer BD, Corbridge TC. Pressure modes of invasive mechanical ventilation. *South Med J*. 2011;104(10):701-709.STUDY QUESTIONS AND ANSWERS

Pressure Support Ventilation

Jeremy B. Richards

LEARNING OBJECTIVES

- Describe ventilator settings for pressure support ventilation.
- Delineate when to use pressure support ventilation for intubated patients.
- Identify the differences between pressure support ventilation and "control" modes of ventilation.
- Determine when and how to adjust ventilator settings for patients treated with pressure support ventilation.
- Describe the limitations of pressure support ventilation for critically ill patients with acute respiratory failure.

INTRODUCTION

Pressure support ventilation (PSV) is a form of mechanical ventilation that delivers a continuous flow of air to the patient through an endotracheal or tracheostomy tube. This mode of mechanical ventilation can help to improve ventilation and oxygenation in select patients with respiratory failure or other respiratory disorders. In a pressure support mode of mechanical ventilation, the patient is able to initiate breaths on their own, and the ventilator provides a set level of pressure to support the patient's inspiratory effort. As such, PSV is appropriate for patients who are able to initiate their inspiratory effort and independently participate in ventilation. This is one of the most comfortable modes of mechanical ventilation for the patient, who assumes control of respiratory rate, tidal volume, inspiratory flow, and inspiratory time. In this chapter, we review the indications for PSV, ventilator settings for this mode of ventilation, and limitations and challenges of PSV in critically ill, mechanically ventilated patients.

INDICATIONS FOR AND PHYSIOLOGY OF PRESSURE SUPPORT VENTILATION

PSV is typically used in patients who are able to initiate breaths but require some level of assistance with ventilation to achieve adequate tidal volume. PSV can be referred to as a "patient-cycled" mode of ventilation, given that all inspiratory efforts are triggered by the patient and not provided by a preset obligatory respiratory rate by the ventilator. With regard to ventilatory mechanics, by providing continuous inspiratory flow at a specific inspiratory pressure, PSV augments the volume and diminishes the patient's respiratory effort for spontaneous breaths, thereby reducing the work of breathing.

PSV may be used in patients with acute respiratory failure, chronic obstructive pulmonary disease (COPD), acute pulmonary edema, or other respiratory disorders. It may also be used in patients who have difficulty coordinating their breaths with the mechanical ventilator or who are ready to or in the process of weaning off of mechanical ventilation and can assume more control achieving the goals of ventilation. Patients with advanced, severe acute respiratory failure with severe hypoxemia, extreme hypercapnia, markedly decreased respiratory system compliance, and/or respiratory controller dysfunction are unlikely to be candidates for PSV; rather, controlled modes of mechanical ventilation (eg, volume assist control or pressure assist control), which assume much more of the work of breathing, are likely to be more appropriate.

Because PSV is a patient-cycled mode of ventilation, the duration of inspiration, duration of expiration, and the total respiratory cycle are determined by the patient; the ventilator merely provides support for inspiratory flow. The inspiratory pressure provided by the ventilator, coupled with the patient's intrinsic inspiratory effort, determines the work of breathing experienced by the patient. Work of breathing can be conceptualized as the product of the inspiratory pressure applied by the ventilator, the mean inspiratory flow (which is determined by the tidal volume divided by the inspiratory time), and the proportion of the inspiratory time to the total respiratory cycle (said differently, how much time during a breath a patient spends inhaling versus exhaling, which directly reflects the patient's respiratory rate and pattern of breathing). Being aware of the patient's work of breathing and the physiologic and mechanical components that contribute to the work of breathing are important in determining if PSV is an appropriate ventilatory mode for a given patient and, if so, whether the ventilatory support provided needs to be adjusted.

PRESSURE SUPPORT VENTILATION—VENTILATOR SETTINGS

There are several key settings that can be adjusted on the ventilator when using PSV. These are described in the following subsections.

Inspiratory Pressure

As noted earlier, the inspiratory pressure is the level of pressure provided by the ventilator to support the patient's inspiratory effort. The units of inspiratory pressure are centimeters of water (cm H_2O), and the inspiratory pressure is generally set *in addition* to the positive end-expiratory pressure (PEEP; eg, if the PEEP is 5 cm H_2O and the pressure support is 10 cm H_2O, the actual inspiratory pressure delivered by the ventilator is 15 cm H_2O). The target inspiratory pressure is typically set at a level that is sufficient to maintain the patient's oxygenation and ventilation, but not so high that it causes discomfort or excessively high tidal volumes.

Acknowledging that the appropriate inspiratory pressure is dependent on a given patient's clinical circumstances and physiology, the inspiratory pressure for a patient on PSV will range typically from 5 to 15 cm H_2O. The appropriate inspiratory pressure for a given patient can be determined by being cognizant of their work of breathing, which entails monitoring both their tidal volume and their respiratory rate, as well as their physical exam (eg, are they using accessory muscles of inhalation). A patient with a low tidal volume (eg, <6 mL/kg of predicted body weight) and/or a high respiratory rate (eg, >25-30 breaths/min) may benefit from a higher inspiratory pressure to decrease their work of breathing. After adjusting the inspiratory pressure provided by the ventilator, the clinician must continue to monitor the patient's tidal volume, respiratory rate, and pulmonary mechanics to determine if the adjusted inspiratory pressure was effective in decreasing the work of breathing.

Patients who require inspiratory pressures higher than 15 cm H_2O may be better served by a control mode of ventilation, in which the ventilator provides a set tidal volume (or inspiratory pressure) at a set respiratory rate (see Chapter 5). Patients who require less than 5 cm H_2O should be assessed for readiness for extubation and liberation from mechanical ventilation (see Chapter 9).

After setting the inspiratory pressure, the clinician should closely monitor the impact of the patient's ventilator settings. Specifically, the set inspiratory pressure delivered by the ventilator coupled with the patient's intrinsic inspiratory effort will affect the patient's inspiratory flow, work of breathing, tidal volume, and respiratory rate (see Section "Pressure Support Ventilation—Clinical Monitoring").

Positive End-Expiratory Pressure

PEEP is the level of pressure that is maintained in the airways during expiration. It can be used to improve oxygenation by decreasing the risk of alveolar collapse during exhalation and minimizing atelectasis. Similar to the inspiratory pressure, PEEP is measured in units of centimeters of water (cm H_2O), and it is adjusted as needed to optimize the patient's respiratory system physiology. The patient's gas exchange, as reflected by their oxygenation (assessed with pulse oximetry and/or arterial blood gas results), is the primary determinant of the PEEP that should be delivered by the ventilator. In patients with severe obstructive lung disease and flow limitation, applied PEEP may be used to offset intrinsic PEEP and make it easier for a patient to trigger the ventilator (see Chapter 7 on PEEP and Chapter 11 on mechanical ventilation in patients with chronic obstructive lung disease).

A typical PEEP for a patient on PSV is 5 to 10 cm H_2O. Patients requiring higher PEEP may be better served by a control mode of ventilation, in which the ventilator controls all aspects of the respiratory cycle. Patients requiring only 5 cm H_2O of PEEP with similarly low inspiratory pressures should be assessed for their readiness to be liberated from mechanical ventilation. Of note, if a patient is not ready to be extubated, the PEEP should generally be maintained no lower than 5 cm H_2O as lower PEEP (or no PEEP) has been associated with adverse outcomes in mechanically ventilated, critically ill patients, including increased mortality in some subgroups of critically ill patients.

Fraction of Inspiratory Oxygen

The fraction of inspired oxygen (F_{IO_2}) is the percentage of oxygen in the gas mixture delivered to the patient. It can be adjusted to ensure that the patient is receiving the appropriate amount of oxygen, as measured by pulse oximetry and/or the partial pressure of arterial oxygen on arterial blood gas analyses. For more details regarding principles of gas exchange and considerations for titrating the F_{IO_2}, please refer to Chapter 3.

PRESSURE SUPPORT VENTILATION—RESPIRATORY RATE

In PSV, the respiratory rate is not directly set as it is in other modes of mechanical ventilation such as assist control ventilation. It is important to note that the respiratory rate in PSV is not fixed and may vary depending on the patient's respiratory effort and lung mechanics—the patient's own respiratory drive determines the respiratory rate; there is no "backup" rate—if the patient becomes apneic, the ventilator will not deliver a breath until a determined duration of apnea occurs (see section that follows). The ventilator provides a continuous flow of air or oxygen at a predetermined pressure, and the patient initiates and terminates each breath either by activating a pressure sensor in the breathing circuit or based on flow-based triggers.

For pressure-triggered breaths, if the patient generates a sufficiently negative intrathoracic pressure when inhaling, the ventilator can detect this pressure change and cycle from providing PEEP to providing the preset inspiratory pressure. A typical threshold for a pressure-triggered cycle is -0.5 to -2 cm H_2O. Reciprocally, if the patient generates positive intrathoracic pressure at the end of exhalation (signaling a forcible expiratory effort), the ventilator will cycle from providing the preset inspiratory pressure to PEEP (see **Figure 6-1A**).

Although pressure-based triggers can determine when the ventilator cycles between providing inspiratory pressure and PEEP, PSV is primarily a flow-cycled or flow-triggered mode of ventilation. Termination of flow-triggered breaths is dependent on changes in flow rather than a specific volume or pressure: a reduction in flow rate by a certain amount from the peak flow during inspiration (typically 1-5 L/min) is the signal for cycling from providing the preset inspiratory pressure to providing PEEP (**Figure 6-1B**). Relatedly, backup flow-based criteria such as cycling from inspiratory pressure to PEEP after a certain duration (eg, 5 seconds) is another way that the ventilator can transition from inspiratory to expiratory pressures. Of note, patients with obstructive airways disease and flow limitation may have auto-PEEP because of incomplete exhalation and air trapping. Such patients must first overcome their auto-PEEP to trigger the ventilator, which can result in excessive work of breathing. In such patients, flow-triggering is advantageous and preferred as compared to pressure-triggered breaths. On inhalation, flow may be relatively low, and decreases in flow may not reach the target to terminate inhalation. Under these circumstances, the ventilator may try to sustain inhalation longer than desired by the patient, leading to dyssynchrony with the ventilator. This finding may be erroneously interpreted as a need for greater levels of pressure support.

As noted earlier, the inspiratory pressure is set by the clinician and determines the amount of pressure provided by the ventilator to assist the patient's inspiratory efforts and to maintain adequate minute ventilation. Regardless of whether breaths are pressure- or flow-triggered, higher pressure support level can help the patient generate a higher tidal volume with a lower respiratory rate, whereas a lower pressure support level may result in a lower tidal volume and higher respiratory rate.

Finally, if a patient does not make any respiratory efforts, the ventilator will detect apnea and transition from PSV to a controlled mode of ventilation (typically volume assist control).

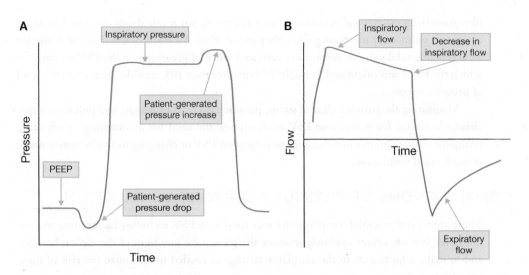

Figure 6-1: Pressure-time tracing. A, The pressure drop generated by a patient during forcible inhalation and the pressure increase generated by active exhalation. **B,** A flow-time tracing in which the ventilator cycles from inspiratory pressure and low to delivering positive end-expiratory pressure (PEEP) after a specific preset decrease in the inspiratory flow rate.

The presets for when a ventilator transitions from PSV to volume assist control vary, but typically a period of apnea of more than 20 seconds will result in the ventilator alarming and initiating a backup respiratory rate.

PRESSURE SUPPORT VENTILATION—CLINICAL MONITORING

It is important to closely monitor patients on PSV to ensure that they are receiving the appropriate level of ventilation and oxygenation. This includes monitoring vital signs, oxygen saturation (Spo_2), and blood gas levels. It is also important to monitor the patient's respiratory status, including their work of breathing, as indicated by the rate and depth of breaths, use of accessory muscles of ventilation, and their qualitative level of discomfort or fatigue.

As noted earlier, the concept of the "work of breathing" is a helpful paradigm for assessing a patient's respiratory effort and respiratory status. Specifically, monitoring the patient's tidal volume and respiratory rate while adjusting PSV settings is critical. The tidal volume and respiratory rate are not set by the ventilator, and as such these values are reflective of the patient's inspiratory effort coupled with the support provided by the ventilator. If the patient's tidal volume is prohibitively low (eg, <6 mL/kg of predicted body weight) and/or if their respiratory rate is too high (eg, >25-30 breaths/min), then they may be receiving inadequate support, and increasing the inspiratory pressure may help to reduce their work of breathing and improve their pulmonary mechanics.

Although monitoring the patient's tidal volume and respiratory rate is important, it can also be useful to calculate the patient's rapid shallow breathing index (RSBI) to obtain an integrative assessment of their pulmonary mechanics. The RSBI is defined as the patient's spontaneous respiratory rate divided by their tidal volume (in liters). The RSBI is typically calculated at the end of a spontaneous breathing trial to assess a patient's readiness for liberation from mechanical ventilation (see Chapter 9), but it can also be used to determine a patient's pulmonary mechanics while they are on PSV. An RSBI of less than 105 indicates an acceptable tidal volume, respiratory rate, and work of breathing on the PSV settings for which the RSBI was calculated. If the RSBI is greater than 105, consider increasing the level of pressure support.

Monitoring the patient's clinical status, parameters of gas exchange, and pulmonary mechanics is critical for patients on PSV to determine the need for maintaining or adjusting ventilator settings, and/or maintaining the patient on PSV or changing to an alternative mode of mechanical ventilation.

COMPLICATIONS OF PRESSURE SUPPORT VENTILATION

There are several potential complications associated with PSV, including barotrauma and volutrauma. It is important to closely monitor the patient for any signs of these complications and to make adjustments to the ventilator settings as needed to minimize the risk of these complications.

Barotrauma

A transpulmonary pressure is a special form of transmural pressure (P_{TM}), that is, the pressure across the wall of a flexible structure. A transmural pressure is defined as the pressure inside the structure minus the pressure outside the structure. The larger the transmural pressure, the greater the size of the flexible structure. Transpulmonary pressure is defined as the pressure in the alveolus, delivered by the ventilator during inspiration, minus the pressure on the other side of the alveolar wall, the pleural pressure, generated by the patient's intrinsic inspiratory effort (see **Figure 6-2**). Because patients on PSV are breathing spontaneously, they can potentially generate high transpulmonary pressures, which can result in barotrauma. A patient's intrinsic inspiratory effort is characterized as a negative intrathoracic pressure, such that the transpulmonary pressure during inspiration can be quite high if a patient is generating significant inspiratory force because of increased work of breathing, discomfort, agitation, or anxiety. Remember: transpulmonary pressure $= P_{alv} - P_{pl}$, and if P_{pl} is negative, one is essentially adding P_{pl} to P_{alv} to determine the transpulmonary pressure.

High transpulmonary pressures can result in injury to the lung parenchyma, which can manifest as micro-anatomic pathology such as interstitial emphysema or macro-anatomic phenomena such as pneumothorax. In addition, and more common than micro- or macro-anatomic injuries, excessive transpulmonary pressure leading to overdistension of alveoli

Transpulmonary pressure

$$T_{TP} = P_{alv} - P_{pl}$$

Figure 6-2: **Transpulmonary pressure is defined as the pressure in the alveolus, delivered by the ventilator during inspiration, minus the pressure on the other side of the alveolar wall, the pleural pressure, generated by the patient's intrinsic inspiratory effort.** In this equation, T_{TP} is the transpulmonary pressure, P_{alv} is the alveolar pressure, and P_{pl} is the pleural pressure.

(volutrauma) can result in systemic inflammation and acute lung injury from immunomodulatory, inflammatory mediators. In extreme cases, acute lung injury can progress to acute respiratory distress syndrome (ARDS) with noncardiogenic pulmonary edema, decreased lung compliance, and impaired gas exchange.

In general, transpulmonary pressures are not directly measured, as this would require placement of an esophageal manometer to measure pleural pressures. In the absence of esophageal manometry and direct measurements of the pleural pressures generated during spontaneous breathing on PSV, clinical monitoring and acumen can serve to alert clinicians to the possibility of barotrauma. Patients with increased work of breathing, as evidenced by high tidal volumes, accessory muscle use, and/or high respiratory rates, may be generating excessively negative intrathoracic pressures during inspiration, resulting in an increased risk for barotrauma. In addition, patients requiring high inspiratory pressures delivered by the ventilator may also be at risk for high transpulmonary pressures and barotrauma.

Volutrauma

Similar to barotrauma, excessively high tidal volumes can result in alveolar stretch and injury. Mechanical injury because of volutrauma includes interstitial emphysema and/or pneumothorax, and indirect injury is due to alveolar stretch and resultant systemic inflammation and acute lung injury. Monitoring for volutrauma is more straightforward than for barotrauma, as exhaled tidal volumes are directly and quantitatively measured and reported by the ventilator.

In general, tidal volumes will vary for patients on PSV as there is no preset, repetitive tidal volume delivered by the ventilator for each breath. As such, the patient intermittently may generate large tidal volumes, which is part of normal respiration (there is variation in the volume of breaths that we take when breathing spontaneously). Intermittent large-volume breaths are unlikely to cause injury or volutrauma. If the patient consistently has excessively large breaths, however, injury from stretch and alveolar damage may occur. In general, tidal volumes greater than 8 mL/kg of predicted body weight are associated with an increased risk of injury, and tidal volumes of 10 to 12 mL/kg of predicted body weight have been shown to cause lung injury in certain patient populations (eg, patients with ARDS).

If a patient's tidal volumes are consistently greater than 8 mL/kg of predicted body weight, then the inspiratory pressure should be decreased to target volumes of 6 to 8 mL/kg of predicted body weight to decrease the risk of the patient developing volutrauma while on PSV.

SUMMARY

PSV is a mode of mechanical ventilation that can be used to provide assistance with ventilation in patients who are able to initiate breaths on their own. It is important to closely monitor the patient to ensure that they are receiving adequate ventilation and oxygenation while on PSV and to carefully adjust the ventilator settings as indicated to decrease the risk of ventilator-associated complications. Understanding the concept and determinants of the "work of breathing" can help clinicians effectively monitor and support patients on PSV, optimizing physiological-based and patient-centered care.

KEY POINTS

- PSV is a mode of mechanical ventilation that delivers a continuous flow of air to the patient, allowing them to initiate breaths on their own while the ventilator provides a set level of pressure support.
- PSV is appropriate for patients who can initiate their inspiratory effort and independently participate in ventilation, and it is comfortable for the patient as they have control over respiratory rate, tidal volume, inspiratory flow, and inspiratory time.
- Indications for PSV include respiratory failure, COPD, acute pulmonary edema, and patients who have difficulty coordinating their breaths with the ventilator or are in the process of weaning off mechanical ventilation.
- Ventilator settings for PSV include inspiratory pressure, PEEP, Fio_2, but not respiratory rate.
- The inspiratory pressure is set to support the patient's inspiratory effort, typically ranging from 5 to 15 cm H_2O, and it should be adjusted based on the patient's work of breathing and overall pulmonary mechanics.
- PEEP is adjusted to optimize respiratory system physiology and can be used to improve oxygenation by preventing alveolar collapse during exhalation. A typical PEEP for PSV is 5-10 cm H_2O.
- Fio2 is adjusted to ensure appropriate oxygenation based on pulse oximetry and/or arterial blood gas results.
- Respiratory rate in PSV is determined by the patient's own respiratory drive, and the ventilator provides support based on pressure or flow triggers. Monitoring the patient's work of breathing, tidal volume, and respiratory rate is important in adjusting PSV settings.
- Complications of PSV include barotrauma and volutrauma, which should be monitored for and managed accordingly.

STUDY QUESTIONS AND ANSWERS

Questions

1. A 55-year-old man with very severe COPD has been intubated and mechanically ventilated in the intensive care unit for the past 8 days. For the past 3 days, he has been on PSV. His current settings are an inspiratory pressure of 5 cm H_2O, a PEEP of 5 cm H_2O, and a Fio_2 of 40%. His tidal volumes on these settings range from 300 to 500 mL (6-8 mL/kg of predicted body weight) with a respiratory rate of 18 to 24 breaths/min. His oxygen saturations, measured by pulse oximetry, have ranged between 90% and 94%. On exam, he is not using accessory muscles of respiration and he is able to answer yes/no questions and follow simple commands.

   Which of the following is the most appropriate next step in his management?

   A. Change from PSV to volume assist control ventilation.

   B. Increase the inspiratory pressure to 10 cm H_2O.

   C. Perform a spontaneous breathing trial.

   D. Decrease the PEEP to 0 cm H_2O.

   E. Extubate the patient.

2. A 23-year-old woman with cystic fibrosis was intubated 3 days ago for acute hypoxic respiratory failure because of bibasilar pneumonia. She was initially on a volume assist control mode of ventilation, but because of persistent dyssynchrony with the ventilator, she was transitioned to PSV overnight. This morning, her ventilator settings include an inspiratory pressure of 20 cm H_2O, a PEEP of 10 cm H_2O, and a FIO_2 of 100%. On these settings, her tidal volumes are 200 to 300 mL (5-6 mL/kg of predicted body weight), respiratory rate is 30 to 35 breaths/min, and oxygen saturation is 88% to 92%. An arterial blood gas on these settings demonstrates a pH of 7.28, a $PacO_2$ of 58 mm Hg, and a PaO_2 of 63 mm Hg.

   Which of the following is the most appropriate next step in her care?

   A. Change back from PSV to volume assist control ventilation.

   B. Increase the PEEP to 14 cm H_2O.

   C. Decrease the FIO_2 to 80%.

   D. Increase the inspiratory pressure to 25 cm H_2O.

   E. Decrease the respiratory rate to 20 breaths/min.

3. A 47-year-old man with cirrhosis was intubated yesterday for altered mental status because of hepatic encephalopathy. He is receiving no sedative medications, but his mental status remains depressed. He is on PSV, with settings of an inspiratory pressure of 10 cm H_2O, PEEP of 5 cm H_2O, and a FIO_2 of 50%. On these settings, his tidal volumes range from 800 to 1200 mL (12-14 mL/kg of predicted body weight), his respiratory rate is 6-10 breaths/min, and his oxygen saturations are 98% to 100%.

   Which of the following is the most appropriate adjustment to his ventilator settings?

   A. Increase the inspiratory pressure to 12 cm H_2O.

   B. Increase the PEEP to 8 cm H_2O.

   C. Increase the FIO_2 to 60%.

   D. Decrease the inspiratory pressure to 5 cm H_2O.

   E. Decrease the PEEP to 0 cm H_2O.

Answers

1. **Answer C. Perform a spontaneous breathing trial**

   Rationale: Based on the degree of support he is requiring and his overall clinical circumstances, it is appropriate to assess his readiness for extubation and liberation from mechanical ventilation by performing a spontaneous breathing trial. As noted in the chapter, if the patient's ventilatory requirements are minimal (eg, an inspiratory pressure of 5 cm H_2O and a PEEP of 5 cm H_2O), it is appropriate to assess their readiness for extubation and liberation, barring other barriers to a spontaneous breathing trial. It is not appropriate to simply extubate the patient; even though the patient is currently on "minimal" settings, a spontaneous breathing trial (typically on no PEEP) should still be done to accurately assess the patient's readiness to be liberated from the ventilator. Given that the patient's tidal volumes and respiratory rates are within acceptable ranges, and given that his work of breathing appears to be acceptable, there is no need to increase the inspiratory pressure (answer B is incorrect). Although a spontaneous breathing trial should be performed on 0 cm H_2O of PEEP, the patient should not be indefinitely exposed to 0 cm H_2O of PEEP. As noted in the chapter, "zero" of PEEP has been associated with adverse outcomes for mechanically ventilated patients. Finally, answer option A is incorrect;

(continued)

the patient appears to be acceptably stable on PSV—consequently, there is no apparent indication to transition to a "full" mode of ventilatory support based on the available information.

2. **Answer A. Change back from PSV to volume assist control ventilation**

   Rationale: This patient is requiring excessive support with regard to both oxygenation and ventilation, the latter leading to a significant respiratory acidosis, and continuing PSV is not appropriate. Given the severity of the patient's respiratory failure, taking full control of her ventilatory parameters is necessary. As such, transitioning back to volume assist control ventilation is indicated, along with increased sedation (and possibly paralysis) to achieve adequate synchrony with the ventilator settings. Increasing the patient's PEEP may help with her oxygenation, but this adjustment is insufficient to address her overall severely compromised respiratory status. In addition, a PEEP of 14 cm H_2O is generally considered to be excessive for a patient on PSV. As such, answer option B is incorrect. Answer option C is also incorrect, as the patient's oxygenation is marginal, as evidenced by a Spo_2 ranging from 88% to 92% and a Pao_2 of only 63 mm Hg. Decreasing the oxygen delivered by the ventilator is not appropriate at this time. As noted in the chapter, an inspiratory pressure of greater than 15 cm H_2O is prohibitive for most patients on PSV, such that answer option D is incorrect. Finally, the respiratory rate is determined by the patient's spontaneous respiratory effort on PSV; it is not set by the ventilator. As such, answer option E is incorrect.

3. **Answer D. Decrease the inspiratory pressure to 5 cm H_2O**

   Rationale: The patient's tidal volumes are excessively high, at 12 to 14 cm H_2O; this can be rectified by decreasing the patient's inspiratory pressure, which is the most appropriate intervention for his ventilator settings. He is at risk for volutrauma in the setting of receiving large tidal volume breaths; consequently, it is appropriate to decrease the inspiratory pressure delivered by the ventilator with the goal of decreasing his tidal volumes. Increasing the inspiratory pressure delivered (answer option A) is incorrect, as this would be expected to result in increased tidal volumes, which is clearly not indicated. Increasing or decreasing the PEEP provided by the ventilator (answer options B and E) is not indicated, because his oxygenation is acceptable (based on his oxygen saturations) and decreasing the PEEP provided to less than 5 cm H_2O is associated with adverse outcomes. Similarly, increasing his Fio_2 is not indicated with acceptable oxygen saturations (answer option C is incorrect). Finally, it may be reasonable to decrease his Fio_2 from 50%, but dropping all the way down to 21% is a significant decrease, and it would be more appropriate to pursue a stepwise approach (eg, decreasing the Fio_2 to 40% or 30%) while following his oxygen saturations.

Suggested Readings

Dekel B, Segal E, Perel A. Pressure support ventilation. *Arch Intern Med*. 1996;156(4):369-373.

Hess D. Ventilator modes used in weaning. *Chest*. 2001;120(6 Suppl):474S-476S.

Hess D. Ventilator waveforms and the physiology of pressure support ventilation. *Respir Care*. 2005;50(2):166-186.

Hurst JM, Branson RD, Davis Jr K. Cardiopulmonary effects of pressure support ventilation. *JAMA Surg*. 1989;124(9):1067-1070.

Singer BD, Corbridge TC. Basic invasive mechanical ventilation. *South Med J*. 2009;102(12):1238-1245.

Wahba RW. Pressure support ventilation. *J Cardiothorac Anesth*. 1990;4(5):624-630.

Positive End-Expiratory Pressure: To PEEP or Not to PEEP?

Richard M. Schwartzstein

LEARNING OBJECTIVES

- Describe the concept of end-expiratory pressure and its relationship to lung volume.
- Explain the relationship between end-expiratory pressure and lung volume.
- Clarify the role of end-expiratory pressure in stabilizing the alveolus, particularly in conditions characterized by reduced respiratory system compliance.
- Differentiate positive end-expiratory pressure (PEEP) that originates from the physiology of the patient (intrinsic PEEP or PEEPi) and PEEP that is applied by the ventilator.
- Explain the physiology underlying the notion of "total PEEP" or measured PEEP when applied PEEP is used in a patient with PEEPi.
- Detail the complications and dangers of PEEP.

INTRODUCTION

Positive pressure ventilation typically focuses on providing assistance during inhalation, particularly in patients with decreased respiratory system compliance or increased airway resistance. In addition, hypoxemia is common in patients with acute respiratory failure; although this is often addressed by increasing the fraction of oxygen in the inspired gas (FIO_2), individuals with pulmonary shunt may benefit from other strategies to open or "recruit" lung units that are collapsed and/or filled with fluid or inflammatory material and not participating in gas exchange. Diseases associated with reduced lung and/or chest wall compliance develop a low functional residual capacity (FRC; see Chapter 2) and are prone to alveolar collapse (eg, interstitial lung disease, congestive heart failure, morbid obesity, acute respiratory distress syndrome [ARDS], kyphoscoliosis). By altering the pressure in the alveolus at the end of exhalation by applying positive end-expiratory pressure (PEEP), we can stabilize alveoli, minimize alveolar collapse, and improve oxygenation and compliance of the lung.

Chronic obstructive pulmonary disease (COPD), particularly emphysema, associated with flow limitation, may develop PEEP that is intrinsic to their abnormal physiology (PEEPi), which leads to hyperinflation and increased work of breathing. When these patients develop acute respiratory failure, applying PEEP with the ventilator may reduce the work associated with initiating an inspiration during mechanical ventilation.

This chapter outlines the physiology underlying these issues and demonstrates how the clinician may use PEEP to enhance the respiratory status of the patient with acute respiratory failure. The chapter also describes some of the pitfalls associated with the use of PEEP and strategies to minimize the complications of this intervention with the ventilator.

FUNCTIONAL RESIDUAL CAPACITY, END-EXPIRATORY LUNG VOLUME, AND POSITIVE END-EXPIRATORY PRESSURE

As discussed in Chapter 2, the FRC is determined by the balance of forces between the chest wall (recoiling outward toward its resting position) and the lung recoiling inward (toward its resting position). FRC, by definition, is the "resting volume" of the respiratory system; ventilatory muscles are not active. The relationship between the forces exerted by the lung and the chest wall is represented in the Rahn diagram (**Figure 7-1**). Conditions that result in reduced compliance of the lung (eg, increased elastic or surface forces such as pulmonary fibrosis and ARDS) lead to reduced FRC; alternatively, increased compliance of the lung is associated with increased FRC. Chest wall abnormalities typically work in the opposite direction because the recoil of the chest wall is in the opposite direction from the lung; decreased compliance of the chest wall results in an elevated FRC and increased compliance is associated with reduced FRC.

At FRC, there is no airflow into or out of the lung; this is the volume at the end of a relaxed exhalation. Because mouth pressure is atmospheric pressure, which by convention is considered zero pressure, the pressure at the alveolus must also be zero; if it were not, there would be flow of gas into or out of the alveolus because flow in a tube is determined by the difference in pressure at the two ends of the tube (see Chapter 2 for more complete description of flow through tubes).

If a patient is being treated with mechanical ventilation and the alveolar pressure during exhalation is not allowed to go below 5 cm H_2O, we say we have applied PEEP of 5 cm H_2O. Under these conditions, end-expiratory volume is now greater than FRC; we are not allowing

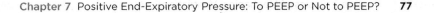

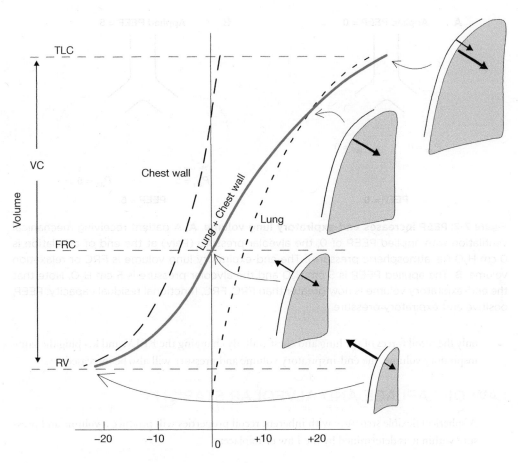

Figure 7-1: Pressure-volume characteristics of the respiratory system. This diagram shows the passive pressure-volume characteristics of the lung and chest wall in isolation, as well as the two integrated together as the respiratory system. Note that the resting position of the lungs is at a volume below the RV, and the resting position of the chest wall is close to the TLC. The schematics of the lung and chest wall show the forces exerted by the lungs and chest wall at the different volumes. At FRC, the forces exerted by the chest wall and the lungs are equal in intensity and opposite in direction. Thus, this is the resting position of the respiratory system. At volumes above FRC, the balance of forces is such that the respiratory system wants to get smaller; at volumes below FRC, the balance of forces pushes the system toward a higher volume, that is, back to FRC. FRC, functional residual capacity; RV, residual volume; TLC, total lung capacity; VC, vital capacity. (From Statics: Snapshots of the Ventilatory Pump. In: Schwartzstein RM, Parker MJ. *Respiratory Physiology: A Clinical Approach.* Wolters Kluwer; 2006:34-60. Figure 3.2.)

the lung volume to get to the relaxed end-expiratory volume (**Figure 7-2**). End-expiratory lung volume (EELV) is a generic term for the volume of the respiratory system at the end of any given exhalation. You can voluntarily change your end-expiratory volume easily by closing your glottis before completing exhalation or starting a new breath before the previous one has been completed. FRC is a specific EELV at which the determinants of the volume are

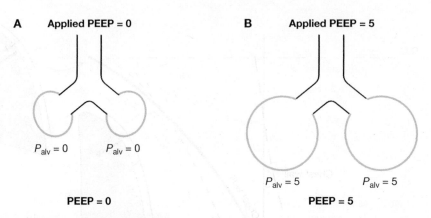

Figure 7-2: PEEP increases end-expiratory lung volume. A, A patient receiving mechanical ventilation with applied PEEP of 0, the alveolar pressure (Palv) at the end of exhalation is 0 cm H_2O (ie, atmospheric pressure). The end-expiratory lung volume is FRC or relaxation volume. **B**, The applied PEEP is 5 cm H_2O and the alveolar pressure is 5 cm H_2O. Note that the end-expiratory volume is now greater than FRC. FRC, functional residual capacity; PEEP, positive end-expiratory pressure.

only the recoil forces of the lung and chest wall. By changing the EELV, and keeping the same inspiratory volume, the end-inspiratory volume and pressure will also be increased.

LAW OF LAPLACE AND ALVEOLAR STABILITY

A spherical flexible structure with inherent recoil properties will produce a volume and pressure within it as determined by the Law of Laplace:

$$P = 2T/r$$

in which P is the pressure within the structure, T is the tension within the wall of the structure, and r is the radius of the structure. The alveolus, although not a perfect sphere, acts in ways consistent with the Law of Laplace (see Chapter 2 for a more complete discussion).

The size of an alveolus is determined in part by the transmural pressure across the wall of the alveolus; transmural pressure equals the pressure inside the alveolus minus the pressure outside the alveolus, which is the pleural pressure ($P_{TM} = P_i - P_o$). At FRC, the pressure in all the alveoli is zero, but the pressure in the pleural space varies from the dependent regions of the lung to the more superior regions because of the impact of gravity and weight of the lung. In the upright person, pleural pressure is more negative at the apex of the lung and more positive at the base. Consequently, alveolar volume at the apex is greater than at the base at FRC (in a supine patient, alveoli in the anterior portion of the chest will have larger volume than those in the posterior regions).

Assuming tension in the wall of the alveolus is constant, the Law of Laplace tells us that the smaller alveoli will have a larger pressure within them than the larger alveoli and gas should flow from the smaller to the larger alveoli, causing the smaller alveoli to collapse (**Figure 7-3**). If the alveolus collapses, there will be reduced ventilation into that unit and V̇/Q̇ mismatch, or shunt, will result (see Chapter 3 for more complete discussion). This effect is minimized because of increased density of surfactant during exhalation, which reduces surface tension

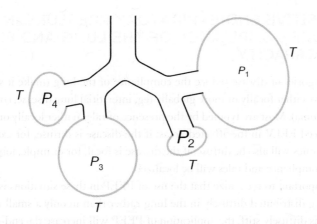

Figure 7-3: Small alveoli are predisposed to collapse. A four-alveolar model of the lungs with the assumption that recoil forces or tension (elastic and surface forces), noted by "T," are the same. The smaller the alveolus, the larger the pressure generated by the recoil forces (Law of Laplace). Gas will flow from higher pressure to lower pressure per Ohm's law, and the smaller alveoli will collapse.

in the air-liquid interface in the alveolus, thereby reducing recoil forces and preventing an increased pressure with the alveolus as it deflates. In disease states with abnormalities in surfactant, such as ARDS, however, the Law of Laplace results in significant increase in alveolar pressure in pathologic regions of lung and predisposition to alveolar collapse and shunt.

In a healthy lung, these areas of collapse are very small and easily reopened when you take a deep breath. If you are sedentary and breathing with relatively small tidal volumes, you may develop small regions of atelectasis at the bases of the lung. This may stimulate mechanoreceptors in the lung, which send a signal to the brain making you feel slightly short of breath and urging you to take a deep breath; this is a hypothesis for why we sigh from time to time. In conditions in which the compliance of the lung is reduced and FRC is abnormally low, there is a greater predilection for units to collapse. When they reopen on the next inhalation, there is a sudden equilibration of pressure between the airway and alveolus, which leads to a popping sound that we report as rales or inspiratory crackles.

In patients with very heavy chest wall (eg, morbid obesity) or abnormal surfactant, the areas of atelectasis may be more significant and not easily reversed. These patients may have reduced lung volume, more atelectasis, and, in the case of ARDS, gas exchange characterized by shunt. The abnormal surfactant in ARDS leads to a significant increase in recoil forces in the lung and difficulty reopening alveoli during inspiration; these units no longer participate in gas exchange and severe hypoxemia ensues.

One way to prevent collapse of lung units is to maintain a higher lung volume during exhalation. With a higher radius (volume) of the alveolus, pressure will be lower per the Law of Laplace and the likelihood of collapsed units during exhalation will be diminished. This is the rationale for the use of applied PEEP for patients treated with a mechanical ventilator. Because the ventilator usually determines the tidal volume and the patient may be sedated, the patient may not be able to take a deep breath (sigh) to open collapsed unit. Even in patients with relatively normal lungs who are managed with mechanical ventilation because of abnormalities with the respiratory control centers (eg, drug overdose), applied PEEP of 5 cm H_2O is commonly used to minimize atelectasis and the associated gas exchange abnormalities.

USE OF POSITIVE END-EXPIRATORY PRESSURE IN DISEASES THAT REDUCE COMPLIANCE OF THE LUNG AND FUNCTIONAL RESIDUAL CAPACITY

Several categories of disease reduce the compliance of the lung (make it stiffer; increase the recoil forces), either focally or more globally (eg, interstitial lung disease, congestive heart failure, pneumonia). Most are typified by the presence of rales (either locally or diffusely) because of the reduced EELV in the affected areas; if the disease is diffuse, for example, pulmonary edema, the rales will also be diffuse; if the disease is focal, for example, lobar pneumonia, the abnormal compliance and rales will be localized.

It is important to recognize that the use of PEEP in these situations is predicated on the disease being distributed diffusely in the lung rather than in only a small region of the lung. If the lung is diffusely stiff, the application of PEEP will increase the end-expiratory volume throughout the lung. In a patient with a very focal process, for example, a lobar pneumonia, and the remainder of the lung demonstrating normal compliance, the effect of the PEEP will be felt primarily in the normal parts of the lung (normal compliance); the normal regions (but not the stiff, abnormal regions) will have an elevated end-expiratory volume (**Figure 7-4**). This outcome in patients with focal disease will not improve oxygenation and may lead to excessive end-inspiratory volume in the normal regions of the lung, thereby increasing the risk of lung damage because of volutrauma.

In patients with focal pneumonia, the interstitial and/or alveolar inflammation reduces compliance in the regions of infection (and as noted earlier would not be helped with the application of PEEP); for diffuse pneumonias, commonly atypical pneumonias, the entire lung may be affected. Surfactant is typically normal or minimally disrupted and the gas exchange abnormality is characterized by $\dot{V}/\dot{Q}$ mismatch.

Cardiogenic pulmonary edema, with increased fluid in the interstitium, makes the lung heavier; consequently, lung volume is reduced, and rales are present. Surfactant is normal and gas exchange abnormalities are also characterized largely as $\dot{V}/\dot{Q}$ mismatch (the fluid in the interstitium compresses small airways, increasing resistance and reducing the ventilation to the

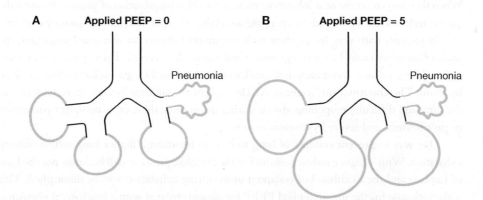

Figure 7-4: PEEP has less effect on abnormal lung in focal lung disease. **A,** Four-alveolar model of the lung with three normal alveoli (normal compliance) and one "stiff" alveolus because of pneumonia (reduced compliance), with applied PEEP of 0. **B,** With applied PEEP of 5, each of the normal alveoli has increased in size, whereas the abnormal alveolus has barely changed. PEEP, positive end-expiratory pressure.

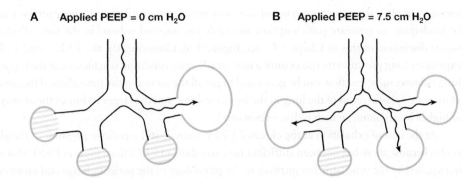

Figure 7-5: PEEP and recruitment of alveoli in ARDS. A, Four-alveolar model of the lung in a patient with ARDS and PEEP of 0. Three of the four alveoli are collapsed and filled with fluid; they are not participating in gas exchange. All of the gas provided by the ventilator is flowing into one alveolus; consequently, that alveolus is quite large at end inspiration. **B,** The same patient after initiation of applied PEEP at 7.5 cm H_2O. Two of the previously collapsed alveoli are now open and receiving gas from the ventilator. The inspired volume is now distributed over many alveoli; consequently, no single alveolus is at risk for overdistension. ARDS, acute respiratory distress syndrome; PEEP, positive end-expiratory pressure.

alveoli distal to those airways). In severe cases, in which alveoli become filled with fluid, shunt physiology may become apparent. The use of PEEP in patients with cardiogenic pulmonary edema may also be beneficial because of the associated decrease in preload and afterload (see Chapter 4 for more complete discussion).

Patients with ARDS have diffuse disease and the most pronounced changes in compliance because of abnormalities in surfactant; consequently, FRC is reduced and alveolar collapse and associated shunt physiology with marked hypoxemia may be found. Although the disease does not affect every alveolus equally, it is a diffuse process amenable to the use of PEEP. Use of applied PEEP in patients with ARDS opens alveoli (a process usually described as "recruiting" lung units) so they may participate in gas exchange (diminish shunt). In addition, because the volume of gas delivered by the ventilator on each breath will now be distributed to more open alveoli, the pressure required to deliver the tidal volume will be reduced and the risk of volutrauma associated with overdistension of alveoli will be diminished (**Figure 7-5**).

Applied PEEP may also be advantageous in ARDS to minimize atelectrauma. Repetitive collapse and reopening of alveoli with positive pressure breathing may cause sheer forces in the alveolus that can cause lung damage. By raising EELV and preventing alveolar collapse, atelectrauma may be minimized (see Chapter 13 for discussion of atelectrauma).

EXPIRATORY RESISTANCE AND APPLIED POSITIVE END-EXPIRATORY PRESSURE

Exhalation at normal levels of ventilation is passive, relying only on the elastic recoil of the lung. For a patient with acute respiratory failure, sedated and treated with positive pressure ventilation, exhalation is also passive. If there is expiratory airway resistance, the flow generated by passive recoil of the lung may not be sufficient to exhale all the air provided during an inhalation initiated at FRC. In patients with severe expiratory resistance and "flow limitation," a condition characterized by the inability to increase flow at a given volume regardless of increases in pleural pressure, even use of accessory muscles of ventilation during exercise may be inadequate to generate sufficient flow to exhale the inspired volume in the time allotted (more discussion of this in Chapter 4—see Figure 4-6). Consequently, the EELV (and end-expiratory lung pressure) increases until a new steady-state condition is achieved; at the higher lung volume, sufficient flow can be generated to get all the air out in the time allotted (because of increased elastic recoil of the lung at the higher volume and the larger radius of the airways at higher lung volume, which reduces resistance).

At the end of exhalation at the elevated EELV, there is still a positive pressure in the alveolus because there has not been sufficient time to exhale to FRC; thus, there is PEEP that is not applied by the ventilator but intrinsic to the physiology of the patient's lungs and airways. We call this PEEPi. For a spontaneously breathing patient not supported by a mechanical ventilator, to get air into the lung, that is, to create a negative pressure in the alveolus, one must first exert a negative pressure in the pleural space sufficient to bring the alveolar pressure from a positive number to zero and then a negative pressure that will create inspiratory flow from the mouth ($P_{mouth} = 0$) to the alveolus. This requires greater work by the inspiratory muscles, which leads to dyspnea and the sensation of increased work or effort of breathing; the presence of PEEPi under these circumstances is sometimes termed a "threshold inspiratory load" on the respiratory system (**Figure 7-6**).

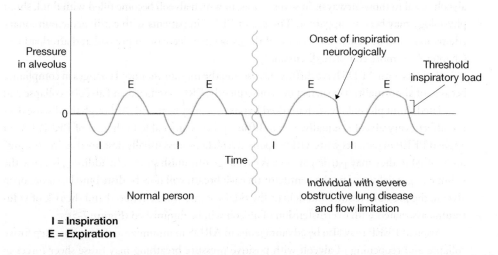

I = Inspiration
E = Expiration

Figure 7-6: Intrinsic PEEP and the threshold inspiratory load. In a healthy, normal individual, inspiration occurs when alveolar pressure is less than zero and exhalation occurs when alveolar pressure is greater than zero. There is a short "expiratory pause" at the end of the expiratory phase of the respiratory cycle, when no flow occurs. In an individual with severe expiratory airway resistance, the brain signals to the inspiratory muscles to begin inspiration before the pressure in the alveolus has returned to zero (ie, there is still positive pressure in the alveolus, intrinsic PEEP, at the time that the inspiratory muscle activity is initiated). The inspiratory muscles are activated and the chest wall begins to expand, but no inspiratory flow occurs until alveolar pressure is less than zero. The intrinsic PEEP is called a "threshold inspiratory load"; the movement of gas into the lung does not begin until the respiratory system overcomes this "threshold" of positive alveolar pressure at the end of exhalation. PEEP, positive end-expiratory pressure.

For the patient with acute respiratory failure because of COPD or acute asthma with flow limitation, the respiratory rate and tidal volume chosen may not allow sufficient time for exhalation of the volume provided by the ventilator; end-expiratory volume and pressure will be elevated—the patient will have PEEPi while receiving mechanical ventilation. For the patient to trigger the ventilator, which typically is set to provide a positive pressure breath when the machine detects negative pressure in the system, the patient must create a negative pressure in the alveolus (and hence at the mouth) to be sensed by the ventilator. Again, as with the spontaneously breathing patient without ventilatory support, this increases the work and effort of breathing. In a patient with acute respiratory failure and severe illness, there may not be sufficient strength to trigger the ventilator, which leads to ventilator dyssynchrony (see Chapter 18).

We measure the PEEPi in patients receiving mechanical ventilation by performing an expiratory hold. The "expiratory hold" or pause is accomplished by closing all the valves at the end of exhalation so no air goes into or out of the patient (**Figure 7-7**). Having established conditions of "no flow" in the system, the pressure at the mouth, which is where the measurement is being made by the ventilator, comes into equilibrium with the pressure at the alveolus (this procedure is analogous to the inspiratory hold or plateau pressure used to assess respiratory system compliance, discussed in Chapter 2).

To address this problem, we use applied PEEP, provided by the mechanical ventilator, to minimize the work of breathing required to initiate a breath. For example, you are treating a patient with acute respiratory failure because of an exacerbation of COPD and the patient has PEEPi of 7 cm H_2O. You set the applied PEEP at 5 cm H_2O; as soon as the patient reduces alveolar pressure below 5 cm H_2O, the ventilator will begin pushing air into the lung. The patient only needs to drop the alveolar pressure (by contracting the inspiratory muscles) by 2 cm H_2O in order to begin getting assistance from the ventilator. This same phenomenon is seen in this type of patient treated with noninvasive positive pressure, either in the bilevel positive airway pressure (BiPAP) or continuous positive airway pressure (CPAP) mode. The measured PEEP after applied PEEP is instituted is commonly higher than the original PEEPi but less than a sum of the applied PEEP and PEEPi.

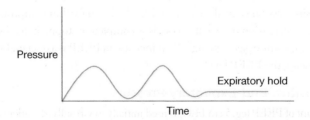

Figure 7-7: Measurement of PEEP in mechanically ventilated patients. For a patient with acute respiratory failure who is intubated and receiving mechanical ventilation, one can measure PEEP with an expiratory pause or hold. The valves of the ventilator are closed and no air may go into or out of the lung. Although the pressure being measured is at the mouth, the initiation of the expiratory hold allows equilibration of pressure from the mouth to the alveoli (analogous to the inspiratory hold used to determine the pressure of the alveolus at the end of inspiration, or plateau pressure—see Chapter 2). The rise in pressure from the beginning to the end of the expiratory hold represents this equilibration process and now represents alveolar pressure at the end of exhalation. PEEP, positive end-expiratory pressure.

DANGERS AND COMPLICATIONS OF POSITIVE END-EXPIRATORY PRESSURE

There are four major complications or dangers associated with the use of PEEP in mechanical ventilation. One primarily involves the respiratory system, and two represent effects that PEEP has on the cardiovascular system (although one of these also has gas exchange consequences).

The first complication is hyperinflation. By definition, the use of PEEP raises the EELV by preventing alveolar pressure from returning to zero during exhalation. If the EELV is elevated and one continues to put in the standard tidal volume, the end-inspiratory volume (and pressure) will be elevated as well. This may lead to lung injury via volutrauma, causing damage to the alveolus leading to capillary leak or pneumothorax. It is difficult to assess lung volume at the bedside with standard monitoring instruments; consequently, we use plateau pressure on the ventilator (see Chapter 2) to infer changes in lung volume, assuming compliance of the lung has not changed from the time of earlier measurements. Ideally, we would like to keep the transpulmonary pressure below 20 to 25 cm H_2O to avoid volutrauma (see Chapter 13). The plateau pressure provides us with a measure of intra-alveolar pressure, but transpulmonary pressure requires us to also know the pressure outside the alveolus, that is, the pleural pressure or intrathoracic pressure. We typically assume the pleural pressure is zero unless the patient's chest wall is heavy (eg, body mass index [BMI] is quite elevated or there is anasarca), there is increased intra-abdominal pressure (eg, ascites), or large pleural effusions. In these circumstances, an esophageal balloon may be placed to allow an estimate to be made of intrathoracic pressure. If intrathoracic pressure is elevated, we may have a higher plateau pressure on the ventilator without risking volutrauma.

Because PEEP increases lung volume and intrathoracic pressure, it reduces venous return to the thorax from the extrathoracic veins. Consequently, ventricular filling is reduced, the patient "moves to the left" on the Starling curve (preload is reduced), and cardiac output may fall (see Chapter 4) with potential for a drop in blood pressure. This is the second potential complication of PEEP.

The third and fourth complications of PEEP relate to its possible effect on the pulmonary blood vessels. The increase in lung volume has an effect on pulmonary vascular resistance (increasing resistance in alveolar vessels), which can further compromise cardiac output. Furthermore, if perfusion of alveolar vessels is completely stopped, dead space will increase, which may compromise gas exchange. If an increase in PEEP is associated with a rise in $Paco_2$, consider reducing the PEEP level.

Setting Positive End-Expiratory Pressure

A small amount of PEEP (eg, 5 cm H_2O) is used initially in virtually all patients placed on mechanical ventilation to minimize the development of atelectasis with constant tidal volume. The two major indications for employing PEEP at higher levels with mechanical ventilation are:

1. hypoxemia because of intrapulmonary shunt from ARDS
2. flow limitation with the presence of PEEPi

For patients with significant pulmonary shunt because of ARDS, one may use tables developed from empiric studies to adjust PEEP based on the level of hypoxemia. Generally, mild to moderate hypoxemia is treated with applied PEEP of 5 to 10 cm H_2O and moderate to severe hypoxemia with applied PEEP of 10 to 15 cm H_2O. Caution is needed, however, because of concerns about volutrauma and hemodynamic complications, as noted earlier (also see Chapter 13). An alternative strategy is to do a "best PEEP" trial by assessing the compliance of the respiratory system starting with low applied PEEP and then gradually increasing the PEEP level with repeated measures of compliance. As noted earlier, patients with significant alveolar collapse may exhibit low lung compliance because the tidal volume delivered by the ventilator is distributed to only a small fraction of the total alveoli. If one is able to recruit a significant portion of these alveoli to participate in gas exchange with applied PEEP, the tidal volume will be distributed across a wider distribution of alveoli, which prevents individual alveoli from becoming overdistended, which would be associated with decreased compliance (the lung units get stiffer or less compliant, with greater elastic recoil, as they are distended to higher volume). Consequently, if you increase applied PEEP and compliance increases, you know you have recruited more alveoli and can try an even higher level of applied PEEP. On the other hand, if compliance falls with the elevation in applied PEEP, you are overdistending lung units and should reduce the applied PEEP.

For patients in whom PEEP is applied to minimize the problems associated with increased airway resistance and flow limitation, the applied PEEP is generally set 1 to 2 cm H_2O below PEEPi.

SUMMARY

FRC is determined by the balance of forces of chest wall and lung recoil. At FRC, alveolar pressure is zero. Based on the Law of Laplace, the smaller the radius of the alveolus, the more likely that an alveolus will collapse, leading to atelectasis in the lung and potential for gas exchange abnormalities. Although healthy individuals vary tidal volume with activity and/or sighs to minimize atelectasis, patients with acute respiratory failure who are treated with mechanical ventilation get a repetitive small tidal volume, which can predispose to the development of atelectasis. When PEEP is applied by the ventilator, EELV is elevated above FRC and the probability of alveolar collapse falls. The use of PEEP to elevate EELV is particularly important in patients with diseases that increase recoil forces in the lung (eg, ARDS) and are associated with very low FRC.

Applied PEEP is also important in patients with obstructive lung disease characterized by flow limitation; these individuals have PEEPi, which increases the work of breathing and may lead to failure to trigger the ventilator. Use of applied PEEP in this setting minimizes the challenges posed by PEEPi.

Applied PEEP may cause harm to the patient by causing hyperinflation and by altering the hemodynamics. In setting applied PEEP, one must use strategies that minimize risk to the patient.

KEY POINTS

- FRC is relaxation volume at the end of a quiet exhalation.
- Diseases associated with reduced lung compliance have a low FRC.
- Reduced FRC leads to greater risk of alveolar collapse based on the Law of Laplace. This is a particular problem in patients with ARDS and abnormal surfactant.
- Collapsed alveoli in ARDS are associated with hypoxemia because of shunt.
- PEEP is useful for patients with diffuse lung disease that results in reduced lung compliance.
- Flow limitation may lead to PEEPi and increased work to initiate inspiration or trigger the mechanical ventilator. Applied PEEP may minimize this problem.

- Applied PEEP can be set in patients with ARDS based upon oxygenation and/or changes in lung compliance; attention should be paid to possible respiratory and cardiovascular complications from applied PEEP that is too high.
- Applied PEEP can be set in patients with increased airway resistance based on the determination of PEEPi; applied PEEP is set at 1 to 2 cm H_2O below PEEPi.

STUDY QUESTIONS AND ANSWERS

Questions

1. You are caring for a 54-year-old man with sepsis who has developed severe hypoxemia requiring intubation and initiation of mechanical ventilation. The chest radiograph shows diffuse alveolar infiltrates and low lung volume. There are no pleural effusions and the heart size is normal. The arterial blood gas shows Pao_2 58 mm Hg, $Paco_2$ 41 mm Hg, and pH 7.36 with Fio_2 0.8. The ventilator is delivering a tidal volume of 450 mL by volume ventilation and plateau pressure is 18 cm H_2O. Applied PEEP is set at 0 cm H_2O. Blood pressure is 105/70. At this point you should:
   A. increase the Fio_2 to 1.0.
   B. increase the applied PEEP to 10 cm H_2O.
   C. diurese the patient.
   D. reduce the PEEP to zero.
   E. increase the PEEP to 15 mm Hg.

2. You are caring for a 70-year-old patient with a long history of COPD who was intubated and treated with mechanical ventilation because of acute pneumonia and hypoxemia. Chest radiograph shows low lung volume with upper lobe bullae and a patchy right lower lobe infiltrate. The present ventilator settings are assist control, volume ventilation with a respiratory rate of 14 breaths/min, and a tidal volume of 6 mL/kg with applied PEEP of 5 cm H_2O. You note that the patient is making inspiratory efforts that do not trigger the ventilator. An "expiratory hold" shows PEEPi of 10 cm H_2O. The arterial blood gas reveals Pao_2 65 mm Hg, $Paco_2$ 50 mm Hg, and pH 7.37. At this time, you should:
   A. raise the applied PEEP to 7 to 8 cm H_2O.
   B. increase the respiratory rate.
   C. increase the tidal volume.
   D. decrease the Fio_2.
   E. raise the applied PEEP to 12 mm Hg.

3. You come on duty and are called to evaluate a 25-year-old woman admitted yesterday with acute respiratory failure because of drug overdose. She has no history of cardiopulmonary disease. She has been ventilated overnight with volume ventilation, an Fio_2 of 0.3, and applied PEEP of 0. The nurse calls you to see the patient because her oxygen saturation has dropped from 95% to 89%. Tidal volume is 7 mL/kg. She is afebrile with a normal white blood cell count. On exam, there are rales at the right base. A chest radiograph is notable for atelectasis in the right lower lobe. At this time you should:
   A. increase the tidal volume.
   B. start pressure ventilation.
   C. increase the respiratory rate.
   D. start applied PEEP at 5 cm H_2O.
   E. increase the respiratory flow.

Answers

1. **Answer B. Increase the applied PEEP to 10 cm H_2O**

   Rationale: The patient's history, chest radiograph, and large intrapulmonary shunt, which you can infer from the low Pao_2 with a very high Fio_2 (the P/F ratio is less than 100), are consistent with ARDS. The low lung volume on chest radiograph suggests a low total lung capacity and likely a low FRC, and the alveolar opacities with normal size heart and absent pleural effusions are indicative of noncardiogenic pulmonary edema. To enhance oxygenation, an increase in applied PEEP is indicated as the next best step to recruit alveoli to participate in gas exchange. Given the plateau pressure of 18 cm H_2O, an increase to 10 cm H_2O rather than 15 cm H_2O is indicated to avoid possible overdistension of the lung, although one would hope that compliance of the lung might increase as alveoli are opened and participate in gas exchange (tidal volume more evenly distributed throughout the lung). Diuresis is not indicated with low suspicion of cardiogenic pulmonary edema (although one tends to aim for a low intravascular volume given the capillary leak associated with ARDS). Remember that an increase in PEEP will diminish venous return and preload for the heart, which can lead to a fall in blood pressure if intravascular volume is too low.

2. **Answer A. Raise the applied PEEP to 7 to 8 cm H_2O**

   Rationale: The patient is acting in a manner consistent with flow limitation with PEEPi and hyperinflation. Because of the high PEEPi, he is having difficulty triggering the ventilator. To make it easier for him to trigger the ventilator, applied PEEP should be targeted just below the level of PEEPi. If applied PEEP is greater than PEEPi, you are likely to cause further hyperinflation and possible lung injury and pneumothorax. An increase in respiratory rate or tidal volume will increase dynamic hyperinflation; both of these will exacerbate the issue of inadequate expiratory flow needed to exhale the amount of gas pushed into the lung on inhalation by the ventilator.

3. **Answer D. Start applied PEEP at 5 cm H_2O**

   Rationale: The patient likely has hypoxemia because of V̇/Q̇ mismatch from atelectasis in the right lower lobe. With constant tidal volume in the normal range, even healthy lungs will be predisposed to some atelectasis. To prevent atelectasis, we use applied PEEP, initially at 5 cm H_2O, to elevate the FRC and reduce the risk of atelectasis as well as recruit the alveoli that have already collapsed. Increasing tidal volume may also help, but the patient is near the upper limit of tidal volume used to minimize the risk of volutrauma. Increasing respiratory rate will increase the total ventilation, which may increase the oxygen saturation, but it will not correct the atelectasis. For this patient, pressure and volume ventilation will likely be very similar and the change to pressure ventilation will not alter the problem.

Suggested Readings

Gattinoni L, Marini JJ. In search of the Holy Grail: identifying the best PEEP in ventilated patients. *Intensive Care Med*. 2022;48:728-731.

Walkey AJ, Del Sorbo L, Hodgson CL, et al. Higher PEEP versus lower PEEP strategies for patients with acute respiratory distress syndrome: a systematic review and meta-analysis. *Ann Am Thorac Soc*. 2017;14:S297-S303.

Setting the Ventilator and Basic Monitoring

Jeremy B. Richards • Diana Bouhassira

LEARNING OBJECTIVES

- Identify the key ventilator settings that are set by the operator and the resulting dependent parameters, which are monitored to assess the impact of the settings.
- Describe the types of lung injury that can be caused by mechanical ventilation.
- Review the data and rationale for low tidal volume ventilation.
- Describe the effects of positive end-expiratory pressure (PEEP) and understand how PEEP is optimized for a given patient.
- Discuss approaches to mechanical ventilation in certain common disease states.

INTRODUCTION

The goal of this chapter is to review the general approach to setting and interpreting the ventilator, provide a brief overview of the types of lung injury that can develop in a mechanically ventilated patient (described further in Chapter 16), and provide an overview of approaches to mechanical ventilation in common disease states, some of which are discussed in more detail in other chapters in the book.

SETTING THE VENTILATOR

When approaching a mechanically ventilated patient, the key factors to consider are which parameters are being set by the ventilator and which parameters are dependent upon the patient's respiratory system mechanics (resistance and compliance) and gas exchanger. When choosing the ventilator mode and settings, there are four key parameters to consider when approaching any intubated and mechanically ventilated patient.

Ventilator Settings Affecting Oxygenation

Two parameters primarily affect the patient's oxygenation and two primarily affect ventilation. When considering the mechanics of mechanical ventilation, it is helpful to keep in mind that unlike normal breathing, which is dependent on generating negative intrathoracic pressure to pull air into the lungs, contemporary mechanical ventilation almost exclusively relies on positive pressure ventilation. In other words, every inspiration is the product of air being forced into the patient by the ventilator, as compared to normal breathing patterns in which air flows into the lungs as a result of decreased intrathoracic pressure following diaphragmatic contraction.

With regard to ventilator settings that affect oxygenation, the relevant parameters one sets on the ventilator are the fraction of inspired oxygen or "F_{IO_2}" and positive end-expiratory pressure or "PEEP." F_{IO_2} simply refers to the proportion or percentage of supplemental oxygen being provided in the air entering the lung via the ventilator. Typically, when patients are first intubated and mechanical ventilation is initiated, they are provided with the maximum amount of F_{IO_2} available (100%), which is then titrated down based on their observed oxygen saturation as measured by pulse oximetry. PEEP is the pressure at the airway opening (or end of the endotracheal tube), maintained by the ventilator at the end of expiration in order to decrease alveolar collapse (see Chapter 7 for a more complete discussion of PEEP). As the radius of the alveolus diminishes during exhalation, the recoil forces of the alveolus may lead to collapse in accord with the Law of Laplace. In spontaneously breathing healthy individuals, we vary our tidal volume (TV) on a regular basis, which opens alveoli that may have collapsed, but in the intubated, sedated patient, the TV is the same on every breath; if an alveolus collapses, it may not reopen.

If alveoli collapsed at the end of every exhalation with positive pressure ventilation, mechanical strain would occur as they were subsequently forced open during the next inspiration. This mechanical strain is referred to as atelectrauma, that is, damage because of repetitive atelectasis and reopening of a lung unit. Atelectasis of the lung leads to ventilation/perfusion mismatch, which contributes to hypoxemia (see Chapter 3); consequently, PEEP is used to avoid worsening hypoxemia. As a general guide for patients without known specific lung pathophysiologic processes, setting the initial PEEP to a pressure of 5 cm H_2O is a reasonable starting point. Later in this chapter, we will discuss strategies for optimizing PEEP based on a patient's specific respiratory system physiology and overall clinical circumstances.

Ventilator Settings Affecting Ventilation

Oxygenation describes the process of oxygen uptake across the alveolar-capillary basement membrane and is assessed with the oxygen saturation (Spo_2) and partial pressure of arterial oxygen (Pao_2). Ventilation refers to the process of moving air in and out of the respiratory system with the goal of optimizing the partial pressure of arterial carbon dioxide ($Paco_2$). Regarding the parameters that affect ventilation, the two primary ventilator settings to consider are TV and respiratory rate or "RR" (sometimes represented as "f" for "frequency"). Because ventilation determines the patient's ability to exhale CO_2, it also regulates the arterial pH; CO_2 in the blood is transformed to carbonic acid, which dissociates to H^+ and bicarbonate. Consequently, low ventilation increases the $Paco_2$ and reduces pH, whereas high ventilation reduces $Paco_2$ and raises pH. A patient's ventilatory status can be monitored via arterial or venous blood gases. Ventilation is specifically a product of how much air is inhaled and exhaled, but gas exchange depends on the proportion of inhaled air that actually interacts with the alveoli (termed "alveolar ventilation") versus the proportion of inhaled air that interacts with dead space (termed "dead space ventilation").

As a general guideline, when using a ventilator mode in which volume is an independent parameter set by the operator, starting with a TV of 6 to 8 mL/kg of ideal body weight (IBW) is appropriate. The RR can be set somewhere between 12 and 20 breaths/min, depending on the patient's clinical circumstances and their acute and chronic respiratory pathophysiology.

Monitoring and Optimization of Ventilator Settings

Optimization of each of the parameters requires careful and frequent monitoring of the patient's oxygen saturation (most easily obtained noninvasively via pulse oximetry) and their ventilation via Pco_2 monitoring in venous or arterial blood gases (ABGs) and/or via end-tidal CO_2 monitoring (which can be measured and reported by many contemporary mechanical ventilators; one must remember, however, that the end-tidal Pco_2 may not accurately assess arterial Pco_2 in patients with diffuse lung disease). ABGs measure the patient's oxygenation as well as ventilation but are technically more difficult to obtain repeatedly as a monitoring metric without an invasive arterial line. ABGs (and arterial lines) are not always necessary for mechanically ventilated patients, because pulse oximetry provides a reliable measure of oxygenation.

Importantly, recent literature suggests that the algorithm used by the pulse oximeter may not be equally accurate in black patients as compared with white patients; specifically, the pulse oximeter may underestimate arterial O_2 saturation in black patients. Venous blood gases are easier to obtain and provide sufficient information about changes in the patient's pH and Pco_2 to manage ventilation, but are not useful for monitoring oxygenation. The severity of certain disease conditions, particularly acute respiratory distress syndrome (ARDS), which is discussed further and in Chapter 14, is characterized by use of the "Pao_2:Fio_2 ratio," or a ratio of arterial partial pressure of oxygen (Pao_2) to the fraction of inspired O_2 (Fio_2), such that ABG monitoring may be more appropriate in these patients. The higher the Fio_2 for any given Pao_2, the worse the gas exchange problem.

With respect to the dependent parameters evaluated on the ventilator, these vary based on which ventilator mode is being used. The commonly used ventilator modes can be categorized into those providing full support to the patient (ie, pressure control or volume control) versus partial support (ie, pressure support ventilation). In the latter mode, the patient is spontaneously breathing but with backup support from the ventilator to ensure they are achieving adequate ventilation. In general, it is the healthcare provider's decision whether to use a volume-dependent mode or a pressure-dependent mode, and this decision relates to the patient's underlying condition and lung mechanics (see Chapter 5).

With respect to pressures measured and reported by the ventilator, peak pressure is the pressure applied during inspiration as gas is pushed into the lung to achieve a certain inspiratory volume, and plateau pressure is the pressure in the lungs at the end of inspiration when all flow has ceased. The peak pressure reflects both the resistance of the airways and

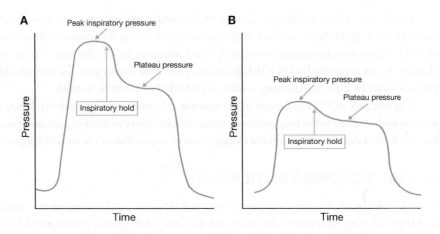

Figure 8-1: Pressure-time tracings depicting different respiratory system pressures after an inspiratory hold for patients with high **(A)** and low **(B)** respiratory system compliance.

the respiratory system compliance, whereas the plateau pressure reflects only the stiffness or recoil forces of the respiratory system. Compliance is a characteristic of both the lung and the chest wall and can be calculated by measuring change in volume (eg, the TV in volume assist control ventilation) divided by change in pressure (eg, the plateau pressure minus the PEEP) (see Chapter 2 for review of the inspiratory hold used to obtain the plateau pressure). A high compliance means that there is a large change in volume for a small change in pressure, whereas low compliance means that there is relatively less change in volume for higher pressures (**Figure 8-1**).

VENTILATOR-ASSOCIATED LUNG INJURY

Before considering specific disease types and related ventilator management considerations, it is worth pausing to discuss the types of injury, known collectively as ventilator-associated (or ventilator-induced) lung injury (VILI), which can be caused by mechanical ventilation.

One type of damage, referred to as atelectrauma, has been noted earlier. To review, atelectrauma refers to damage to the alveoli because of mechanical shearing forces generated by repeated recruitment and decruitment (or expansion and collapse), which occurs when sufficient PEEP is not applied and alveoli collapse at the end of exhalation. To conceptualize this type of damage, picture the process of blowing up a deflated balloon. You have probably had the experience of starting to blow up a balloon and noticing that it requires significantly more force to get the first bit of air into it and then requires much less force once the balloon has started to fill up. Now imagine that there was already a little bit of air in the balloon before you started blowing up the balloon—this would allow you to expand the balloon to full capacity without nearly as much force, as compared to starting with a completely empty balloon. As discussed earlier, the use of applied PEEP from the ventilator prevents the lung from fully emptying during exhalation, thereby reducing the chance of alveolar collapse.

Volutrauma is the result of cyclic alveolar overdistension because of excessive TVs. This form of trauma to the alveoli leads to damage to the capillary and alveolar endothelium, resulting in microvascular leakage and pulmonary edema and ultimately ARDS-like pathophysiology.

Barotrauma refers to damage because of elevated peak and plateau pressures experienced by the lung. However, animal studies have suggested that the primary pathophysiology of VILI relates to volutrauma, and that elevated pressures in the absence of large-volume changes do not generally lead to VILI. When the chest wall is very stiff, for example, plateau pressures may be high, but the lung volume at end inhalation can be normal.

Any category of VILI can result in the systemic release of inflammatory cytokines, which mediate both damage to the lung and cause inflammatory injury to other organs and tissues. See later for further discussion of ventilator management strategies that can be used to mitigate VILI.

LOW TIDAL VOLUME VENTILATION

Considerable data from over 20 years of large, well-designed studies support the conclusions that large TVs are injurious to the lungs and that low tidal volume ventilation (LTVV) decreases morbidity and mortality in patients with ARDS. Specifically, the paradigm-shifting ARDSNet trial was a large randomized controlled trial that demonstrated that patients randomized to a TV of 6 to 8 mL/kg IBW and a goal plateau pressure less than 30 cm H_2O had an overall mortality rate of 31% as compared to 39.8% in patients randomized to a TV of 10 to 12 mL/kg IBW and a goal plateau pressure of less than 50 cm H_2O ($P = 0.007$).

Since that time, further trials and studies have demonstrated that LTVV is an appropriate and potentially beneficial strategy in almost all patients, including those without known lung injury, who require mechanical ventilation. Thus far, there is no evidence suggesting that LTVV is harmful in any population requiring full ventilatory support.

LTVV is generally defined as TVs of 6 to 8 mL/kg IBW with a resultant goal plateau pressure of less than 30 cm H_2O. In order to maintain this goal pressure, the TV can be reduced to 4 mL/kg IBW if needed. PEEP is usually maintained at 5 cm H_2O or more in order to prevent atelectasis. Given smaller TV, adequate minute ventilation is maintained by increasing RR (generally to 20-35 breaths/min). For patients with ARDS, the goal oxygenation is generally a peripheral oxygen saturation (Spo_2) level of 88% to 95%, or an arterial Po_2 of ~60 to 80 mm Hg.

Initial concerns about the use of LTVV included questions about whether LTVV would result in increased Pco_2 and acidosis, but generally minute ventilation can be appropriately maintained by increasing RR. Another concern is whether LTVV requires increased need for sedation and analgesia to maintain patient comfort and synchrony with the vent. If significant dyssynchrony is noted despite deep sedation, short-term neuromuscular blockade can be considered.

OPTIMIZING POSITIVE END-EXPIRATORY PRESSURE

As noted earlier, PEEP refers to a minimum baseline pressure that is applied by the ventilator throughout the ventilatory cycle, including at the end of expiration when intrathoracic and airway pressures are lowest, in order to maintain alveolar recruitment. Regardless of the specific disease state resulting in respiratory failure and the need for mechanical ventilation, the goal of optimizing PEEP is to maximize the portion of the lung that is successfully ventilated and to reduce trauma to alveoli by reducing the degree of cyclic opening and closing, which may lead to lung injury. PEEP may additionally improve oxygenation in the setting of pulmonary edema by reducing airway narrowing from the interstitial fluid and consequent $\dot{V}/\dot{Q}$ mismatch.

Excess PEEP, however, can also result in lung injury via alveolar overinflation, as well as in strain on the right heart if overdistension results in stretching of the perialveolar vessels with a resultant increase in pulmonary vascular resistance. In patients who have excessive auto-PEEP (see Chapter 7), like those with obstructive lung disease described earlier, or in those who have inadequate preload because of intravascular volume depletion, PEEP can contribute to elevated intrathoracic pressure and result in hypotension secondary to reduced venous return to the right side of the heart.

There are several methods by which one can determine the optimal PEEP for a given patient. One method, known as the "best PEEP trial," involves first increasing PEEP to a predetermined maximum, generally leading to end-inspiratory pressures around 38 to 40 cm H_2O unless there are contraindications to such high pressures, such as hypotension or air leak/bronchopulmonary fistula. Subsequently, PEEP is reduced in increments of 2 to 3 cm H_2O while measuring oxygenation, peak pressures, and mean arterial blood pressures at each new PEEP level. The "best PEEP" is the one that maximizes oxygenation while minimizing deleterious effects on peak pressures and mean arterial pressures. Alternatively, one begins with a low PEEP and assesses the compliance of the lung every few minutes with successively increasing levels of PEEP. The PEEP level that results in the best compliance is the preferred PEEP; the best compliance indicates you have balanced minimization of atelectasis with avoidance of overdistension of lung during inhalation. Remember that increases in PEEP do not always lead to comparable increases in end-inspiratory pressures if lung units are opened and the inspiratory volume is distributed over a larger number of alveoli.

At some medical centers, esophageal manometry is available, and the effect of PEEP on pleural and transpulmonary pressures can be directly measured, which may be useful when standard measures may be inaccurate because of large patient body mass index (BMI) and/or chest wall mass. The goal is to achieve a transpulmonary pressure at end exhalation of approximately +2 cm H_2O. Thus far, however, data have not supported any difference in mortality or duration of mechanical ventilation attributable to use of esophageal manometry as compared with standard methods of PEEP titration. More detail regarding esophageal manometry is available in Chapter 17.

INITIAL SEDATION AND PATIENT-VENTILATOR DYSSYNCHRONY

Initial sedation of a mechanically ventilated patient requires both pain management and sedation. General practice may vary between institutions, but continuous infusion of an opiate medication such as fentanyl in combination with a sedative such as propofol is an appropriate place to start. Sedation is titrated using the Richmond Agitation Sedation Scale (RASS), with a general goal of the patient being at a RASS score of 0 to –2 (0 meaning alert and calm, and –2 meaning that they briefly awaken to voice [eyes open for less than 10 seconds]). Analgesia is used to address the discomfort of the endotracheal tube and to treat dyspnea that typically is present from the cardiopulmonary process precipitating respiratory failure and that may be exacerbated by the ways in which we set the ventilator, for example, restricting TV when the drive to breathe is elevated.

A common problem that may arise and require troubleshooting is patient dyssynchrony with the mechanical ventilator, or the patient "fighting the ventilator." Patient dyssynchrony can lead to increased work of breathing and patient distress, and it is important to determine any underlying triggers for dyssynchrony. Two important etiologies to consider are hypoxemia and acidosis. If neither of these is present, other possible etiologies include discomfort with the RR and/or TV set on the ventilator, mucus plugging, bronchospasm, and mainstem intubation, among others (see Chapter 20 for in-depth discussion of ventilator dyssynchrony). If the patient is "overbreathing" the ventilator (triggering many additional breaths beyond the set rate), increasing the RR, if appropriate, may improve synchrony. It is important, however, to remember that this will increase ventilation and, if the patient is experiencing a reversible cause for the high rate, it is better to address the underlying problem triggering the increased RR (such as acidosis, pain, or anxiety).

MECHANICAL VENTILATION IN SPECIFIC DISEASE CONDITIONS

Specific clinical conditions or disease states require special consideration when determining, monitoring, and adjusting ventilator settings. Approaches to ventilator settings for ARDS, obstructive lung disease, and interstitial lung disease (ILD) are discussed in the next subsections.

Acute Respiratory Distress Syndrome

In the era of COVID-19, ARDS has become ubiquitous in intensive care units (ICUs) around the world. ARDS is defined as acute onset (<7 days) of bilateral, noncardiac pulmonary edema causing profound deficits in oxygenation (Pao_2:Fio_2 ratio of <300; see **Table 8-1**). Because ARDS is a syndrome, it can be the result of any inflammatory process, infectious or otherwise, and can occur because of direct pulmonary injury (eg, pneumonia or aspiration pneumonitis, among others) or extrapulmonary inflammation (eg, trauma or pancreatitis, among others). ARDS is classically characterized as having an initial inflammatory phase lasting 7 to 10 days and a subsequent fibroproliferative phase. The effect of ARDS on the lungs is often heterogeneous, leading some areas of the lung to become densely consolidated and unable to participate in gas exchange, some areas of the lung collapsed but recruitable, and other areas of the lung to be relatively normal. This heterogeneity of lung injury and pathophysiology poses challenges to the provider when working to identify and maintain optimal ventilator settings.

Specifically, an unfortunate consequence of the heterogeneous inflammation observed in ARDS is that ventilation may be unevenly distributed, causing overdistension in alveoli that are the least consolidated (and most compliant), potentially leading to VILI and exacerbating the inflammatory process. Because of this risk, LTVV is a core principle of management; we

TABLE 8-1	Clinical Definition of ARDS Using the Berlin Criteria
Parameter	**Description**
Pao_2:Fio_2 ratio of <300	A Pao_2:Fio_2 ratio of 200-300 defines mild ARDS, 100-200 is moderate, and 0-100 is severe ARDS.
Bilateral consolidations on chest x-ray	Bilateral "alveolar" consolidations not fully explained by effusions, lung collapse, and/or nodules are necessary to define ARDS, as this indicates diffuse involvement of the pulmonary parenchyma.
Acute onset of respiratory symptoms	Timing is within 1 week of known clinical insult or worsening respiratory symptoms.
Noncardiogenic origin of pulmonary edema	Objective assessment of the cause of pulmonary edema, such as echocardiography, is a component of this criteria for defining ARDS.

ARDS, acute respiratory distress syndrome.

also use the plateau pressure to ensure that we are not exceeding a transpulmonary pressure that would overdistend even normal alveoli. The severe hypoxemia seen in ARDS is due to intrapulmonary shunting and ventilation-perfusion mismatch in the setting of exudative alveolar fluid and inflammatory debris, which leads to a decrease in surfactant thereby causing increased alveolar surface tension and collapse, such that optimization of PEEP to maintain open alveoli is another core principle of mechanical ventilation in ARDS.

A third key aspect of ARDS management is the positioning of patients in a prone position. Prolonged (>12 hours) prone positioning of patients with moderate to severe ARDS (defined as $Pao_2:Fio_2$ <150) has been shown to reduce mortality. By placing the position in the prone position, one alters the weight of the chest wall on the lungs, which results in better aeration and ventilation of normally dependent regions. The primary risks associated with proning include increased probability of endotracheal tube obstruction or dislodgment and pressure sores. Chapter 14 provides more details about mechanical ventilation and respiratory support for patients with ARDS.

Obstructive Lung Disease

The obstructive lung diseases (chronic obstructive pulmonary disease [COPD], asthma, tracheobronchomalacia, and others) are treated very differently with mechanical ventilation as compared to ARDS. These diseases are characterized by expiratory obstruction of airways, which leads to an inability to fully exhale the volume of air that is inhaled if expiratory time is constrained, leading to dynamic hyperinflation, an inability to effectively eliminate CO_2, and a phenomenon called auto-PEEP or intrinsic PEEP (see Chapter 11). As mentioned earlier, the volume of air moving in and out of the lungs multiplied by the rate at which a patient is breathing determine total or minute ventilation. If minute ventilation is reduced, it may lead to accumulation of carbon dioxide and, as a result, respiratory acidosis. Severe respiratory acidosis may result in systemic complications including encephalopathy, cardiac arrest, and even death.

Auto-PEEP or intrinsic PEEP refers to an increased end-expiratory pressure in the lungs as a result of the patient's inability to completely exhale (ie, to exhale to the functional residual capacity [FRC]) prior to initiating the next inhalation. If the patient starts the breath at a lung volume greater than FRC, this increase in end-expiratory volume and pressure may lead to an increase in end-inspiratory pressure, which can result in volutrauma with overdistension of alveoli, pneumothorax, or cardiovascular collapse from reduced venous return to the heart in the setting of very high intrathoracic pressures. High levels of auto-PEEP can additionally lead to patient dyssynchrony with the ventilator and increase the amount of patient effort required to trigger the ventilator in a mode where the patient is initiating breaths.

Auto-PEEP can be detected by looking at the waveforms on the ventilator. Specifically, auto-PEEP can manifest as the initiation of the inspiratory portion of the respiratory cycle before expiratory flow has completely returned to zero (stated differently, a patient normally should completely finish exhaling, that is, alveolar pressure falls to zero, before inspiration is initiated; see **Figure 8-2**). In order to quantify the degree of auto-PEEP, an expiratory hold maneuver can be performed to assess the pulmonary pressure at the end of exhalation.

For patients with obstructive lung disease who require mechanical ventilation, a patient's obstructive pathophysiology can be counteracted by controlling the duration of inspiration and expiration. The ventilator parameter that controls the duration of inhalation and exhalation is called "I:E time" or the "I:E ratio" and is the ratio of inspiratory time to expiratory time. By setting the I:E time to allow a prolonged expiratory time beyond what a spontaneously breathing and awake patient might otherwise be able to tolerate, sufficient time can be provided for the

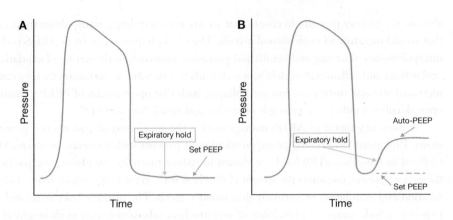

Figure 8-2: Pressure-time tracing depicting an expiratory hold maneuver for a patient with normal expiratory flow **(A)** and for a patient with increased auto-PEEP **(B)**. The rise in the pressure when the expiratory hold is initiated represents equilibration of the pressure from the alveolus to the mouth/end of endotracheal tube. What is shown as "auto-PEEP" represents the "measured" PEEP with this maneuver, which reflects the interaction of the patient's intrinsic PEEP and applied PEEP from the ventilator. PEEP, positive end-expiratory pressure.

patient to exhale the air in their alveoli and airways to achieve an end-expiratory volume closer to FRC, thereby reducing auto-PEEP and improving ventilation. Reducing the RR is an additional, and simpler, method that can be attempted to allow for longer expiratory time, more complete exhalation, and diminished auto-PEEP in patients with severe airway obstruction.

Apart from supporting the patient via appropriate ventilator strategies, the key to managing patients with COPD is to address the underlying obstruction with bronchodilators, steroids, and appropriate systemic medical management. Patients experiencing severe bronchospasm may require heavy sedation to tolerate the settings needed to maintain appropriate ventilation. Paralytics may be required in severe cases, such as for patients with status asthmaticus, to obligate ventilator synchrony and to achieve a decreased RR.

Finally, many patients with long-standing COPD may live with chronic hypercapnia and an associated compensatory metabolic alkalosis. In these individuals, ventilation should be targeted to the patient's baseline $Paco_2$ thereby maintaining a normal pH for that patient, which will not occur at a "normal $Paco_2$" of 40 mm Hg. More details about ventilator management and monitoring for patients with COPD are available in Chapter 11.

Interstitial Lung Disease

Ventilatory approaches for patients with ILD are discussed in detail in Chapter 15, but basic approaches and general considerations for optimal ventilator management of patients with ILD are reviewed here. The primary pathophysiologic manifestation of patients with ILD is decreased respiratory system compliance, attributable to increased lung stiffness from parenchymal scarring and fibrosis. Similar to ARDS, decreased respiratory system compliance results in high airway pressure (both the peak and plateau inspiratory pressures) in response to a given TV. As such, targeting a low TV approach to mechanical ventilation is critical for patients with ILD, and frequent monitoring of the peak inspiratory and plateau pressures is necessary to guide the need for adjustments to the delivered TV.

Advanced ILD is also characterized by an increased dead space to TV ratio (referred to as "V_d/V_t"). Functionally, this means that a patient's alveolar volume is reduced in proportion to their overall TV, such that gas exchange is impaired, resulting in hypoxemia and decreased elimination of carbon dioxide. As such, for patients with advanced, severe ILD, close monitoring of their oxygenation and ventilation is critical to guide the need for adjustments to PEEP, F_{IO_2}, and RR. Assessing a patient's baseline $Paco_2$ can help to inform what Pco_2 should be targeted while a patient is intubated and mechanically ventilated.

SUMMARY

Although the approach to setting, monitoring, and adjusting mechanical ventilator settings can seem overwhelming, it can be helpful to appreciate that mechanical ventilation is simply a means of supporting oxygenation and ventilation. Oxygenation is characterized as delivery of oxygen to the alveoli and transfer of oxygen across the alveolar-capillary basement membrane; the ventilator parameters of F_{IO_2} and PEEP are the primary means of influencing and optimizing oxygenation. Ventilation is the process of moving air in and out of the lungs (specifically, perfused alveoli) during inspiration and expiration, which results in elimination of carbon dioxide from the body. Ventilation is affected by the RR and the TV (achieved directly by setting the TV in volume control modes of ventilation or achieved indirectly by setting in the inspiratory pressure in pressure control modes of ventilation). Monitoring the effects of mechanical ventilation, from following a patient's oxygenation parameters (eg, Spo_2 and/or Pao_2), ventilatory parameters (eg, $Paco_2$ or $ETco_2$), and pulmonary mechanics (eg, the pulmonary pressures for a patient on a volume control mode of ventilation) can inform the need for adjustments to a patient's ventilatory settings. Overall, an understanding of physiology and pathophysiologic mechanisms can help make ventilator settings less intimidating and more approachable and can contribute to optimized patient care.

KEY POINTS

- Ventilator settings affecting oxygenation include F_{IO_2} and PEEP. F_{IO_2} is adjusted based on oxygen saturation, and PEEP helps prevent alveolar collapse at end exhalation.
- Ventilator settings affecting ventilation include TV and RR. TV is set based on ideal body weight, and RR is adjusted based on the patient's clinical condition and respiratory physiology.
- Close monitoring of oxygen saturation (via pulse oximetry) and CO_2 levels (via arterial or venous blood gases) is necessary. Arterial blood gases provide more comprehensive information but are more invasive.
- Ventilator modes can provide full support (pressure control or volume control) or partial support (pressure support ventilation). The mode selection depends on the patient's physiology (and pathophysiology) and lung mechanics.
- Peak pressure reflects airway resistance and compliance, while plateau pressure indicates respiratory system stiffness. Compliance can be calculated by measuring change in volume (V_t) and change in pressure (plateau pressure minus PEEP).
- VILI can occur because of atelectrauma (alveolar collapse and reopening), volutrauma (alveolar overdistension), and barotrauma (elevated pressures). Inflammatory cytokines released during VILI can cause damage to the lungs and other organs.
- LTVV with tidal volumes of 6-8 mL/kg IBW and lower plateau pressures (<30 cm H_2O) reduces morbidity and mortality in patients with ARDS. LTVV is generally beneficial for all patients requiring mechanical ventilation.
- PEEP maintains alveolar recruitment and reduces cyclic opening and closing of alveoli. Optimizing PEEP aims to improve ventilation and oxygenation while avoiding over-inflation and strain on the right heart. Various methods can help determine the optimal PEEP for individual patients.

Questions

1. A 35-year-old man with asthma is admitted to the ICU with acute hypercapnic respiratory failure after having been intubated and initiated on mechanical ventilation in the emergency department. He initially presented with 1 day of wheezing, chest tightness, and severe short-ness of breath. His Spo_2 was 80% on ambient air on presentation, with an RR of 38 breaths/min. An ABG demonstrated a pH of 7.24, $Paco_2$ of 62 mm Hg, and Pao_2 of 70 mm Hg. He received succinylcholine and etomidate for paralysis and sedation and was intubated without immediate complications.

   On arrival to the ICU, the respiratory therapist reports that he is on a volume assist con-trol mode of ventilation with the following settings: TV 400 mL (7 mL/kg of IBW), RR 24 breaths/min, PEEP 5 cm H_2O, and Fio_2 of 100%. The respiratory therapist also reports that his peak pressure is 40 cm H_2O, plateau pressure is 25 cm H_2O, and the measured end-expiratory pressure is 15 cm H_2O, with a postintubation ABG demonstrating pH of 7.32, $Paco_2$ of 50 mm Hg, and Fio_2 of 420 mm Hg.

   Which of the following is the most appropriate next step in his management?

   A. Decrease the RR to 18 breaths/min.

   B. Increase the TV to 500 mL (8 mL/kg of IBW).

   C. Place the patient in prone position.

   D. Decrease the PEEP to 0 cm H_2O.

2. You are called to evaluate a patient with ARDS because of COVID-19 pneumonia. The pa-tient was admitted 2 days ago, and after initially having been managed with high-flow nasal cannula, he was intubated and initiated on mechanical ventilation yesterday. He has been on volume assist control ventilation with the following settings: TV 420 mL (6.5 mL/kg of IBW), RR of 26 breaths/min, PEEP of 8 cm H_2O, and Fio_2 of 60%. With these settings, his peak inspiratory pressure is 34 cm H_2O and his plateau pressure is 30 cm H_2O. His most recent ABG demonstrates a pH of 7.30, $Paco_2$ of 52 mm Hg, and a Pao_2 of 55 mm Hg. The respiratory therapist asks if you'd like to make any adjustments to his ventilator settings based on the most recent ABG results.

   A. Increase the TV to 480 mL (7 mL/kg of IBW).

   B. Increase the PEEP to 12 cm H_2O.

   C. Increase the Fio_2 to 80%.

   D. Increase the RR to 32 breaths/min.

3. You are asked to evaluate a patient who is dyssynchronous with the ventilator. Specifically, the patient is breathing above the set RR—the set rate is 20 breaths/min, and the patient is consistently breathing at 24 to 26 breaths/min. The patient was intubated for multifocal pneumonia 3 days ago and remains critically ill with vasopressor-dependent shock and mul-tiorgan system failure. She has been on volume assist control ventilation, with the following settings: TV 360 mL (6.5 mL/kg of IBW), RR of 20 breaths/min, PEEP of 8 cm H_2O, and Fio_2 of 50%. Her most recent ABG demonstrated a pH of 7.33, $Paco_2$ of 44 mm Hg, and Pao_2 of 90 mm Hg (on a Fio_2 of 50%). On exam, she is sedated on propofol, with a RASS score of −3. Which of the following is the next most appropriate step in her care?

   A. Increase her TV to 500 mL (8 mL/kg of IBW).

   B. Increase her PEEP to 12 cm H_2O.

   C. Increase her Fio_2 to 70%.

   D. Increase her RR to 25 breaths/min.

Answers

1. **Answer A. Decrease the RR to 18 breaths/min**

   Rationale: The patient has evidence of auto-PEEP as demonstrated by the increased end-expiratory pressure of 15 cm H_2O, which indicates incomplete exhalation in the setting of severe airways obstruction and increased airways resistance. In this setting, decreasing the RR to allow for more complete exhalation is indicated. The patient also has a persistent acute respiratory acidosis, although his pH and $Paco_2$ are improved from presentation. Decreasing the RR will decrease both overall ventilation and alveolar ventilation, such that monitoring the patient's acid/base status while decreasing his RR is important; further interventions, such as increasing his TV, may be necessary; a larger TV, however, for any given expiratory time could lead to higher intrinsic PEEP. At this time, however, increasing his TV is not immediately indicated as his acute respiratory acidosis is improved from presentation and his plateau pressure is already close to 30 cm H_2O. Regarding placing him in prone position, he does not have ARDS and his $Pao_2:Fio_2$ ratio is far above 150, such that there is no indication for proning. Finally, decreasing his PEEP is not indicated because it will increase the work needed to trigger the ventilator (see Chapter 11 for a more complete discussion). Furthermore, studies have demonstrated that zero applied PEEP (ZEEP) is associated with worse clinical outcomes as compared to providing PEEP for mechanically ventilated patients.

2. **Answer C. Increase the Fio_2 to 80%**

   Rationale: Of the available options, increasing his Fio_2 is the most appropriate next step given that his Pao_2 is very low at 55 mm Hg—addressing hypoxemia is a mandate in managing a patient with acute hypoxemic respiratory failure, and increasing the Fio_2 is a direct and effective manner to achieve this goal. Increasing the PEEP could also help to optimize oxygenation, but in his case the plateau pressure is already elevated at 30 cm H_2O, and increasing the PEEP could further increase the plateau pressure. thereby raising his risk for volutrauma and associated adverse outcomes, including increased mortality (one caveat here—in some patients, an increase in PEEP might improve compliance by opening up collapsed alveoli and distributing the inspired volume among a larger number of alveoli, thereby not leading to an increase in the plateau pressure, but this must be done with caution in this scenario). Similar to increasing the PEEP, increasing the tidal volume is not indicated as that would result in an increase in pulmonary pressures and increase his mortality risk. Finally, although increasing his RR would address his elevated $Paco_2$ and acute respiratory acidosis and might have a marginal impact on oxygenation, this is less important than addressing hypoxemia more directly. As such, increasing his Fio_2 is a straightforward and important intervention given his current clinical circumstances.

3. **Answer D. Increase her RR to 25 breaths/min**

   Rationale: As noted in the chapter, it is important to determine any underlying triggers for ventilator dyssynchrony. Two important etiologies to consider are hypoxemia and acidosis. If neither of these is present, other possible etiologies include discomfort with the RR set on the ventilator, mucus plugging, bronchospasm, and mainstem intubation, among others. In the absence of obvious pain or other processes contributing to ventilator dyssynchrony, if patient is "overbreathing" the vent, increasing the RR if appropriate may improve synchrony to better match the patient's endogenous respiratory drive with the ventilator's set rate.

Suggested Reading

Acute Respiratory Distress Syndrome Network; Brower RG, Matthay MA, et al. Ventilation with lower tidal volumes as compared with traditional tidal volumes for acute lung injury and the acute respiratory distress syndrome. The Acute Respiratory Distress Syndrome Network *N Engl J Med*. 2000;342:1301-1308.

Beitler JR, Sarge T, Banner-Goodspeed VM, et al. Effect of titrating positive end-expiratory pressure (PEEP) with an esophageal pressure-guided strategy vs an empirical high PEEP-Fio2 strategy on death and days free from mechanical ventilation among patients with acute respiratory distress syndrome: a randomized clinical trial. *JAMA*. 2019;321(9):846-857. doi:10.1001/jama.2019.0555

Champion L, Cardinal P, Hodder R. Chapter 12 introduction to mechanical ventilation. In: Neilipovitz D, ed. *Acute Resuscitation and Crisis Management*. 2005:107.

Kilickaya, O, Gajic, O. Initial ventilator settings for critically ill patients. *Crit Care*. 2013;17(2):123.

Munshi L, Del Sorbo L, Adhikari NKJ, et al. Prone position for acute respiratory distress syndrome: a systematic review and meta-analysis. *Ann Am Thorac Soc*. 2017;14:S280-S288. doi:10.1513/AnnalsATS.201704-343OT

Sjoding MW, Dickson RP, Iwashyna TJ, Gay SE, Valley TS. Racial bias in pulse oximetry measurement. *N Engl J Med*. 2020;383:2477-2478. doi:10.1056/NEJMc2029240

Liberating the Patient from Mechanical Ventilation

Sarah Ohnigian • Ali Trainor • Jeremy B. Richards

LEARNING OBJECTIVES

- Delineate clinical criteria for performing a spontaneous awakening trial for a mechanically ventilated patient.
- Describe specific strategies for performing a spontaneous awakening trial for a mechanically ventilated patient.
- List the physical signs and clinical findings that determine whether a patient has "passed" or "failed" a spontaneous breathing trial.
- Identify physical exam findings that indicate increased work of breathing and diminished neuromuscular reserve for critically ill, mechanically ventilated patients.
- Describe the steps for and the meaning of a "cuff leak test" in determining readiness for extubation for a mechanically ventilated patient.

INTRODUCTION

Given the risks of prolonged mechanical ventilation, it is important to ensure that critically ill patients are liberated from mechanical ventilation as soon as it is safe to do so. Determining the safest, most appropriate time for extubation and liberation from mechanical ventilation is crucial, as postextubation failure and subsequent reintubation are associated with increased morbidity and mortality. Therefore, using a multifaceted approach to optimally determine a patient's pretest probability of being successfully extubated is important in assessing when and whether to liberate a patient from mechanical ventilation.

This approach to liberating patients from the ventilator hinges on assessing three important factors of the patient's respiratory and clinical status: (1) the brain as the "respiratory controller," (2) the airway and lungs as the "ventilatory pump," and (3) the alveolar-capillary interface as the "gas exchanger." Assessing and characterizing the patient's overall clinical state, which holistically incorporates several elements of the respiratory system, is an important component of determining a patient's readiness for extubation and liberation.

With regard to the "respiratory controller," the patient must be alert enough, with sufficient central nervous system processing, to send the appropriate signals to drive the respiratory system and to receive, synthesize, and process signals from the respiratory system. Therefore, as a critical component of assessing the patient's readiness for extubation, it is important to assess a patient's level of sedation and key respiratory reflexes, such as the cough reflex.

With regard to the "ventilatory pump," the patient must have functional airways to facilitate adequate flow of gas to support oxygenation and ventilation, without excessive airways resistance or obstruction. Similarly, the patient's neuromuscular status must be adequately intact, such that they can breathe independently, gag when liquids or solids are near the epiglottis, and generate an adequate cough to clear secretions. Determining the status of a patient's "ventilatory pump" requires analysis of their current ventilator settings, blood gas results, volume status, and underlying pulmonary function.

With regard to the "gas exchanger," the patient must have adequate oxygenation, such that withdrawing positive pressure ventilation and/or high F_{IO_2} delivered by the ventilator will not result in precipitous desaturation and critical hypoxemia. In addition, alveolar ventilation must be adequate to provide an appropriate $Paco_2$ to support acceptable acid-base balance and neurologic function.

Overall, to be ready for extubation and liberation from mechanical ventilation, a patient must have a stable and improved clinical state including acceptable hemodynamics, adequate organ function, and reasonable functional status. In this chapter, we review how to assess each of the three respiratory system domains and to evaluate whether a patient can be safely liberated from mechanical ventilation.

ASSESSMENT OF THE CONTROLLER

The central nervous system controls the respiratory system, potentiating the drive to breathe and monitoring the status and function of the neuromuscular system and lungs during inspiration and expiration. In almost all cases, intubated patients are given "analgosedation" (ie, analgesia to ensure comfort for the patient with respect to pain and dyspnea, and sedation to minimize anxiety and traumatic memories) to allow them to breathe comfortably with the assistance of the ventilator. In some cases, patients also may be incapacitated by disease states and/or toxic processes that impact their neurologic status. Although it is well known that sedation causes many detrimental consequences, including altered mentation, delirium, suppression of the respiratory drive, and muscle weakness, sedation remains a core component of the care of mechanically ventilated patients to achieve ventilator synchrony and to address dyspnea and breathlessness associated with acute respiratory failure and mechanical ventilation (see Chapter 19). As sedation directly impacts the ability of a patient to spontaneously breathe, it is necessary to actively and conscientiously manage sedation in anticipation of extubation and liberation from mechanical ventilation.

To assess the level of sedation of critically ill patients, the Richmond Agitation and Sedation Scale (RASS) is a widely used clinical tool. The level of alertness (or sedation) is measured

RASS score

Score	Richmond Agitation & Sedation Scale		CAM-ICU
Score		Description	
+4	Combative	Violent, immediate danger to staff	
+3	Very agitated	Pulls at or removes tubes, aggressive	RASS ≥ −2 Proceed to CAM-ICU assessment
+2	Agitated	Frequent non-purposeful movements, fights ventilator	
+1	Restless	Anxious, apprehensive but movements not aggressive or vigorous	
0	Alert & calm		
−1	Drowsy	Not fully alert, sustained awakening to voice (eye opening & contact > 10 secs)	
−2	Light sedation	Briefly awakens to voice (eye opening & contact < 10 secs)	Voice
−3	Moderate sedation	Movement or eye-opening to voice (no eye contact)	
−4	Deep sedation	No response to voice, but movement or eye opening to physical stimulation	Touch RASS < −2 STOP Recheck later
−5	Un-rousable	No response to voice or physical stimulation	

Figure 9-1: **The scores and related descriptions of the Richmond Agitation and Sedation Scale.** (From Nickson C. *Five tips for ICU sedation.* March 19, 2015. Intensive website. Accessed February 15, 2023. https://intensiveblog.com/five-tips-for-icu-sedation/. Table 1.)

based on the patient's clinical status—patients are evaluated for their ability to open their eyes, purposefully make eye contact, respond to stimuli, as well as their general appearance including movements and subjective measures of anxiety and agitation (**Figure 9-1**).

In addition, to assess the status of a patient's respiratory controller, it is useful to test a patient's cough reflex. This is achieved by deep tracheal suctioning, which should irritate the airway epithelium thereby activating airway irritant receptors and triggering a cough reflex. This is a highly reproducible stimulus, and if a patient does not cough, it is an indication that they are too sedated to safely pursue extubation. Of note, though the gag reflex is also commonly tested, it is an unreliable indicator given that it carries significant variability between people. In fact, after being intubated even for only 24 to 48 hours, the gag reflex can be attenuated.

For patients who may be ready for extubation and liberation, it is imperative to assess a patient's neurologic status without sedation at least once daily to evaluate their readiness for and ability to be liberated from the ventilator. This evaluation is known as a spontaneous awakening trial (SAT), where all analgosedation is turned off and the patient's mental status is assessed. This sedation liberation protocol has been rigorously studied and results in a shorter duration of mechanical ventilation, a shorter intensive care unit (ICU) length of stay, and decreased mortality in mechanically ventilated patients.

To assess whether a patient is appropriate for an SAT, first, one should screen a patient for safety prior to performing an SAT. The patient must not have evidence of active seizures, must not have escalating sedative doses because of agitation, must not be receiving neuromuscular blockade, must not have had myocardial ischemia in the last 24 hours, must not have increased intracranial pressure, and must not be experiencing active alcohol or benzodiazepine withdrawal (**Table 9-1**). If it is deemed to be safe to do so, the next step in an SAT is to turn off all sedatives and analgesics. It is important to emphasize that these medications are completely turned off rather than slowly decreased over time or downtitrated. After stopping all sedative and analgesic infusions, these medications should remain off for up to 4 hours.

TABLE 9-1 Contraindications to Performing a Spontaneous Awakening Trial
Active seizures/status epilepticus
Escalating sedative doses because of agitation
Administration of neuromuscular blockade
Myocardial ischemia within the past 24 h
Increased intracranial pressure
Active withdrawal from alcohol and/or benzodiazepines

The patient's mental status should then be assessed. A patient "passes" an SAT if the patient is able to open their eyes to stimuli and if they tolerate stopping sedatives without major issues. It is also helpful to assess if a patient is able to follow commands, such as move their extremities, stick out their tongue, open or close their eyes in response to verbal prompting. A patient is deemed to have "failed" the SAT if the patient has sustained anxiety, agitation, severe pain, respiratory rate over 35 breaths/min for greater than 5 minutes, oxygen saturation less than 88% for 5 minutes or longer, arrhythmia, or increased work of breathing. If a patient fails the SAT, analgosedation should be reintroduced at half of the prior dose and titrated to goal RASS, the team should analyze factors that may have contributed to the failure and design a plan to correct them, and the appropriateness of repeating an SAT should be assessed going forward on a daily basis.

The final assessment of the respiratory controller, determination of whether or not the patient can initiate their own breaths with an appropriate tidal volume, requires a spontaneous breathing trial (SBT), which is described later.

INTEGRATED ASSESSMENT OF THE VENTILATORY PUMP, GAS EXCHANGER, AND RESPIRATORY CONTROLLER

To assess the patient's ventilatory pump, holistic assessment of their respiratory status is appropriate. Specifically, one should determine what mode of ventilation the patient is receiving and what specific ventilator settings they are requiring. A patient who is on a "controlled" mode of ventilation, with a set respiratory rate and set tidal volume, may be in a different clinical state than a patient treated with a "support" mode of ventilation, and their relative readiness for extubation and liberation may be different; the degree of assistance provided by the ventilator is different with different modes and settings. Relatedly, patients with high positive end-expiratory pressure (PEEP) and/or high F_{IO_2} may not be appropriate candidates for pursuing an SBT. Prior studies have demonstrated that patients who "pass" an SAT, with a F_{IO_2} of less than or equal to 50% and a PEEP of less than or equal to 8 to 10 cm H_2O, can be safely considered for an SBT. In addition, an SBT should not be pursued for patients who are clinically unstable, as characterized by active myocardial ischemia within the past 24 hours, hemodynamic instability requiring significant vasopressor or inotropic support (eg, norepinephrine at or above 2 µg/min and/or dobutamine at or above 5 µg/kg/min), and/or increased intracranial pressure.

Spontaneous Breathing Trial

For patients who "pass" an SAT who have acceptable PEEP, F_{IO_2}, and clinical stability, pursuing a daily SBT is appropriate. There are different strategies for performing an SBT, with local practice patterns and institutional culture influencing the type of support provided during an SBT. In general, some degree of inspiratory pressure is provided, ranging from 5 to 8 cm H_2O, although some advocate for performing SBTs with no inspiratory pressure (eg, 0 cm H_2O). Whether to provide PEEP during an SBT is also debated, with some individuals and institutions advocating for no PEEP (eg, 0 cm H_2O), whereas others recommend providing minimal (eg, 5 cm H_2O) PEEP during an SBT. In general, less support during an SBT will increase the specificity of predicting postextubation success, such that a patient who "passes" an SBT on minimal or no support will be more likely to independently breathe after extubation and liberation than someone who appears to be doing well with pressure support ventilation (PSV) of 5 cm H_2O and PEEP of 5 cm H_2O.

The appropriate duration of an SBT has also been assessed by randomized controlled trial—a shorter duration (30 minutes) has been demonstrated to be noninferior to a longer duration (120 minutes) in a heterogeneous population of critically ill, mechanically ventilated patients who were determined to be "ready to wean" by their healthcare providers. A longer SBT may still be appropriate for selected patients, particularly those with chronic respiratory diseases (eg, severe chronic obstructive pulmonary disease [COPD]) or malnourished, debilitated patients whose ability to breathe on their own may be particularly uncertain. It is important to note that when longer SBTs are determined to be appropriate for a given patient, there is no evidence supporting SBTs longer than 120 minutes.

Patients should be monitored throughout the SBT, with close attention on both their overall clinical status as well as specific respiratory parameters. A patient is determined to have "failed" an SBT if they develop significant and refractory anxiety, diaphoresis, and/or a greater than 20% to 25% increase in heart rate to above 140 beats/min. Additionally, if a patient experiences a sustained increase or decrease in their heart rate of greater than 20% from their baseline (prior to starting the SBT), then the SBT should be terminated. Hemodynamic fluctuations, such as an increase in the systolic blood pressure to greater than 180 mm Hg or to less than 90 mm Hg, are signs that a patient is not tolerating an SBT, and that the SBT should be aborted. If the patient has ventilatory pump dysfunction during an SBT, then the test should be stopped—examples of ventilatory pump dysfunction include increased accessory muscle use, dyspnea, a respiratory rate of greater than 35 breaths/min, and/or a respiratory rate of less than 8 breaths/min.

Gas exchanger dysfunction during an SBT is also an indication to abort the test, specifically if the patient's oxygen saturation decreases to less than 90% or if it decreases by more than 5% from their pre-SBT baseline (eg, a decrease in the oxygen saturation from 98% at the beginning of the SBT to 91% during the SBT indicates a "failed" SBT). Finally, although checking an arterial blood gas after an SBT is not always indicated, if it is determined to be appropriate for a given patient, evidence of an acute respiratory acidosis (eg, a pH of 7.30 or less with a $Paco_2$ of 50 mm Hg or higher) at the end of an SBT indicates that the patient has "failed" and should not be extubated.

Rapid Shallow Breathing Index

In addition to the abovementioned clinical assessments, the rapid shallow breathing index (RSBI) is an important clinical assessment to calculate at the end of an SBT; it is a critical element in the determination of the readiness of a patient for extubation. The RSBI is calculated by dividing the patient's unassisted respiratory rate by tidal volume (in liters). An RSBI of less than 105 suggests spontaneous breathing is likely to be successful, and that the patient may be safely extubated and liberated from mechanical ventilation (assuming other assessments of the controller, ventilatory pump, and gas exchanger are appropriate). It is important to emphasize that the RSBI is *one* component of assessing a patient at the end of an SBT—a holistic approach to patient assessment is critical, with the RSBI as one piece of the overall assessment. The trend in the RSBI can also be useful (eg, if the RSBI increases significantly during an SBT, even if it is not greater than 105 at the end of the test, it may indicate that a patient is at increased risk of fatigue and is not yet ready to be extubated). The RSBI may be less useful in patients with COPD and in patients older than 65 years, given these patients may have decreased neuromuscular function and at baseline demonstrate higher respiratory rate and lower tidal volumes.

An additional important component of assessing a patient's readiness for extubation is the presence of secretions. Airway secretions are very common in intubated patients, and the endotracheal tube itself can cause irritation of the airway epithelium and cause secretions. Determining the presence, volume, and consistency of secretions is important, and assessing for the presence and strength of a patient's cough is critical in deciding whether a patient can be extubated. It is possible that a patient who passes an SAT and SBT may not be able to be extubated because of copious and tenacious secretions, particularly if they seem to have trouble generating an adequate cough to clear the secretions.

Cuff Leak Test

It is common to assess for the presence of laryngeal edema prior to extubation by performing a "cuff leak" test. Laryngeal edema is more likely to occur in patients who underwent traumatic intubation (or who have had to be reintubated), who have been intubated for more than 6 days, and who have a large endotracheal tube in place. In addition, female sex is associated with increased prevalence of airway edema, most likely because a larger endotracheal tube relative to airway caliber has been placed.

A "cuff leak" is typically performed by simply deflating the pilot balloon on the endotracheal tube and listening for air leaking around the tube (usually heard as a "gurgle" or sonorous upper airway rhonchi). Most accurately referred to as a "qualitative" cuff leak (**Figure 9-2**), this test is neither sensitive nor specific with regard to predicting postextubation success or failure. A "quantitative" cuff leak is performed by setting a patient to a volume assist control mode of ventilation, with a set tidal volume, and then deflating the cuff and measuring the amount (or volume) of air that leaks around the endotracheal tube. The "quantitative" cuff leak test is more accurate with regard to predicting postextubation laryngeal edema as compared to a qualitative cuff leak, although it's laborious to perform and may involve having to re-sedate or even paralyze a patient to obtain an accurate quantitative cuff leak.

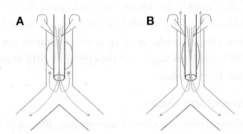

Figure 9-2: A, The airflow when the balloon or "cuff" of an endotracheal tube is inflated—the air stays within the airways because the inflated cuff keeps air from flowing up around the tube. **B,** Airflow when the cuff is deflated—some air stays within the lungs but some escapes around the endotracheal tube, passing through the vocal cords and past the arytenoids. Gurgling can be heard when the cuff is deflated and air passes through the secretions that have pooled at the level of the vocal cords and arytenoids. This "gurgling" represents a "positive" cuff leak test.

If a patient fails a cuff leak test, then common practice is to provide systemic steroids for at least 4 hours before extubation. There are many different glucocorticoid regimens for steroids to decrease the risk of postextubation laryngeal edema, without one regimen having been demonstrated to clearly be better than others.

Neuromuscular Status

Although aspects of the abovementioned pre-extubation assessments incorporate a patient's neuromuscular function, directly determining a patient's neuromuscular status is important prior to pursuing extubation and liberation from mechanical ventilation. If a patient is able to lift their head up off of the bed and hold it up for 10 seconds, that indicates adequate core strengths and correlates with an ability to independently ventilate. Related to this maneuver, healthcare providers can also assess for sternocleidomastoid contraction as a sign of increased work of breathing (and the patient's overall neuromuscular status). Visible sternocleidomastoid contraction is a sensitive indicator of increased work of breathing and diminished neuromuscular reserve. One can also palpate the sternocleidomastoid during the respiratory cycle to assess for phasic contraction of the muscle during respiration; if present, the strength of sternocleidomastoid contraction can be described semiquantitatively as mild, moderate, or severe in nature.

Another physical finding indicative of increased work of breathing and diminished neuromuscular status is the "tracheal tug." A provider can place their finger over the patient's thyroid cartilage, and if the thyroid cartilage demonstrably moves downward during inhalation, it is a clear sign of increased work of breathing (the downward "tugging" is a result of forceful diaphragmatic contraction pulling the entire mediastinum, including the trachea, downward during contraction). Tracheal tug is not present during comfortable, normal breathing.

Another important consideration relative to patients' neuromuscular status is early mobility. Early mobility in mechanically ventilated patients is generally considered to help decrease exposure to sedative medications, improve patients' mental status, and decrease the risk of neuromuscular deterioration during critical illness.

Procedures

A final consideration with regard to determining a patient's readiness for extubation and liberation from mechanical ventilation is whether they have to undergo any procedures or tests that require that they be intubated, sedated, and mechanically ventilated. For example, for a patient who needs to undergo a test such as a magnetic resonance imaging (MRI), the healthcare team may decide to wait to extubate the patient until after the study is performed. Relatedly, a patient who underwent surgery and is going to return to the operating room (OR) the next day may remain intubated and ventilated between surgeries. Once it is determined that there are no more relevant diagnostic tests and/or therapeutic interventions to be performed, then pursuing SAT, SBT, and extubation and liberation may be appropriate.

High-Risk Patients

The risks of extubation failure and subsequent need for reintubation have been associated with increased morbidity and mortality. Even though the guidelines have been studied and provide guidance for how to evaluate a patient for ventilator liberation, every clinical context is unique. In fact, SBTs are not always reliable, with about 10% to 25% of patients developing postextubation respiratory failure after passing their SBT. Given these serious consequences, it is necessary to consider certain high-risk patients where extra caution and consideration should be taken. Some of the known high-risk patient features are: age over 65 years, coexisting COPD, coexisting chronic heart failure (CHF), hypercapnia during SBT, more than one failed SBT, high severity of illness, upper airway stridor, weak cough, impaired neurologic status, increased secretions, RSBI > 105, positive fluid balance, and neuromuscular disease.

If a patient has a particularly high risk for extubation failure, clinicians should consider optimizing those factors amenable to interventions while also considering extubating to non-invasive ventilation. This strategy can be particularly helpful for patients with COPD, CHF, hypercapnia, and positive fluid balance. In patients with chronic hypoventilation (eg, patients with severe or very severe COPD), extubating to continuous positive airway pressure (CPAP) or bilevel positive airway pressure (BiPAP) has been associated with improvements in rates of successful extubation, ICU length of stay, and in short-term and long-term mortality. In addition, extubating to high-flow nasal cannula has also been shown to be helpful.

SUMMARY

One of the best practices for care of the critically ill patient is routine evaluation for the safety of liberating from the ventilator. Given that extubation failure as well as prolonged intubation both have detrimental consequences, clinicians must follow a clear daily assessment of the major drivers of spontaneous breathing including: neurologic status, respiratory system, and overall clinical status. This includes RASS monitoring, daily SAT, and a holistic assessment of the patient's overall clinical status. It is important to note that clinicians should interpret these recommendations and consider each patient individually when considering liberation from mechanical ventilation, including patient values and preferences. If every patient whom you extubate succeeds, you may be waiting too long to pursue an extubation and prolong intubation for some of your patients and contributing to complications associated with prolonged intubation; on the other hand, if you have a high "failure" rate, then you may not be making appropriate assessments of your patient's readiness for extubation, which is also associated with increased morbidity and mortality. Finding that "sweet" spot is one of the great challenges of critical care medicine.

STUDY QUESTIONS AND ANSWERS

Questions

1. A 74-year-old man with very severe COPD was intubated 5 days ago in the setting of an acute exacerbation. After treatment with bronchodilators, glucocorticoids, and azithromycin, his clinical status has improved. He is currently sedated with propofol via continuous infusion, and he is minimally responsive—he opens his eyes to voice, but is not following any commands. He is on a pressure support mode of ventilation, with an inspiratory pressure of 10 cm H_2O, PEEP of 5 cm H_2O, and a FIO_2 of 40%. His most recent arterial blood gas from 2 hours ago demonstrated a pH of 7.35, $Paco_2$ of 52 mm Hg, and a Pao_2 of 94 mm Hg. His heart rate is 94 beats/min, blood pressure 142/80 mm Hg, respiratory rate 12 breaths/min, and oxygen saturation 98%. Which of the following is the most appropriate next step in determining if he is ready to be extubated and liberated from mechanical ventilation?

A. Decrease his inspiratory pressure from 10 to 8 cm H_2O.

B. Stop the propofol infusion.

C. Decrease the FIO_2 to 21%.

D. Decrease the dose of the propofol infusion by half.

E. Transition from pressure support to volume assist control ventilation.

2. A 43-year-old woman was intubated 3 days ago for management of acute hypoxic respiratory failure because of aspiration pneumonia in the setting of an opiate overdose. A successful SAT was performed this morning, followed by an SBT with an inspiratory pressure of 5 cm H_2O, a PEEP of 0 cm H_2O, and a FIO_2 of 40%. After breathing spontaneously for 30 minutes on these settings, her heart rate is 100 beats/min, which increased from 85 beats/min at the beginning of the SBT, and her systolic blood pressure is 150 mm Hg, increasing from 130 mm Hg at the beginning of the SBT. Her respiratory rate is 36 breaths/min, with tidal volumes of ~320 mL, and an RSBI of 103. Her oxygen saturation is 92%, decreased from 96% at the beginning of the SBT. Which of the following findings indicate that she is *not* ready to be extubated and liberated from mechanical ventilation?
   A. RSBI of 103.
   B. Increase in her heart rate from 85 to 100 beats/min.
   C. Systolic blood pressure of 150 mm Hg at the end of the SBT.
   D. Respiratory rate of 36 breaths/min at the end of the SBT.
   E. Decrease in her oxygen saturation from 96% to 92% during the SBT.

3. A 55-year-old man was intubated 21 days ago with acute respiratory distress syndrome (ARDS) because of COVID-19 pneumonia. He was extubated 3 days ago (18 days after first being intubated), but had to be reintubated because of difficulty handling his secretions, aspiration events, and recurrent hypoxic respiratory failure. Today, he passed an SAT and SBT and the respiratory therapist tells you that his qualitative cuff leak test was positive (eg, throat gurgling was heard when the balloon on the endotracheal tube was deflated). Which of the following parameters is a risk factor for this patient developing postextubation laryngeal edema?
   A. Being reintubated 3 days ago
   B. Prolonged intubation
   C. Male sex
   D. Positive cuff leak test
   E. A and B

Answers

1. **Answer B. Stop the propofol infusion**
   Rationale: The most appropriate next step in determining his readiness for extubation and liberation from mechanical ventilation is to perform an SAT, which is accomplished by stopping all sedative and analgesic medications to assess the patient's underlying mental status. An SAT is performed by stopping all sedatives; slowly decreasing or downtitrating sedative infusions results in oversedation and prolongs the duration of mechanical ventilation. If he successfully tolerates an SAT, then pursuing an SBT is warranted; an SBT cannot be performed without first performing an SAT to assess the patient's underlying mental status. Simply decreasing the inspiratory pressure from 10 to 8 cm H_2O will not meaningfully determine the patient's readiness for extubation and liberation, and although minimizing the patient's FIO_2 is reasonable overall, it is not a critical intervention at this time and will not meaningfully help to determine the patient's readiness for extubation.

(continued)

2. **Answer D. Respiratory rate of 36 breaths/min at the end of the SBT**

   Rationale: Her respiratory rate of 36 breaths/min at the end of the SBT is concerning and is above the putative upper limit of an acceptable respiratory rate of 35 breaths/min. Her tachypnea may not be sustainable without ventilatory support, and her healthcare providers should determine why she is tachypneic, and whether it represents a concerning, serious, and/or reversible process that needs to be addressed prior to extubation. Her RSBI is close to, but under, the upper limit of 105 and is not in itself a contraindication to considering extubation and/or liberation. As a reminder, the RSBI is one component of a holistic assessment of determining if a patient is ready to be extubated or not—it should not be used in isolation as the sole determinant of a patient's readiness for extubation and liberation. An increase in a patient's heart rate by 20% to 25% (or to a heart rate of >140 beats/min) indicates prohibitive hemodynamic instability, and extubation should not be performed under those settings. A systolic blood pressure of greater than 180 mm Hg or less than 90 mm Hg is a sign that a patient is not tolerating an SBT and that the SBT should be aborted. And, with regard to oxygenation, if a patient's oxygen saturation decreases to less than 90% or if it decreases by more than 5% from their pre-SBT baseline (eg, a decrease in the oxygen saturation from 98% at the beginning of the SBT to 91% during the SBT), it indicates a "failed" SBT. In this patient's case, the only parameter that clearly indicates that she is not ready for extubation and liberation is her elevated respiratory rate.

3. **Answer E. Being reintubated 3 days ago and prolonged intubation**

   Rationale: Prolonged intubation and having to be reintubated are risk factors for laryngeal injury, with trauma, irritation, injury, and edema of the vocal cords and arytenoids occurring because of mechanical trauma from contact with the endotracheal tube. In general, being intubated for more than 6 days is considered a risk factor for laryngeal edema, as is having to pass an endotracheal tube through the larynx more than once. Female, not male, sex is associated with increased risk of laryngeal edema, because healthcare providers tend to place a large endotracheal tube in proportion to the patient's body habitus for women as compared to men. And, although it is not particularly sensitive or specific, a positive cuff leak test is considered to be a sign that there is no significant or clinically prohibitive laryngeal edema. In this setting, if the concern for laryngeal edema is sufficiently high, direct visualization (via fiberoptic laryngoscopy or video laryngoscopy) could be considered to further assess for the presence and degree of laryngeal swelling *or* a short course of glucocorticoids could be empirically provided to decrease laryngeal swelling and inflammation prior to extubation.

Suggested Readings

El-Khatib MF, Bou-Khalil P. Clinical review: liberation from mechanical ventilation. *Crit Care.* 2008;12(4):221. doi:10.1186/cc6959.

Esteban A, Alía I, Tobin MJ, et al. Effect of spontaneous breathing trial duration on outcome of attempts to discontinue mechanical ventilation. Spanish Lung Failure Collaborative Group. *Am J Respir Crit Care Med.* 1999;159(2):512-518. doi:10.1164/ajrccm.159.2.9803106.

Esteban A, Frutos F, Tobin MJ, et al. A comparison of four methods of weaning patients from mechanical ventilation. Spanish Lung Failure Collaborative Group. *N Engl J Med*. 1995;332(6):345-350. doi:10.1056/NEJM199502093320601.

Fan E, Zakhary B, Amaral A, et al. Liberation from mechanical ventilation in critically ill adults. An Official ATS/ACCP Clinical Practice Guideline. *Ann Am Thorac Soc*. 2017;14(3):441-443. doi:10.1513/AnnalsATS.201612-993CME.

Girard TD, Alhazzani W, Kress JP, et al.; ATS/Chest Ad Hoc Committee on Liberation from Mechanical Ventilation in Adults. An official American Thoracic Society/American College of Chest Physicians clinical practice guideline: liberation from mechanical ventilation in critically ill adults. Rehabilitation protocols, ventilator liberation protocols, and cuff leak tests. *Am J Respir Crit Care Med*. 2017;195(1): 120-133. doi:10.1164/rccm.201610-2075ST.

Girard TD, Kress JP, Fuchs BD, et al. Efficacy and safety of a paired sedation and ventilator weaning protocol for mechanically ventilated patients in intensive care (Awakening and Breathing Controlled trial): a randomised controlled trial. *Lancet*. 2008;371(9607):126-134. doi:10.1016/S0140-6736(08)60105-1.

Ouellette DR, Patel S, Girard TD, et al. Liberation from mechanical ventilation in critically ill adults: an official American College of Chest Physicians/American Thoracic Society Clinical Practice Guideline: inspiratory pressure augmentation during spontaneous breathing trials, protocols minimizing sedation, and noninvasive ventilation immediately after extubation. *Chest*. 2017;151(1):166-180. doi:10.1016/j.chest.2016.10.036.

Tobin MJ. Why physiology is critical to the practice of medicine: a 40-year personal perspective. *Clin Chest Med*. 2019;40(2):243-257. doi:10.1016/j.ccm.2019.02.012.

Yang KL, Tobin MJ. A prospective study of indexes predicting the outcome of trials of weaning from mechanical ventilation. *N Engl J Med*. 1991;324(21):1445-1450. doi:10.1056/NEJM199105233242101.

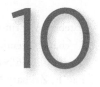
Noninvasive Mechanical Ventilation and High-Flow Nasal Cannula

Elias Baedorf Kassis • Ryan Kronen

INTRODUCTION

Although invasive mechanical ventilation provides the most control and highest level of respiratory support in patients with respiratory failure, there are potential complications associated with the use of invasive (ie, intubated) mechanical ventilation (see Chapter 15). These complications include trauma and hemodynamic instability during intubation, infection because of loss of natural airway defense mechanisms, and direct injury to the lung through volutrauma, barotrauma, and atelectrauma, as well as detrimental consequences related to failed extubation and tracheostomy. In many cases, noninvasive ventilation (NIV) and high-flow nasal cannula (HFNC) offer an effective alternative for patients with relatively milder degrees of respiratory failure who may be spared these complications. Particularly in the early stages of respiratory failure, these forms of respiratory support may buy time for pharmacologic treatments to work, thereby sparing the patient invasive mechanical ventilation. The correct application of these noninvasive modalities is dependent upon the unique patient characteristics and the proper use of the mode itself. This chapter discusses the mechanics, physiologic principles, and clinical applications of NIV and HFNC in respiratory failure.

ETIOLOGIES OF RESPIRATORY FAILURE

To begin, we briefly review the framework for classification and etiologies of respiratory failure that you should consider when choosing respiratory support options, including NIV and HFNC. Respiratory disease is often divided by clinicians into two main groups based on gas exchange derangements: hypoxemic and hypercarbic, defined as Spo_2 less than 90% and Pco_2 greater than 45 mm Hg, respectively. Remember, however, as outlined in Section 1 that a physiologic approach to respiratory disease and respiratory failure entails an understanding of the roles of the controller, the ventilatory pump, and the gas exchanger. When thinking about diseases associated with gas exchange abnormalities, one may start with conditions that lead to dysfunction of the lung parenchyma, including the alveoli, leading to abnormalities in ventilation-perfusion matching (see Chapter 3 for more details). These diseases, which include pneumonia, acute respiratory distress syndrome (ARDS), pulmonary edema, and other processes that contribute to alveolar collapse and filling, may result in significant hypoxemia. As will be reviewed in further detail in this chapter, HFNC and noninvasive continuous positive airway pressure (CPAP) are modalities that provide high oxygen flow and positive inspiratory and end-expiratory pressure, respectively, and tend to be the first-line choices for hypoxemic respiratory failure secondary to parenchymal lung pathologies.

The combination of peripheral nerves, neuromuscular junctions, respiratory muscles, and the airways can be conceptualized as the ventilatory "pump." Failure of the ventilatory pump, or in other words, diseases that prevent adequate movement of air and ventilation to occur (see Chapters 1 and 2), may be secondary to airways disease, which involves either the upper or lower airways, or extrapulmonary causes including cardiovascular disease, muscular or diaphragmatic weakness, skeletal abnormalities, obesity, and peripheral nervous system dysfunction. The third element of the respiratory system, the controller, can also lead to hypoventilation and hypoxemia (see Chapters 1 and 3) as a consequence of reduced alveolar ventilation. Failure of this pump function most commonly leads to hypercapnic respiratory failure because of inadequate ventilation; remember, however, that severe parenchymal disease can reduce alveolar ventilation to the point that hypercapnia may result despite an increase in total ventilation if there is sufficient mismatch of ventilation and perfusion in the lung.

Bilevel positive airway pressure (BiPAP) offers ventilatory assistance by providing variable amounts of inspiratory pressure support (PS) and is the preferred modality for mild to moderate respiratory failure because of hypoventilation or "pump" failure. When managing respiratory failure, the type, etiology, and other contributing factors should all be considered in order to make informed treatment decisions. This can help you choose the optimal modality for the patient based upon the specific pathophysiology and reason for respiratory failure.

INTRODUCTION TO CONTINUOUS POSITIVE AIRWAY PRESSURE AND BILEVEL POSITIVE AIRWAY PRESSURE

NIV is composed of two distinct entities: BiPAP and CPAP. Both work by applying supra-atmospheric pressure (ie, positive pressure) to the airways. CPAP provides a constant set pressure throughout the respiratory cycle, providing equal amounts of positive end-expiratory pressure (PEEP) during inspiration and expiration (**Figure 10-1A**). In contrast, BiPAP delivers different levels of pressure during the inspiratory and expiratory cycle (**Figure 10-1B**): inspiratory positive airway pressure (IPAP) and expiratory positive airway pressure (EPAP, which is essentially the same as PEEP). Being able to independently set IPAP and PEEP enables you to provide additional support during inspiration compared to CPAP because the latter is limited by the amount of PEEP one can use for a particular patient (excessive PEEP can lead to hyperinflation or overdistension of the lung). The PS component of BiPAP is the difference between IPAP and EPAP. Thus, PS is the additional pressure above EPAP provided during inspiration. Typically, BiPAP pressure levels are reported as IPAP over EPAP. This should be distinguished from PS with invasive mechanical ventilation, for which the traditional nomenclature reports PS over PEEP; a noted earlier, functionally, EPAP and PEEP are equivalent.

There are multiple CPAP and BiPAP machines available for clinical and home use. Although models may differ, the general components of a CPAP/BiPAP machine are relatively constant and include the pump (either a portable compressor or flow generator), tubing, and machine-patient interface. Several interfaces (the connection between the machine's tubing and the patient) are available including nasal pillows, nasal masks, oral mouthpieces, oronasal masks (or full-face masks), total face masks (covering the eyes, nose, and mouth, aka scuba masks), and helmet masks (**Figure 10-2**). Masks limited to the nose may be more comfortable and less anxiety-inducing for patients but have higher rates of air leak and require adequate nasal breathing. Full-face masks may produce a sense of claustrophobia in some patients. Oral mouthpieces and helmets are rarely used in the United States, although helmet systems gained use at some sites during the COVID pandemic. To the degree that the patient-machine interface can produce a closed system, that is, reduce the amount of ambient air being mixed with the machine delivered gas on each breath, one can deliver a higher and more consistent FIO_2. Of note, critical care ventilators can also be used for the "pump function" of BiPAP or CPAP.

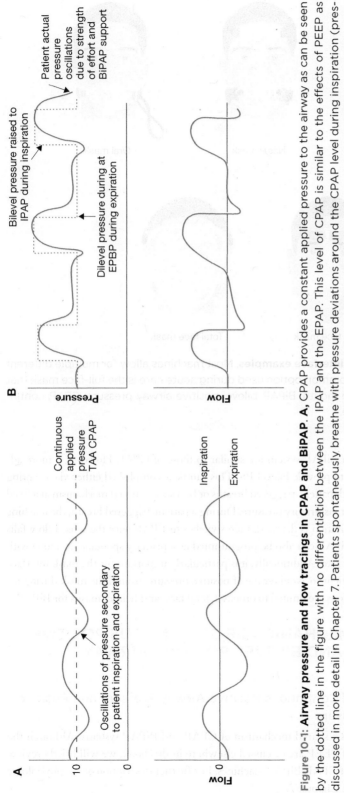

Figure 10-1: Airway pressure and flow tracings in CPAP and BiPAP. A, CPAP provides a constant applied pressure to the airway as can be seen by the dotted line in the figure with no differentiation between the IPAP and the EPAP. This level of CPAP is similar to the effects of PEEP as discussed in more detail in Chapter 7. Patients spontaneously breathe with pressure deviations around the CPAP level during inspiration (pressure lower than the set pressure because of the patient's inspiratory effort leading to "negative" force) and expiration (pressure higher than the set pressure because of the "positive" recoil force of the lungs) as seen by the solid line in the figure. During inspiration, the inspiratory effort lowers the airway pressure, and as the CPAP machine attempts to maintain a continuous pressure, inspiratory flow may be augmented. CPAP is particularly useful acutely in patients with congestive heart failure, where the CPAP decreases preload and afterload on the heart. **B,** BiPAP provides two levels of pressure for patients with a higher level of applied pressure during inspiration (IPAP) and a lower level of applied pressure during expiration (EPAP) as seen by the dotted line in the figure. The difference in the IPAP and the EPAP is similar to the level of pressure support applied during invasive mechanical ventilation. Note that the IPAP during BiPAP is set as the total pressure though and not the additional pressure support above EPAP, so equivalent levels of support would be reported differently. The resulting pressure waveforms (*solid line*) are in this case a result of the combination of patient effort and the level of applied pressure from the IPAP. Note that in a patient with large inspiratory efforts, the visualized pressure may never actually rise to the level of the applied IPAP during inspiration, but with more modest efforts the IPAP level may be achieved by the end of inspiration. BiPAP, bilevel positive airway pressure; CPAP, continuous positive airway pressure; EPAP, expiratory positive airway pressure; IPAP, inspiratory positive airway pressure; PEEP, positive end-expiratory pressure.

115

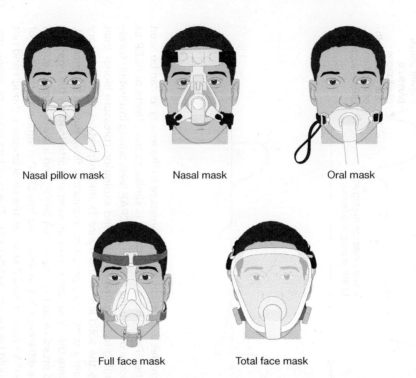

Nasal pillow mask   Nasal mask   Oral mask

Full face mask   Total face mask

Figure 10-2: BiPAP and CPAP interface examples. Most machines allow for multiple different interface options. The most common option used during acute care is the full-face mask that covers both the nose and the mouth. BiPAP, bilevel positive airway pressure; CPAP, continuous positive airway pressure.

The components of a BiPAP system are similar to those of CPAP. However, a more advanced pump is required to provide bilevel PS. This can be accomplished either via a sensing mechanism to coincide with patient-triggered breaths or by a simple timed mechanism at a fixed respiratory rate with target inspiratory pressure. During a patient-triggered breath, the machine provides IPAP when inspiration is detected, then switches to EPAP once the sensed flow falls below a threshold level. BiPAP can also be programmed as a primary spontaneous mode with a backup fixed respiratory rate. Additionally, it is particularly important for the mask interface to form a seal with the patient to avoid escape of positive pressure around the mask during inspiration. Thus, mask options are limited to oronasal, total face, and helmet masks for BiPAP.

PHYSIOLOGY AND MECHANICS OF CONTINUOUS POSITIVE AIRWAY PRESSURE AND BILEVEL POSITIVE AIRWAY PRESSURE

Beneficial Effects of Continuous Positive Airway Pressure and Positive End-Expiratory Pressure

The provision of PEEP is a shared mechanism of CPAP and BiPAP systems. Although the physiology and benefits of PEEP are discussed elsewhere in this book, we will briefly review them here in the context of CPAP/BiPAP machines. For further description of the physiologic effects of PEEP, please see Chapter 7.

PEEP and CPAP, by definition, provide positive pressure during the expiratory phase. The same pressure is applied during the inspiratory phase in CPAP. Because the inspiratory support is relatively small with a low CPAP level, the main potential benefit of CPAP on the respiratory system is to raise the end-expiratory lung volume and prevent alveolar collapse (see Chapter 7), which improves oxygenation and lung compliance and reduces the work of breathing and the probability of alveolar trauma. Recruitment of additional alveoli during the expiratory phase (ie, prevention of alveolar collapse thereby allowing the alveoli to participate in gas exchange on the next breath) decreases shunting and improves ventilation-perfusion matching, thereby improving oxygenation.

Lung mechanics are also affected. Alveoli are more likely to remain open with a positive transpulmonary gradient (the pressure difference between the alveolar pressure and intrapleural pressure), thus reducing atelectrauma and derecruitment caused by collapsed alveoli and the stresses associated with forcibly opening them on inspiration. PEEP provided by CPAP additionally can be used to titrate the set point at which the lungs exist along the pressure-volume curve (see Chapter 20 for more details on how this is done). This can be used to optimize compliance by improving recruitment of alveoli (the inspired volume is now distributed over a larger number of alveoli, which results in better compliance of the lung) and moving the functional lung volumes during tidal inflation into a more optimal location along the pressure-volume curve.

CPAP can reduce the work of breathing, particularly in patients with obstructive airway disease and expiratory flow limitation leading to auto-PEEP (also known as intrinsic PEEP; see Chapter 11 for more details on the physiology of this process). In these patients, exhalation is unable to be completed during the expiratory phase. As a result, more air than usual remains within the alveoli, leading to positive alveolar pressures at the end of exhalation in contrast to an alveolar pressure that equals zero in a healthy individual. In order to bring additional air into the lungs during inspiration, the patient must first overcome these elevated alveolar pressures (ie, create a negative alveolar pressure) to create a pressure gradient from the mouth to the alveoli (remember, pressure at the mouth normally is zero, ie, atmospheric pressure). With CPAP, in contrast, the machine provides positive pressure at the mouth and inspiratory flow begins as soon as the alveolar pressure is reduced to less than the PEEP setting rather than less than zero. Consequently, this initial pressure gradient required to generate inspiratory flow is easier to overcome, reducing the patient's work with each inspiration. Additionally, CPAP is often said to maintain airway patency and flow by maintaining a positive transmural pressure across the airway wall during expiration, although this only occurs if CPAP is greater than the intrinsic PEEP. It should be noted that in patients with heterogeneous parenchymal lung disease, CPAP may have a detrimental effect including barotrauma and overdistension.

Continuous Positive Airway Pressure and the Cardiovascular System

PEEP provided through CPAP can substantially impact the cardiovascular system through multiple mechanisms (see Chapter 4 for more detail), which may be advantageous for patients with pulmonary edema. First, PEEP decreases preload by increasing intrathoracic pressures, thereby impeding systemic venous return to the right ventricle (RV) during expiration. Second, PEEP decreases left ventricular (LV) afterload, which can be conceptualized as follows. LV afterload may be thought of as wall stress, which is proportional to intraventricular pressure as dictated by the Law of Laplace. The increased pressure around the heart generated by PEEP requires the heart to generate less wall stress to meet the same pressure goal needed to eject blood into the aorta (the positive intrathoracic pressure can be thought of as assisting the contraction of the cardiac muscle by "squeezing" the heart).

Afterload may also be altered by the effect of PEEP on the pulmonary vasculature. PEEP may either increase or decrease pulmonary vascular resistance (PVR). PVR will be decreased if PEEP improves alveolar recruitment and thereby decreases hypoxic pulmonary vasoconstriction, and/or if PEEP shifts lung volumes upward toward functional residual capacity (FRC), where PVR is lowest. However, PVR will be increased if lung volumes are pushed above FRC, at which point intra-alveolar vessels are constricted and resistance rises. RV afterload, which is generated in part by the degree of PVR, may thus be either increased or decreased by PEEP depending on the lung volume relative to FRC and the ability of PEEP to improve derecruitment. In practice, PEEP often increases RV afterload. This becomes a particularly troubling clinical scenario as both the increase in RV afterload and decrease in RV preload may impair ventricular function, which can lead to a fall in RV stroke volume and rapid decompensation of a patient with a poorly functioning RV.

Potential Harmful Effects of Continuous Positive Airway Pressure

Although there are many benefits from PEEP during CPAP, there may be negative effects in some patients as well, which are important to recognize. As described earlier, increased intrathoracic pressure decreases venous return. Although we typically think of venous return as representing the flow of blood from the lower portion of the body, the cerebral circulation also empties into the vena cava. Consequently, PEEP can also decrease cerebral venous return, thereby increasing intracranial pressures. Consequently, PEEP must be used cautiously in patients in whom increased intracranial pressure would be detrimental, such as seen with intracerebral bleeding or mass effect.

Because of effects on preload, CPAP can reduce cardiac output and worsen hypotension; consequently, it should be used cautiously in patients who are not at or near the plateau of their Starling curve; have RV dysfunction, pulmonary vascular hypertension, low intravascular volume; and in patients who are already hypotensive.

As noted earlier, CPAP may also be less useful in patients with heterogeneous or focal parenchymal lung disease such as pneumonia. In these patients, CPAP can have the paradoxical effect of worsening hypoxemia. This is thought to be due to compression of intra-alveolar capillaries in the normal or uninvolved lung, which is more compliant and receives a greater portion of the inspired volume, thereby diverting blood flow to the injured lung and potentially worsening shunt physiology. Finally, for practical purposes, neither CPAP nor BiPAP should be used in patients who are either uncooperative or have reduced consciousness, as the risk of aspiration is high. This is due both to gastric distension (some of the positive pressure in the posterior pharynx may result in air entering the esophagus and stomach) leading to higher risk of regurgitation and positive pressure in the posterior pharynx pushing secretions into the lung.

Beneficial Effects of Pressure Support Provided by Bilevel Positive Airway Pressure

In addition to PEEP, BiPAP provides additional PS during the inspiratory phase of each breath. As described previously, this is created by two different levels of pressure applied to the patient during inspiration (IPAP) and expiration (EPAP).

BiPAP therefore benefits the patient via several mechanisms. First, minute ventilation is increased by enhancing the patient's intrinsic tidal volume. With the additional pressure and flow applied to airways during inspiration, the patient is able to take larger breaths without additional effort. This is in contrast to CPAP, where the low pressures during inspiration have minimal ventilatory supportive effect. Increased minute ventilation leads to improved alveolar ventilation (barring marked expansion in dead space because of overdistension of alveoli from the larger tidal volume) with more rapid removal of carbon dioxide and heightened oxygen delivery.

By mounting higher tidal volumes and pressures during inspiration, PS further optimizes alveolar recruitment during this segment of the respiratory cycle. Engagement of more alveolar units may also contribute to improved gas exchange.

Additionally, BiPAP has the benefit of reducing the work of breathing. Increased work of breathing and dyspnea commonly derive from increased resistance of the airways, reduced compliance of the respiratory system, or muscle weakness. BiPAP augments the patient's intrinsic pressure generation and tidal volume as described earlier, with subsequent offloading of respiratory muscle work and eased sensations of dyspnea. This may halt the progressive respiratory muscle fatigue associated with a variety of respiratory diseases and circumvents the need for intubation and increased mechanical support. Reduced work also translates to decreased metabolic demand, which is reflected by decreased oxygen consumption and carbon dioxide production. Therefore, hypercapnia is acted upon synergistically (reduced production of CO_2 and enhanced elimination), and overall gas exchange equilibrium is improved.

CLINICAL APPLICATIONS OF CONTINUOUS POSITIVE AIRWAY PRESSURE AND BILEVEL POSITIVE AIRWAY PRESSURE

In the clinical setting, CPAP and BiPAP are most commonly used for chronic obstructive pulmonary disease (COPD) and heart failure exacerbations, with more limited evidence for use in other disease states (**Table 10-1**). The theoretical benefits and evidence base will be described here.

TABLE 10-1 Reviewing the Specific Uses of CPAP and BiPAP	
NPPV	
BiPAP	**CPAP**
☐ Exacerbation of COPD with respiratory acidosis	☐ Cardiogenic pulmonary edema
☐ Type II respiratory failure with chest wall deformity or neuromuscular disease	☐ Obstructive sleep apnea
☐ Failure of CPAP	☐ Chest wall trauma if hypoxic on adequate analgesia
☐ Pneumonia with respiratory acidosis	
☐ Therapeutic trial with a view to intubation if it fails	☐ Pneumonia
☐ Others (ARDS, post-op respiratory failure, to buy time prior to intubation)	

ARDS, acute respiratory distress syndrome; BiPAP, bilevel positive airway pressure; COPD, chronic obstructive pulmonary disease; CPAP, continuous positive airway pressure; NPPV, noninvasive positive pressure ventilation.

Noninvasive Ventilation Use in Chronic Obstructive Pulmonary Disease

The use of BiPAP for COPD exacerbations has been well studied. The pathophysiology and treatment of respiratory failure because of COPD with mechanical ventilation is discussed elsewhere in this book (see Chapter 11), but will be briefly reviewed here in order to emphasize the physiologic basis for the effectiveness of BiPAP.

COPD encompasses multiple diseases, including emphysema, chronic bronchitis, some cases of asthma, and bronchiectasis. However, all of these conditions share the following characteristics: alterations in the lung architecture and airways that ultimately lead to increased airflow resistance in the small conducting airways with progressive, poorly reversible airflow obstruction, increased lung compliance (in emphysema), and air trapping. During an exacerbation, airflow obstruction is magnified by acute inflammation, mucus hypersecretion, edema, and/or bronchoconstriction, all of which further narrow the airways and increase resistance, with resultant decreased ventilation and/or increased work of breathing. Additionally, ventilation/perfusion mismatch and gas exchange are worsened in severe exacerbations. Finally, respiratory muscle fatigue occurs because of a combination of increased airway resistance, increased work to expand the thoracic cage because of hyperinflation, and decreased efficiency of gas exchange with each breath, which necessitates an increase in total ventilation. Ultimately, the patient may develop hypercapnic respiratory failure because of this extra load on the system and consequent "pump failure."

BiPAP combats this series of events through a number of mechanisms, which involve both benefits from EPAP or PEEP and PS. First, PS during inspiration improves alveolar ventilation and therefore mitigates CO_2 retention. Second, PS reduces the work of breathing by supporting respiratory muscles, which secondarily reduces CO_2 production by reducing metabolic demand. PEEP is also beneficial by improving alveolar recruitment and/or by reducing the work of breathing associated with auto-PEEP as discussed earlier and in Chapter 7.

As a result of these mechanisms, BiPAP has been consistently shown to reduce hospital and intensive care unit (ICU) length of stay, intubation rates, complications of therapy (eg, ventilator-associated pneumonia), and mortality across multiple randomized controlled trials (RCTs; grade 1A evidence). A recent Cochrane review demonstrated a number needed to treat (NNT) of only 12 patients to avoid one death, and an NNT of only 5 patients to avoid one intubation. BiPAP remains a first-line treatment for patients presenting with moderate-to-severe acute exacerbations of COPD complicated by respiratory acidosis when there is no immediate indication for intubation. Given the potential benefits of PEEP, CPAP may also provide benefit in COPD exacerbations but is less effective than BiPAP. In patients without acidosis (ie, mild COPD exacerbation), the overall benefit of NIV is less pronounced. BiPAP and CPAP may also be considered in the setting of ambulatory care of COPD patients, although this indication is outside the scope of the discussion in this book.

Noninvasive Ventilation Use in Congestive Heart Failure

Both CPAP and BiPAP should also be considered in the management of acute congestive heart failure (CHF). CHF leads to respiratory failure primarily through the development of pulmonary edema. Increased left-sided cardiac pressures are transmitted to the pulmonary capillaries, causing increased hydrostatic pressure, which shifts fluid initially into the interstitium. The rate of transvascular infiltration of fluid overcomes lymphatic drainage rates with subsequent compression of small airways and disruption of alveolar membrane junctions and flooding into the alveolar spaces. Consequently, gas exchange is impaired leading to worsening $\dot{V}/\dot{Q}$ mismatch and, in some cases, pulmonary shunt. Pulmonary vascular pressure is also increased, which can lead to worsening RV strain, compromise of LV filling because of bowing of the interventricular septum, and further reduction in LV cardiac output. Overall lung compliance is reduced which, along with the reduced efficiency of each breath (ie, decreased alveolar ventilation), leads to increased work of breathing, thereby exacerbating the supply/demand relationship of oxygen for ventilatory muscles. Notably, only a subset of these patients will develop hypercapnia and respiratory acidosis.

Positive pressure is beneficial in this scenario for several reasons. First, the increase in intrathoracic pressure and decreased venous return to the heart may reduce LV end-diastolic volume and pressure, which will reduce pulmonary capillary pressure and transudation of fluid into the lung. Additional alveolar units are recruited, reducing shunt and improving $\dot{V}/\dot{Q}$ matching. Pulmonary compliance will improve as a result of this process and via optimization of the pressure-volume relationship from PEEP as discussed earlier (also see Chapter 20). Improved oxygenation reduces hypoxic pulmonary vasoconstriction and PVR, thereby offloading the RV. Second, as described earlier, PEEP reduces preload and LV afterload which, in the setting of acute CHF, reduces LV wall stress and may improve cardiac function by reducing myocardial oxygen demand. Finally, in the case of patients with concomitant hypercapnia, the additional benefit of PS during the inspiratory cycle will increase minute ventilation and reduce hypercapnia as well as work of breathing.

In contrast to the case of COPD exacerbations, both BiPAP and CPAP are considered first-line treatments for CHF exacerbations (grade 1A evidence). Both have been shown in multiple randomized trials to improve clinical outcomes including reductions in mortality and intubation rate compared to standard oxygen therapy. A recent Cochrane review suggested an NNT of 17 patients to prevent one hospital death, and an NNT of 13 patients to prevent one intubation, with no significant difference detected between BiPAP and CPAP.

Although BiPAP may improve oxygenation more rapidly and theoretically reduces the work of breathing and hypercapnia more effectively than CPAP, multiple studies have shown no significant difference in clinical outcomes between the two. It is unclear at this point whether BiPAP is superior to CPAP in the subset of patients with acute CHF and hypercapnic respiratory failure. Both are recommended in the treatment of acute CHF in patients with respiratory distress, although guidelines differ on whether respiratory acidosis should be part of the eligibility criteria. There is also some evidence to suggest that NIV may be useful in the setting of chronic CHF to improve pulmonary function and exercise tolerance, but more research is needed in this area before definitive recommendations can be made.

Use of Bilevel Positive Airway Pressure During Asthma Exacerbations

Given some of the overlap in pathophysiology between COPD and asthma (airway obstruction secondary to inflammation, excessive secretions, and bronchial hyperresponsiveness), the use of NIV in asthma exacerbations has been of interest and is becoming more commonplace, although this indication is not as thoroughly studied. The clear benefits seen in COPD in terms of mortality and intubation rates have not been matched in the asthmatic population, although this may be due to lack of data. There are some small RCTs to suggest improvement in pulmonary functioning as well as some clinical outcomes including reductions in hospital admission, but these studies are generally of poorer quality because of small sample size, lack of generalizability, and low event rates. A Cochrane review determined that NIV for asthma remained controversial because of a paucity of rigorous studies. More recent investigations suggest reductions in intubation and mortality rates, but these data are retrospective and observational.

The potential benefits of NIV in asthma patients include reduction of work of breathing associated with intrinsic PEEP, improved V̇/Q̇ matching, augmented ventilation with decreased work of breathing and support of the respiratory muscles, mechanical dilation of airways leading to decreased airway resistance and obstruction, and dispersal of bronchodilators to more distal airways.

However, there are several potential situations in which NIV could cause harm. First, because of hyperinflation, patients with acute asthma are already at risk of barotrauma and pneumothorax, which could be exacerbated by the use of positive pressure. Second, inadvertent application of PEEP that is higher than auto-PEEP could worsen hyperinflation. Notably, this risk of hyperinflation may be present with COPD exacerbations as well. Finally, patients should be carefully selected; those who are responding well to traditional therapies will likely not gain additional benefit from NIV, and those who are severely decompensated may be harmed by a trial of NIV which would delay intubation.

Bilevel Positive Airway Pressure Use With Other Forms of Hypercapnic Respiratory Failure

Hypercapnic respiratory failure is also a prominent feature of many other disease states including obesity hypoventilation syndrome (OHS), chronic restrictive diseases, and neuromuscular diseases. The benefit of BiPAP and/or CPAP in these situations is less clear, mostly because of a dearth of evidence. However, there is theoretical benefit based on the known physiology. Both obesity and restrictive chest wall and lung diseases are characterized by increased inward-directed forces leading to a low FRC and a propensity for alveolar collapse because of reduced alveolar radius (recall the Law of Laplace); atelectasis may ensue and there is an increased work of breathing because of the weight of the chest wall. The effects of the chest wall on breathing are complex; for further information see Chapter 18. PEEP in this setting would potentially be able to offset the excess external pressure on the airways associated with obesity and the intrinsic lung recoil of pulmonary fibrosis, thereby increasing FRC and reducing atelectasis.

The majority of patients with OHS also exhibit concomitant sleep-disordered breathing, for which CPAP is the first-line treatment in the chronic setting (the PEEP will reduce the probability of collapse of upper airways during exhalation). PS with BiPAP would additionally reduce the work of breathing and augment weak respiratory muscles (a common impairment in individuals with obesity), thereby improving ventilation and reducing respiratory acidosis. There is insufficient evidence to clearly delineate improved clinical outcomes with NIV (either CPAP or BiPAP) during acute illness for patients afflicted by these conditions despite the excellent physiologic rationale. Evidence is accumulating to support the use of home NIV in patients with chronic hypercapnia to reduce mortality.

In the case of progressive neuromuscular diseases, nighttime NIV is often a component of the standard of care—it is usually initiated during sleep once forced vital capacity is less than 50% of predicted and can be titrated to longer periods as the disease progresses. However, the effect of NIV during acute exacerbations in this scenario is not well studied.

TITRATION OF BILEVEL POSITIVE AIRWAY PRESSURE AND CONTINUOUS POSITIVE AIRWAY PRESSURE

Appropriate titration of CPAP and BiPAP by a trained provider is essential to its practical application in the clinical setting.

First, when evaluating a patient for BiPAP or CPAP, care should be taken to choose a mask interface that provides optimal fit with minimal air leak and is comfortable for the patient. Initial BiPAP settings are typically IPAP of 10 cm H_2O and EPAP of 5 cm H_2O with the goal of achieving tidal volumes of 5 to 7 mL/kg. In general, the difference between IPAP and EPAP should not be less than 4 cm H_2O. Of note, settings less than 8 cm H_2O/4 cm H_2O will likely be inadequate to achieve the desired ventilation and support of ventilatory muscles for most patients. Fraction of inspired oxygen (F_{IO_2}) is initially set at 1.0 or 100%. Subsequent titration is based on oxygen saturation, serial arterial blood gas (ABG) measurements for oxygenation, and use of either venous or ABGs for assessment of adequacy of ventilation (CO_2 removal) at approximately 1- to 2-hour intervals until target gas levels are achieved.

For persistent hypercapnia, IPAP should be increased in increments of 2 cm H_2O. For persistent hypoxemia, both IPAP and EPAP can be increased in increments of 2 cm H_2O. Simultaneously, F_{IO_2} should be decreased to the lowest setting possible that achieves goal Pao_2 or Spo_2. Maximal IPAP and EPAP are reached at approximately 25 and 15 cm H_2O, respectively, at or above which patients can develop discomfort at the mask interface and are at risk for gastric distension. Most BiPAP machines will additionally have an option for timed cycles, which allows for provision of IPAP and EPAP at a set rate regardless of patient respiratory rate. This "backup" rate is usually set at 12 to 16 breaths/min, or 2 breaths/min below the patient's intrinsic respiratory rate.

Initiation of CPAP entails similar mask preparation as earlier and setting initial pressures relatively low, usually starting at 5 cm H_2O. Subsequent titration can be achieved through manual or automatic titration (auto-titrating). Auto-titrating occurs when the CPAP machine senses airway pressures and uses an internal algorithm to adjust applied pressure on a breath-by-breath basis, with the goal of maintaining airway patency. This technique is most frequently applied in the setting of obstructive sleep apnea (OSA). Manual titration will follow a similar algorithm as for BiPAP (earlier) to reach a goal Pao_2 while avoiding pressures exceeding 15 cm H_2O.

Patients on NIV should be closely monitored to enable you to achieve optimal settings and for evaluation of treatment failure. This is typically performed in an ICU or step-down unit where nurse-to-patient ratios are lower. As earlier, serial blood gas measurements should be obtained to ensure appropriate gas exchange. Clinical respiratory status, including patient respiratory rate, tidal volume, lung sounds, accessory muscle use, and other clues to work of breathing should be evaluated frequently. Additionally, mental status should be closely followed, as NIV should not be applied to patients who are somnolent and/or cannot protect their airway from aspiration (impaired gag and cough). In the case of agitated patients, the decision to discontinue NIV or supplement care with sedating medications should be made on a case-by-case basis.

The process for weaning of NIV depends on the clinical scenario. For patients whose condition improves markedly over a short period of time (eg, rapidly improving pulmonary edema), NIV can be stopped abruptly followed by close monitoring. In other cases, stepwise discontinuation is more appropriate. This usually entails periodic trialing off of NIV during the day (eg, off during mealtimes or for several hours at a time). Daytime weaning is preferred given need for close monitoring and lower likelihood of developing hypercapnia because of sleep apnea or impaired mental status at night.

INTRODUCTION TO HIGH-FLOW NASAL CANNULA

Supplemental oxygen has been the standard of care for decades yet has significantly limited capacity to deliver high levels of concentrated oxygen to the alveoli due largely to delivery systems that allow mixing of supplemental oxygen with a substantial amount of ambient air, thereby diluting the delivered oxygen. HFNC, originally introduced at the turn of the 21st century, has since gained widespread clinical application as a much more potent and consistent source of oxygen supplementation and respiratory support. The past decade in particular has seen exponential growth in the use of HFNC worldwide for a broad array of pulmonary diseases.

HFNC is an oxygen supply system that is capable of providing supplemental oxygen at a range of F_{IO_2} up to and including 1.0 at flow rates of up to 60 L/min. The main components of HFNC are a flow generator, an air-oxygen blender, and a humidifier connected to tubing, usually with nasal prongs as the machine-patient interface (**Figure 10-3**). HFNC is most commonly used in a critical care setting given need for close monitoring, similar to NIV.

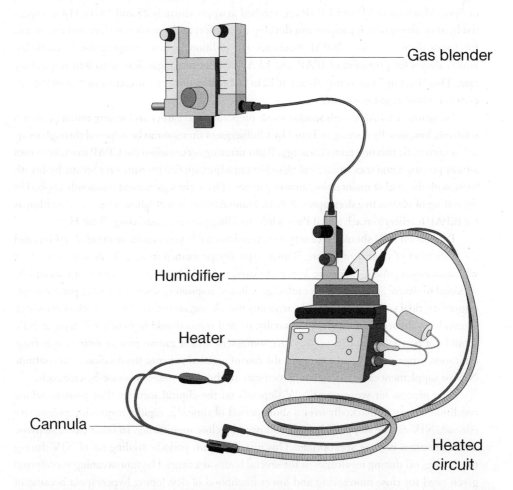

Gas blender

Humidifier

Heater

Cannula

Heated circuit

Figure 10-3: Schematic of the high-flow setup. High-pressure oxygen and air are mixed in a blender to target precise levels of F_{IO_2} at a specific high flow rate. The gas is humidified via the humidifier and warmed via a heating circuit before being delivered to the patient.

PHYSIOLOGY OF HIGH-FLOW NASAL CANNULA

High-Flow Nasal Cannula as Compared to Standard Oxygen Therapy

Traditional supplemental oxygen via nasal cannula or a loose-fitting mask delivers 100% oxygen from the source, but the oxygen inhaled by the patient is diluted by ambient air because inspiratory flow exceeds the flow provided from the oxygen source. Efforts to increase the flow from the oxygen source are thwarted by the drying and cooling effects associated with delivering classical oxygen. Use of tight-fitting masks with CPAP and BiPAP enables delivery of oxygen closer to an F_{IO_2} of 1.0.

HFNC overcomes these problems by providing heated, humidified oxygen up to an F_{IO_2} of 1.0 (ie, 100%) and flow of 60 L/min, with capabilities for tight titration. The main benefits of HFNC compared to standard or low-flow nasal cannula are derived from the ability to accurately titrate F_{IO_2} and provide up to 1.0 F_{IO_2} (compared to a maximum of about 0.55 F_{IO_2} via standard oxygen therapy) and to provide high flows (60 L compared to a maximum of ~15 L with standard oxygen therapy). Maximum flow for standard oxygen therapy is limited by both the internal diameter of the nasal cannula and by the lack of humidification, which at high flows leads to respiratory epithelial injury and patient discomfort. The high flows in HFNC are also responsible for the ability to reach an F_{IO_2} of 1.0 by providing flows in excess of patient ventilation, matching the patients' desired inspiratory flow rates and thereby minimizing entrainment of surrounding air and the resulting dilution of delivered oxygen that occurs with standard delivery options.

Mechanisms of Benefit

There are several mechanisms that are thought to explain the beneficial effects of HFNC above and beyond simply higher oxygen concentration delivery. HFNC delivers modest amounts of PEEP, which is generated by high flow rates with each 10 L/min of flow generating around 0.35 to 0.7 cm H_2O for a maximum of about 6 cm H_2O (depending on whether the mouth is open or closed). As in the case of NIV earlier, PEEP recruits alveoli, improves oxygenation, opens airways and reduces resistance, may reduce hyperinflation states, and may improve compliance. The high flow rates used for HFNC also marginally reduce dead space by providing a volume of air that exceeds the amount the patient is ventilating on their own, thus displacing CO_2 and increasing passive minute ventilation. As a result of this increased alveolar flow, there is higher alveolar P_{O_2} and therefore improved arterial oxygenation. Heated humidification may also be beneficial not only in improving patient comfort and therefore tolerance of the device but also by increasing the water content in mucus and facilitating clearance of secretions, although this effect has yet to be demonstrated in human studies. Finally, HFNC has been shown to decrease the work of breathing, as measured by patient vital signs and respiratory mechanics, likely for multiple reasons as mentioned earlier. Exploratory studies have demonstrated an inverse linear association between the work of breathing and flow rate, whereby higher flow rates are directly correlated with decreased work of breathing.

CLINICAL APPLICATIONS OF HIGH-FLOW NASAL CANNULA

HFNC is utilized in a variety of settings, but is perhaps best studied in the setting of acute hypoxemic respiratory failure because of pneumonia, ARDS, and exacerbations of interstitial lung disease. HFNC for this indication has been shown to reduce mortality, intubation rates (although this remains controversial) and time on the ventilator, and improved patient comfort and work of breathing. Some studies suggest that HFNC may be superior to NIV in this situation.

Other potential scenarios of benefit include preintubation oxygenation, postextubation oxygenation (discussed later), during bronchoscopy, immunocompromised patients, hypoxemia secondary to severe interstitial lung disease, hypercapnic respiratory failure, hypoxemia secondary to heart failure, and OSA. The main mechanism of benefit in the latter three instances is most likely because of PEEP provided by HFNC, as well as improved patient comfort compared to other NIV modalities (tight-fitting masks for CPAP and BiPAP may cause significant patient discomfort). As one escalates oxygen supplementation, HFNC has been found to improve oxygenation rates over a non-rebreather mask and may also be beneficial (and logistically straightforward to implement) in the setting of oxygen supplementation in concert with other instrumentation such as bronchoscopy. As discussed earlier, immunocompromised patients comprise a special population of patients in whom to consider HFNC because of the higher potential risk of infectious complications associated with invasive mechanical ventilation in these individuals. To the extent that HFNC may forestall intubation and mechanical ventilation, HFNC should be considered in these patients to address severe hypoxemia.

Trials comparing HFNC to standard oxygen therapy or NIV have shown mixed results, with some suggesting a benefit of HFNC over NIV and standard therapy in terms of intubation and mortality rates, but others actually demonstrating worse outcomes with HFNC. Unfortunately the evidence here is poor quality. Finally, HFNC may be of use in patients at the end of life in terms of alleviating dyspnea while causing minimal discomfort.

FAILURE OF NONINVASIVE VENTILATION AND HIGH-FLOW NASAL CANNULA

Although NIV and HFNC can often abort the need for mechanical ventilation, many patients will fail noninvasive measures and deteriorate to the point of requiring intubation. Patients requiring NIV are typically in a tenuous respiratory status and have diminished physiologic reserve; consequently, they are at higher risk of life-threatening respiratory compromise and must be monitored closely. For patients who eventually require mechanical ventilation, delays in intubation are associated with increased mortality. For these reasons, close monitoring is critical to determine if the intervention is achieving its goals; if not, proceed expeditiously to intubation and institution of full mechanical ventilation.

NIV and HFNC may fail for several reasons. First, patients may require higher levels of mechanical support than can be provided by noninvasive means (ie, their respiratory failure may be due to a problem with the ventilatory pump in addition to the gas exchanger). These patients can be identified by ongoing evidence of respiratory distress (eg, tachypnea, accessory muscle use, fatigue, and dyspnea) or inability to reach target gas exchange goals despite appropriate application and titration of NIV or HFNC. Second, in the case of CPAP and BiPAP, patients may simply not tolerate the mask apparatus, either because of discomfort or encephalopathy, which manifests as agitation or somnolence with inability to protect the airway. For patients receiving either NIV or HFNC, concern for inability to protect the airway should prompt reevaluation and, in most cases, intubation.

One tool that may be helpful to delineate between patients who would benefit from continued HFNC versus prompt intubation is the ROX index. The ROX index is defined by the ratio of oxygenation (represented as pulse oximetry [Spo_2/Fio_2]) to respiratory rate, where a higher score is associated with a lower risk of intubation. In one validation study of patients with pneumonia treated with HFNC, a score greater than or equal to 4.88 was associated with a lower risk of intubation, whereas a score of less than 2.85, less than 3.47, and less than 3.85 at 2, 6, and 12 hours after HFNC initiation, respectively, predicted HFNC failure and need for intubation. Although the ROX index is not commonly implemented in the clinical setting, it may be a useful adjunct to one's general clinical gestalt in cases that lack clarity.

Prior to declaring failure of treatment, providers should ensure that the equipment had been set up correctly and is working properly (eg, oxygen tubing is secure without avoidable air or pressure leaks). Proper mask fit should be reevaluated in the case of NIV. In the case of the agitated patient, sedation may be considered but is controversial.

NONINVASIVE VENTILATION AND HIGH-FLOW NASAL CANNULA AFTER EXTUBATION

Recurrent respiratory failure following extubation requires reintubation; this is a phenomenon occurring in up to 20% of extubated patients. Both HFNC and NIV have been studied for their potential use in this population to prevent reintubation and are frequently employed clinically in high-risk patients. Patients recently extubated commonly experience respiratory compromise from muscular weakness as well as decreased respiratory drive and difficulty clearing secretions, all of which can contribute to progressive hypoxemia and/or hypercapnia and eventual need for reintubation. The proposed mechanisms of benefit for application of NIV or HFNC immediately after intubation include correction of gas exchange abnormalities and reduced work of breathing. Overall, HFNC and NIV appear to be similar in terms of reducing reintubation rates and mortality compared to standard oxygen therapy, with the most benefit achieved in high-risk patients (eg, prior failed extubation or failed weaning trials, obesity, chronic hypercapnia, CHF). Importantly, NIV and HFNC applied to patients at some interval postextubation in the setting of worsening respiratory distress rather than in the immediate postextubation period have not been shown to reduce reintubation, and could even be deleterious if reintubation is consequently delayed.

SUMMARY

Invasive mechanical ventilation is the gold standard for ventilating patients with respiratory failure, but carries many downsides including possible lung injury and infectious complications. Over the past several decades, NIV and HFNC have become prominent alternatives to reduce the need for invasive mechanical ventilation and improve patient outcomes. In particular, both modalities can be beneficial for patients with COPD, heart failure, and in the postextubation period. NIV may be beneficial for other forms of hypercapnic respiratory failure, whereas HFNC should be considered in states leading to severe hypoxemia. At the same time, there are many disease states for which the potential of NIV and HFNC has yet to be determined, and research is ongoing.

KEY POINTS

- Modes of NIV include CPAP and BiPAP, which provide PEEP and, in the case of BiPAP, inspiratory PS.
- NIV is well studied and has a grade 1A recommendation for use in COPD and heart failure exacerbations, whereas its use in asthma, other forms of hypercapnic respiratory failure, and immunocompromised patients is controversial.

- HFNC is a humidified oxygen supply system that can provide high F_{IO_2} and high flows exceeding the capabilities of standard oxygen therapy.
- HFNC has clear benefit in the setting of hypoxemic respiratory failure, with unclear benefit in immunocompromised patients, hypercapnic or mixed respiratory failure, heart failure, OSA, and periprocedurally.
- Both NIV and HFNC may be beneficial in the immediate postextubation period, particularly in patients at high risk of reintubation.

STUDY QUESTIONS AND ANSWERS

Thought Questions

1. What differentiates BiPAP from CPAP?
2. What are the mechanisms by which NIV improves pulmonary function?
3. What are the mechanisms by which HFNC improves pulmonary function?
4. For what acute clinical indications is NIV recommended?
5. For what acute clinical indications is HFNC recommended?
6. What are the potential deleterious effects of NIV?

Thought Question Answers

1. Both CPAP and BiPAP provide PEEP. CPAP provides this same level of pressure throughout the respiratory cycle. In contrast, BiPAP provides a higher level of pressure during inspiration, known as IPAP, compared to EPAP, which is the equivalent of PEEP. This bilevel pressure delivery requires more advanced equipment including, in most cases, the ability to sense the patient's intrinsic respiratory cycle. Finally, because of the higher pressures typically being administered and the need to avoid air leak, BiPAP masks are limited to those that can provide a tight seal.
2. Both PEEP (CPAP and BiPAP) and PS (BiPAP) improve pulmonary function. PEEP improves oxygenation via alveolar recruitment and higher partial pressures of oxygen at the alveolar surface. PEEP also improves lung compliance, prevents atelectrauma, and reduces the work of breathing by optimizing pressure gradients and stenting open airways. PS in BiPAP increases tidal volume and therefore minute ventilation with subsequent reductions in $Paco_2$, improves gas exchange through alveolar recruitment, and reduces the work of breathing by offloading respiratory muscles.
3. HFNC provides high flows of concentrated oxygen which not only improve hypoxemia but also enhance CO_2 elimination. The high flows also generate modest amounts of PEEP and may decrease the work of breathing. Humidification may facilitate clearance of secretions and improve patient comfort.
4. BiPAP is most effective for COPD exacerbations, whereas both CPAP and BiPAP are effective in CHF. BiPAP may also be beneficial in asthma and other causes of hypercapnia such as neuromuscular disease, OHS, and restrictive diseases. Either BiPAP or CPAP may have a role in preventing intubation in selected populations. Additionally, either modality may be beneficial in the immediate postextubation period, particularly in patients with high reintubation risk or underlying hypercapnic respiratory failure.

5. HFNC is most studied in the setting of acute hypoxemic respiratory failure, which encompasses many etiologies. It may also be useful for preoxygenation of patients prior to intubation, to support individuals immediately postextubation, as well as for hypercapnic respiratory failure, immunocompromised patients, during bronchoscopy, and during end-of-life care.

6. Without close monitoring, NIV may lead to unnecessary delays in intubation. It also poses an aspiration risk for the patient with somnolence, reduced gag reflex, and weak cough. PEEP, in particular, has several potential harmful effects including decreased preload and hypotension, increased RV afterload, increased intracranial pressure, hyperinflation, barotrauma, and rarely iatrogenic pneumothorax.

Multiple Choice Questions

1. A 55-year-old male patient with a history of systolic heart failure presents with dyspnea and weight gain. His chest x-ray is notable for diffuse fluffy infiltrates and small bilateral pleural effusions. His vital signs reveal Spo_2 90% on 2 L, blood pressure 150/100, and respiratory rate 28 breaths/min. On exam, he is mildly tachypneic and is not able to speak in complete sentences because of his respiratory distress. He is alert and oriented. He has diffuse crackles on pulmonary exam and 2+ pitting edema to the knees. Venous blood gas (VBG) is notable for pH 7.36 and Pco_2 47. In addition to diuresis, what options would you consider for management of this patient's respiratory failure?

    A. CPAP

    B. BiPAP

    C. Either CPAP or BiPAP

    D. HFNC

2. Why might CPAP and BiPAP be equally efficacious for heart failure, whereas BiPAP is superior to CPAP for COPD exacerbations?

    A. Positive pressure with both CPAP and BiPAP reduce preload and afterload.

    B. BiPAP helps augment minute ventilation and CO_2 clearance.

    C. Both A and B.

3. What are the potential benefits associated with HFNC?

    A. Humidification improves comfort and reduces epithelial injury of the nasopharynx.

    B. High flow rates match patient demand and improve oxygenation by reducing the amount of entrained room air.

    C. High flow can generate small amounts of PEEP.

    D. All of the above

4. A 42-year-old woman with a history of kidney transplant currently on immunosuppressive therapy presents to the hospital with community-acquired pneumonia. She is initiated on antibiotics, receives intravenous fluids, and is given supplemental oxygen via nasal cannula. Overnight on hospital day 1 she has an increasing oxygen requirement and worsened dyspnea. On your evaluation, her Spo_2 is 94% receiving supplemental oxygen via a non-rebreather mask and blood pressure is 90/60. She is mildly tachypneic and has crackles at the right base and mid-lung. Repeat chest x-ray shows

(continued)

multifocal consolidative opacities in the right middle and lower lobes as well as scattered ground-glass opacities. ABG is notable for pH 7.45, P_{CO_2} 35, P_{O_2} 60. In addition to diagnostic studies and broadening antibiotics, what is your next step in managing her respiratory failure?

A. Start CPAP.
B. Start BiPAP.
C. Intubate.
D. Initiate HFNC.

5. You are evaluating a 65-year-old woman for asthma exacerbation. She has a history of hypertension and gastroesophageal reflux disease (GERD). On exam, you note diffuse expiratory wheezing and accessory muscle use. The patient is somnolent but awakens to sternal rub. Her S_{PO_2} is 92% on 4 L. A VBG is performed, which shows pH of 7.3 and P_{CO_2} of 52. She has already received multiple nebulizers and steroids. What is your next step in the management of her respiratory status?

A. Start CPAP.
B. Start BiPAP.
C. Intubate.
D. Initiate HFNC.

Multiple Choice Question Answers

1. **Answer C. Either CPAP or BiPAP**

   Rationale: This patient would benefit from NIV. Both CPAP and BiPAP have been shown to be effective in the management of pulmonary edema from a heart failure exacerbation. There is currently no clear evidence of superiority for one over the other, thus either could be considered for this patient. However, in the setting of increased work of breathing and mild hypercapnia, some would argue for the use of BiPAP for its ventilatory support over CPAP.

2. **Answer C. Both A and B**

   Rationale: The primary cause of respiratory failure from left-sided heart failure is pulmonary edema. PEEP, which is supplied by both CPAP and BiPAP, reduces pulmonary edema and improves $\dot{V}/\dot{Q}$ matching while also potentially reducing afterload of the left heart. Only a subset of patients with a heart failure exacerbation also experience hypercapnia. In contrast, a COPD exacerbation is manifested by airflow obstruction and decreased ventilation with subsequent hypercapnia in many patients. Although external or machine PEEP may reduce the work of breathing associated with intrinsic PEEP in these patients, only BiPAP provides PS during the inspiratory cycle and therefore augments minute ventilation; CPAP has a minimal role to play in reversing the pathophysiology of COPD.

3. **Answer D. All of the above**

   Rationale: Unlike HFNC, standard oxygen delivery systems are not humidified. Without humidification, air delivered to the nasopharynx at high flow levels leads to epithelial injury and patient discomfort. Without the ability to provide high flows, the patient may entrain air at a faster rate than can be delivered by the oxygen delivery system, thus diluting F_{IO_2}. High flow also provides a small degree of PEEP.

4. **Answer D. Initiate HFNC**

   Rationale: This patient likely has worsening pneumonia with escalating oxygen require-ments and will benefit from HFNC and ICU transfer. Her presentation is consistent with hypoxemic respiratory failure without hypercapnia or evidence of severe respiratory dis-tress. HFNC has been shown to be more effective than non-rebreather mask at improving hypoxemia and can be titrated more precisely, in addition to being more comfortable for the patient. CPAP and BiPAP would likely be less helpful in this scenario and would not be the first choice unless the patient had superimposed COPD. We would likely trial high flow before considering intubation.

5. **Answer C. Intubate**

   Rationale: This patient will likely require intubation. Although NIV such as BiPAP is a consideration for asthmatic patients because of potential beneficial effects on the work of breathing and obstruction, this patient has evidence of severe exacerbation with increased work of breathing, ongoing obstruction despite bronchodilators, and hypercapnia. In addi-tion, her altered mental status is a relative contraindication to the use of BiPAP given high risk of aspiration. HFNC would likely not be beneficial given relatively mild hypoxemia and clear need for some level of respiratory muscle support.

Suggested Readings

Berbenetz N, Wang Y, Brown J, et al. Non-invasive positive pressure ventilation (CPAP or bilevel NPPV) for cardiogenic pulmonary oedema. *Cochrane Database Syst Rev.* 2019;4(4):CD005351. doi:10.1002/14651858.CD005351.pub4.

Boccatonda A, Groff P. High-flow nasal cannula oxygenation utilization in respiratory failure. *Eur J Intern Med.* 2019;64:10-14. doi:10.1016/j.ejim.2019.04.010.

Comellini V, Pacilli AMG, Nava S. Benefits of non-invasive ventilation in acute hypercapnic respiratory failure. *Respirology.* 2019;24(4):308-317. doi:10.1111/resp.13469.

Del Sorbo L, Jerath A, Dres M, Parotto M. Non-invasive ventilation in immunocompromised patients with acute hypoxemic respiratory failure. *J Thorac Dis.* 2016;8(3):E208-E216. doi:10.21037/jtd .2016.02.11.

Esquinas AM, Benhamou MO, Glossop AJ, Mina B. Noninvasive mechanical ventilation in acute ventilatory failure: rationale and current applications. *Sleep Med Clin.* 2017;12(4):597-606. doi:10.1016/j.jsmc.2017.07.009.

Ferreyro BL, Angriman F, Munshi L, et al. Association of noninvasive oxygenation strategies with all-cause mortality in adults with acute hypoxemic respiratory failure: a systematic review and meta-analysis. *JAMA.* 2020;324(1):57-67. doi:10.1001/jama.2020.9524.

Helviz Y, Einav S. A systematic review of the high-flow nasal cannula for adult patients. *Crit Care.* 2018;22(1):71. doi:10.1186/s13054-018-1990-4.

Lim WJ, Mohammed Akram R, Carson KV, et al. Non-invasive positive pressure ventilation for treat-ment of respiratory failure due to severe acute exacerbations of asthma. *Cochrane Database Syst Rev.* 2012;12:CD004360. doi:10.1002/14651858.CD004360.pub4.

MacIntyre NR. Physiologic effects of noninvasive ventilation. *Respir Care.* 2019;64(6):617-628. doi:10.4187/ respcare.06635.

Osadnik CR, Tee VS, Carson-Chahhoud KV, Picot J, Wedzicha JA, Smith BJ. Non-invasive ventilation for the management of acute hypercapnic respiratory failure due to exacerbation of chronic obstructive pul-monary disease. *Cochrane Database Syst Rev.* 2017;7(7):CD004104. doi:10.1002/14651858.CD004104.pub4.

Chronic Obstructive Pulmonary Disease and Mechanical Ventilation

Chronic Obstructive Lung Disease

Richard M. Schwartzstein

LEARNING OBJECTIVES

- Describe the pathophysiology of chronic obstructive pulmonary disease (COPD) and the link between problems with the ventilatory pump, the respiratory controller, and the gas exchanger in patients with COPD and acute respiratory failure.
- Explain the role of intrinsic positive end-expiratory pressure (PEEPi) in patients with COPD and the use of applied PEEP to minimize issues of ventilatory dyssynchrony.
- Clarify the etiology and implications of chronic hypercapnia in COPD for the patient with acute respiratory failure.
- Outline the options for ventilating patients with COPD and acute respiratory failure.
- Explicate the significance of respiratory rate, duty cycle, and dynamic hyperinflation in patients with COPD and acute respiratory failure.
- Explain the challenges associated with pressure support ventilation in patients with COPD.

INTRODUCTION

Chronic obstructive pulmonary disease (COPD) is a general term applied to a category of diseases characterized by increased airway resistance during exhalation. Included in this category are problems as diverse as emphysema, chronic bronchitis, asthma, bronchiectasis, and bronchiolitis. COPD is now the third leading cause of death in the United States and commonly leads to episodes of acute respiratory failure when other processes, such as infection, are superimposed on the chronic state. Patients with COPD often have derangements of all three elements of the respiratory system—the respiratory controller, the ventilatory pump, and the gas exchanger—outlined in Chapter 1. Acute respiratory failure complicating asthma is addressed in detail in Chapter 12. In this chapter, we focus primarily on emphysema, recognizing that most patients with cigarette-induced COPD have a mixture of both emphysema and chronic bronchitis pathologically.

OVERVIEW OF THE PATHOPHYSIOLOGY OF CHRONIC OBSTRUCTIVE PULMONARY DISEASE

COPD is largely a complication of the inhalation of toxins in smoke emanating from combustion, for example, cigarette smoke, air pollution, cooking and heating from wood burning stoves. The toxins may lead to inflammation of airways and lung parenchyma, leading to narrowing of airways and destruction of lung tissue. Physiologically, one sees increased airway resistance manifest as reduced expiratory flow (eg, decrease in forced expiratory volume in 1 second [FEV1]) and increased lung compliance because of destruction of collagen leading to reduced elastic recoil. The latter also contributes to increased expiratory airway resistance during forceful exhalation because of the collapse of small airways tethered open by surrounding lung tissue.

The Ventilatory Pump

Increased airway resistance and diminished elastic recoil contribute to dynamic hyperinflation, particularly when respiratory rate is increased and expiratory time is reduced. With inadequate time to exhale the volume of gas inhaled, end-expiratory lung volume (EELV) increases until the resulting end-inspiratory volume is sufficient to produce the driving force and enlarged airways (with increased radius and reduced resistance) to allow for a new equilibrium to be established between the volume of gas inhaled and exhaled (see Chapter 2 and **Figure 11-1**). Dynamic hyperinflation (the increase in the lung volumes at which one is breathing because of expiratory resistance and insufficient time for exhalation) is associated with greater recoil force of the lungs and less efficient contraction of the inspiratory muscles, which results in increased work of breathing and dyspnea.

Because dynamic hyperinflation signifies that EELV is elevated above functional residual capacity (FRC), the pressure in the alveolus is positive at the time that the next inspiration begins (intrinsic positive end-expiratory pressure [PEEP] or PEEPi). Recall that FRC is defined as relaxation volume for the respiratory system, at which time the outward or expanding forces of the chest wall are equal to the inward or collapsing forces of the lung, and the alveolar pressure is zero (see Chapter 2). To initiate an inhalation under conditions of elevated EELV, the inspiratory muscles must overcome the PEEPi and establish a negative pressure in the alveolus before inspiratory flow will result (see **Figure 11-2** and Chapter 7). This further increases the work of breathing and dyspnea. Studies have shown that the majority of

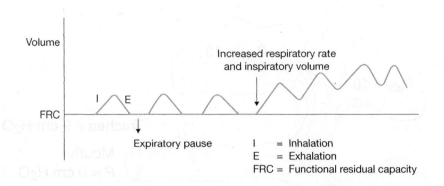

Figure 11-1: **Dynamic hyperinflation in COPD.** During resting breathing, the expiratory portion of the respiratory cycle is typically longer than inspiration ($I/E = 1/2$). During part of the expiratory phase, the expiratory pause, there is no flow in or out of the lungs. As an individual begins to "exercise," which may just be walking for a patient with COPD, the respiratory rate and the inspiratory volume increase. When we increase respiratory rate, we must shorten the time for the respiratory cycle. There are limits (based on inspiratory flow and the inspiratory volume desired) on how much we can shorten inspiratory time; thus, most of the shortening occurs during the expiratory phase. If the patient is flow limited and cannot increase expiratory flow, they may not be able to exhale all of the inspired volume in the time available for exhalation. Thus, the end-expiratory lung volume begins to rise from the functional residual capacity. This process (more air comes in on inhalation than goes out on exhalation) continues until the lung volume has increased sufficiently that the driving pressure (now increased because of the greater recoil forces of the lung at higher volume) and the resistance of the airways (now decreased because of the larger radius of the airways at higher lung volume) have changed sufficiently to increase expiratory flow to the point that the volume of gas exhaled equals the volume of gas inhaled. A new equilibrium is established at a higher lung volume. COPD, chronic obstructive pulmonary disease.

patients with COPD complain about breathing "in" not "out" despite the fact that we describe their condition as a problem with expiratory flow. Because expiratory flow is typically passive during resting ventilation, however, the work associated with breathing is experienced as "inspiratory" effort as a consequence of dynamic hyperinflation and PEEPi.

Gas Exchanger and Respiratory Controller in Chronic Obstructive Pulmonary Disease

COPD, like most respiratory diseases, is a heterogeneous process; some areas of the lung are normal, whereas other regions are mildly affected, and others are severely damaged. Because both airway resistance and recoil forces of the lung are important contributors to ventilation, ventilation/perfusion mismatch ($\dot{V}/\dot{Q}$ mismatch) is present, which leads to hypoxemia. As ventilation to a given region of lung is reduced, the oxygen in the alveolus diffuses into the blood and is not replenished adequately because of the diminished ventilation. Hypoxic pulmonary vasoconstriction, which normally should occur to redirect blood flow to well-ventilated units, is impaired because of the disease process and blood continues to flow to the hypoxic alveolus (see Chapter 3 and **Figure 11-3**). Hypoxemia because of $\dot{V}/\dot{Q}$ mismatch is usually overcome relatively easily by the administration of supplemental oxygen.

Mild-to-moderate degrees of $\dot{V}/\dot{Q}$ mismatch do not lead to hypercapnia because of the linear relationship between $Paco_2$ and ventilation but may occur if the mismatch is severe or the respiratory controller is blunted, and hyperventilation does not occur. In addition, if the

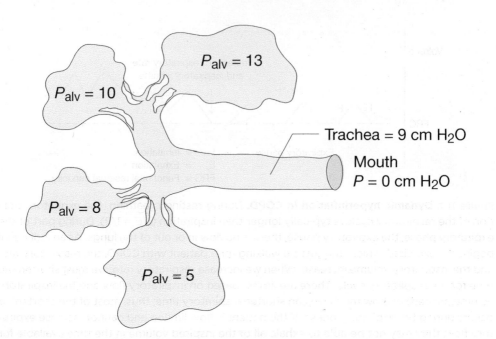

$P_{alv} = 13$

$P_{alv} = 10$

Trachea = 9 cm H_2O

Mouth
$P = 0$ cm H_2O

$P_{alv} = 8$

$P_{alv} = 5$

Figure 11-2: Intrinsic PEEP (PEEPi). The figure depicts the lungs as four "compartments" with variable compliance (recoil force) and variable resistance of the airways leading to that compartment. The pressure in each alveolus is alveolar pressure (P_{alv}) in cm H_2O. Because of the range of recoil forces and resistance in the different compartments, they empty at different rates during exhalation and do not get to an alveolar pressure of zero (atmospheric pressure) by the end of exhalation. The pressure in the trachea, if you do an expiratory pause, is the average of the four compartments. As inspiration begins on the next breath, the chest wall moves out and begins to reduce the pressure in the thorax. P_{alv} begins to fall, but because the pressures in the alveoli are positive (not zero, as it would be at end exhalation in a healthy person), no air goes into the lung until the chest wall has expanded enough to drop P_{alv} below zero. This leads to increased work of breathing. PEEP, positive end-expiratory pressure.

patient has an associated problem that interferes with the normal function of the controller, for example, sleep apnea, chronic hypercapnia may ensue. Chronic hypercapnia is evidenced by the elevated $Paco_2$ with associated chronic elevation of serum bicarbonate, which represents renal compensation for the respiratory acidosis. Some patients with chronic hypercapnia may have a superimposed acute hypercapnia because of the presence of a secondary problem, such as acute bronchitis or pneumonia, or because of inspiratory muscle fatigue prompted by the increased work associated with acute changes in airway resistance and worsening dynamic hyperinflation.

Although administration of supplemental oxygen usually corrects the hypoxemia due to $\dot{V}/\dot{Q}$ mismatch in patients with COPD, it may worsen hypercapnia. The poorly ventilated units, with low alveolar Po_2 (PAo_2), are still getting some ventilation and the supplemental oxygen will raise the PAo_2, reverse the hypoxic pulmonary vasoconstriction, and send more blood to what is still a poorly ventilated lung unit (remember, $Paco_2$ is inversely proportional to alveolar ventilation); consequently, $\dot{V}/\dot{Q}$ mismatch will worsen and $Paco_2$ will rise

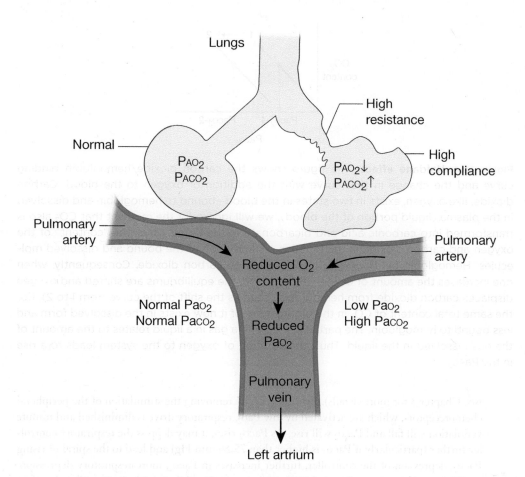

Figure 11-3: **Ventilation/perfusion mismatch.** The figure depicts a two-alveolar model of the lung. One alveolus is normal and the other represents the lung with emphysema; the lung compliance is high (reduced elastic recoil) and the resistance in the airway to that region is high as well. The combination of high compliance and high resistance leads to reduced ventilation to that lung unit (less air going in and out of that region of lung). Because that unit has less ventilation, the alveolar Po_2 (PA_{O2}) will fall as oxygen diffuses from the alveolus into the pulmonary capillary and is not replenished in the alveolus by more ventilation; the result is a fall in Pa_{O2}. Similarly, CO_2 diffuses from the blood to the alveolus but is not removed at a normal rate because of the decreased ventilation, and alveolar CO_2 (PA_{CO2}) rises, which ultimately means that the blood coming to the alveolus will not be able to release its CO_2 and the Pa_{CO2} will rise. As the blood leaving each of the alveoli mixes, the content of carbon dioxide in the blood will be higher and the content of oxygen will be lower, leading to reduced Pa_{O2} and elevated Pa_{CO2}.

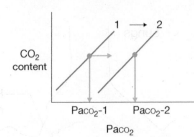

Figure 11-4: Haldane effect. The figure shows the carbon dioxide/hemoglobin binding curve and the change in that curve with the addition of oxygen to the blood. Carbon dioxide, like oxygen, exists in two states in the blood—bound to hemoglobin and dissolved in the plasma (liquid portion of the blood); we will ignore for the moment that CO_2 also is transformed into carbonic acid and bicarbonate in the blood. Thus, the "content" of the oxygen and carbon dioxide in the blood is a summation of the bound and dissolved molecules. Hemoglobin binds oxygen preferentially to carbon dioxide. Consequently, when one increases the amount of oxygen in the blood, the equilibriums are shifted and oxygen displaces carbon dioxide from hemoglobin (seen as the shift of the curve from 1 to 2). For the same total content of CO_2 in the blood, more of it now exists in the dissolved form and less bound to hemoglobin. The partial pressure of a gas in a liquid relates to the amount of the gas dissolved in the liquid. Thus, the addition of oxygen to the system leads to a rise in the $Paco_2$.

(see Chapter 3 for more details). Additionally, by removing the stimulation of the peripheral chemoreceptors, which are activated by low Pao_2, respiratory drive is diminished and minute ventilation will fall and $Paco_2$ will rise. As $Paco_2$ rises, it may depress the respiratory controller further (particularly if $Paco_2$ is higher than 75-80 mm Hg) and lead to the spiral of rising $Paco_2$, depression of the controller, further increases in $Paco_2$, more respiratory depression, etc. This may be a cause of acute hypercapnic respiratory failure in the nonventilated patient and can lead to progressively worsening hypercapnia in the mechanically ventilated patient who is receiving a set rate and tidal volume. Finally, administration of supplemental oxygen may also worsen hypercapnia via the Haldane effect (oxygen supplants CO_2 bound to hemoglobin, putting more CO_2 into solution in the blood, which raises the $Paco_2$); see **Figure 11-4**.

MECHANICAL VENTILATION AND THE CHRONIC OBSTRUCTIVE PULMONARY DISEASE PATIENT

A typical clinical scenario might be characterized by the following: a patient with COPD and dyspnea precipitated by mild-to-moderate exertion develops an acute pulmonary infection superimposed on their chronic lung disease. The inflammatory process typically worsens the airway resistance (mucus production) and gas exchange (worsening $\dot{V}/\dot{Q}$ mismatch); tachypnea is common, which reduces time for exhalation, thereby making dynamic hyperinflation more severe. Although adequate oxygenation is achieved with noninvasive means, the patient's ventilatory pump is failing, evidenced by the use of accessory muscles of ventilation. Dyspnea is severe, and acute on chronic hypercapnia is also a problem.

Because most of the airway resistance is typically on exhalation, initiation of mechanical ventilation is relatively easy and well tolerated by the patient. In order to manage the $Paco_2$, one typically sets a rate and tidal volume; volume or pressure ventilation should be relatively equivalent in their effect. Because the compliance of the respiratory system is normal or elevated and, except for patients with acute bronchospasm or acute/chronic bronchitis, inspiratory resistance is either normal or mildly increased, one should not have a major issue with high airway pressure (either peak or plateau pressure).

One must pay attention, however, to the time allotted for exhalation, which can be affected by respiratory rate and/or the duty cycle (the fraction of total respiratory time spent in inspiration, ie, T_i/T_{tot}). For any given respiratory rate, one wants to maximize the expiratory time to minimize dynamic hyperinflation. To achieve a longer expiratory time (T_e) for a given respiratory rate, one must increase inspiratory flow. This will cause peak airway pressure to be elevated, but if plateau pressure is acceptable (eg, less than 25 cm H_2O), this is not a major source of concern because the peak pressure is being experienced in the larger airways, not in the alveoli; consequently, you will not cause overdistension of alveoli. If dynamic hyperinflation is worsening, one will see evidence of this in a rising plateau pressure; remember, as lung volume increases, the lungs and chest wall become "stiffer," that is, compliance goes down. Hence, the same tidal volume will require higher pressures.

Chronic Obstructive Pulmonary Disease, Intrinsic Positive End-Expiratory Pressure, and the Ventilator

As noted in the previous section, many patients with COPD, particularly those with acute respiratory failure, will have some degree of PEEPi. In the spontaneously breathing patient before mechanical ventilation is started, this contributes to the work of breathing. In the patient treated with mechanical ventilation in a mode in which the patient must trigger the ventilator, PEEPi is still a potential problem. One can assess for PEEPi by doing an expiratory hold at the end of exhalation on the ventilator (**Figure 11-5**).

The patient must trigger the ventilator by creating a negative pressure or inspiratory flow before the ventilator will deliver a breath or provide inspiratory assistance. Consequently, if one does not recognize the presence of PEEPi on the ventilator, the work of breathing to initiate a

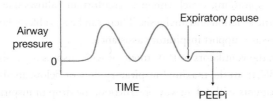

Figure 11-5: Intrinsic PEEP (PEEPi). The figure shows airway pressure as a function of time in a patient receiving positive pressure ventilation. As the ventilator pushes air into the lungs, pressure rises with a subsequent fall during exhalation. At the end of the second exhalation, the inspiratory and expiratory valves are closed and no additional air goes into or out of the lungs; this is called an expiratory "pause" or "hold." Normally, at the end of exhalation, the alveolar pressure should be zero (the same as atmospheric pressure) if the end-expiratory volume is at relaxation volume or FRC. If the patient has not had time to exhale fully to FRC, the alveolar pressure will be higher than zero. The small "bump" upward in pressure during the expiratory hold represents equilibration of the pressure between the mouth (where the pressure is being measured) and the alveolus. There is evidence of positive pressure at the end of exhalation (PEEP) that is intrinsic to the patient (note that applied PEEP is zero). Consequently, we describe the patient as having PEEPi. FRC, functional residual capacity; PEEP, positive end-expiratory pressure.

breath with the ventilator will be similar to that associated with spontaneous breathing without mechanical assistance. If the patient is unable to trigger the ventilator, it will appear that the patient is dyssynchronous with the ventilator, or "fighting the ventilator"; the patient will be seen to try to initiate a breath but one will not be delivered (see Chapter 18 for more details).

To alleviate this problem, one typically sets applied PEEP on the ventilator (see Chapter 7 for a more complete discussion). For example, if the PEEPi is 7 cm H_2O, and there is no applied PEEP, the patient will have to generate an inspiratory force sufficient to drop the alveolar pressure from +7 cm H_2O to zero or below zero to trigger the ventilator. If one sets applied PEEP on the ventilator to 5 cm H_2O, however, the patient only needs to generate an inspiratory force sufficient to drop alveolar pressure from 7 to 5 cm H_2O at which point the ventilator will begin to provide assistance on the inspiration. Typically, applied PEEP is set at approximately 80% of the PEEPi. The institution of applied PEEP may cause measured PEEP (and end-expiratory volume) to rise, but the measured PEEP will be lower than the sum of the PEEPi and applied PEEP in patients with heterogeneous lung disease.

Supplemental Oxygen and Chronic Obstructive Pulmonary Disease

Supplemental oxygen is supplied to achieve blood oxygen saturation of 89% to 92%. Higher Pao_2 is not shown to help patients who do not have acute myocardial ischemia and may worsen hypercapnia by one or more of the following mechanisms: worsening $\dot{V}/\dot{Q}$ mismatch, removing the hypoxic drive to breathe, and displacing CO_2 from hemoglobin into solution in the liquid portion of the blood (Haldane effect) as described above.

Pressure Support Ventilation and Chronic Obstructive Pulmonary Disease

Because most patients with COPD and acute respiratory failure require primarily assistance with inspiration, pressure support ventilation (PSV), as described in detail in Chapter 6, may be a useful mode of ventilation for these individuals. It generally permits the patient to choose their tidal volume, respiratory rate, inspiratory flow, and timing of the respiratory cycle (inspiration and expiration), which enhances comfort and allows one to manage the patient with relatively little sedation and analgesia. There can be a problem, however, with the termination of the pressure support inspiratory assistance.

Historically, the ventilators in PSV mode provide inspiratory assistance until inspiratory flow drops by 25% from the maximal inspiratory flow or below an absolute inspiratory flow of 5 L/min. In patients without airway obstruction, the drop in inspiratory flow occurs fairly rapidly as inspiration reaches its end. In COPD patients, however, the rate of fall in inspiratory flow toward the end of inhalation is less steep. Consequently, the patient may wish to terminate the inspiration, but the ventilator is still attempting to push air into the lungs. This may result in expiratory dyssynchrony, with the patient recruiting expiratory muscles in an effort to push air out while the ventilator is still trying to push air into the patient (see Chapter 18). If the origins of this type of patient discomfort are not recognized, many clinicians will increase the level of PSV, thinking that the problem is not enough support for the patient's inspiration. This will, paradoxically, lead to greater discomfort because it will prolong inspiration even further.

Chronic Hypercapnia, Chronic Obstructive Pulmonary Disease, and the Ventilator

For the patient with COPD who has chronic hypercapnia and develops acute respiratory failure, how does one choose the target $Paco_2$? This is an example of a situation is which a normal value is not actually "normal" for the patient. As discussed in Chapter 3, an elevated $Paco_2$ may minimize the work of breathing for a patient, assuming that the renal system has been able to compensate for the chronic respiratory acidosis and the blood pH is above 7.30. Recall the relationship between alveolar ventilation, CO_2 production, and $Paco_2$:

$$Paco_2 \; \alpha \; \dot{V}co_2 / \dot{V}A$$

This can be transposed to focus on alveolar ventilation:

$$\dot{V}A \; \alpha \; \dot{V}co_2 / Paco_2$$

Thus, the higher the $Paco_2$ for any given amount of CO_2 being produced by the body, the lower the alveolar ventilation needs to be to eliminate all the CO_2 being made as a by-product of metabolism. With a reduced need for alveolar ventilation, total ventilation will be lower as well. If the patient does not have to generate as great a minute ventilation, the work of breathing is reduced, which facilitates weaning the patient from ventilatory support.

SUMMARY

Patients with acute respiratory failure because of COPD can usually be managed fairly easily with mechanical ventilation, but one must be vigilant for a number of issues. Either pressure or volume ventilation is typically acceptable, but one must be vigilant for dynamic hyperinflation. Allowing sufficient time for exhalation, either by reducing respiratory rate or shortening the inspiratory time, is a good strategy for minimizing this problem. If, despite those efforts, dynamic hyperinflation and associated PEEPi result, applied PEEP should be used (at roughly 80% of the PEEPi) to minimize the work associated with inspiration and possible dyssynchrony because of inability to trigger the ventilator.

Ventilation/perfusion mismatch is common in patients with COPD and is typically associated with hypoxemia that is fairly easy to normalize with the use of low-to-moderate levels of supplemental oxygen; one should provide only as much oxygen as needed to maintain O_2 saturation of 89% to 93%. Administration of oxygen, however, may worsen $\dot{V}/\dot{Q}$ mismatch and lead to hypercapnia if total ventilation is fixed. In patients with chronic hypercapnia, one should ventilate the patient in a way that targets $Paco_2$ at or slightly above the patient's baseline level. This will facilitate the patient's ability to breathe off the ventilator after the acute respiratory problem has resolved. PSV is often used to transition patients from ventilatory support to extubation; beware of possible dyssynchrony in these patients because of delayed termination of inhalation.

KEY POINTS

- Be alert for dynamic hyperinflation in patients with COPD and acute respiratory failure.
- Use ventilator strategies that maximize expiratory time to reduce dynamic hyperinflation.
- If PEEPi is present, consider applied PEEP at 80% of the PEEPi to facilitate triggering of the ventilator.
- Use supplemental oxygen to maintain O_2 saturation of 89% to 93%.
- In patients with chronic hypercapnia, target a $Paco_2$ with the ventilator that is equal to or slightly above the patient's baseline $Paco_2$.

STUDY QUESTIONS AND ANSWERS

Questions

1. You are caring for a patient with COPD and acute bronchitis who was intubated and ventilated because of worsening hypercapnia. The chest radiograph shows very large lung volumes and no infiltrate or effusions. The patient is receiving volume ventilation. PEEPi is measured and is found to be 7 cm H_2O. Applied PEEP is set at 5 cm H_2O and the set respiratory rate is 24 breaths/min. O_2 saturation is 90% with F_{IO_2} of 0.4. At this point, what you should consider?
   A. Increase the respiratory rate.
   B. Increase the tidal volume.
   C. Increase the PEEPi.
   D. Decrease the respiratory rate.
   E. Increase the F_{IO_2}.

2. You are caring for a patient with COPD and acute respiratory failure. She is breathing spontaneously with volume ventilation. The respiratory rate is 18 to 22 but she is failing to trigger the ventilator on many of her efforts and is now using accessory muscles of ventilation. What should you now consider?
   A. Assess PEEPi.
   B. Sedate the patient.
   C. Increase the tidal volume.
   D. Increase the backup rate on the ventilator so it is higher than the patient's spontaneous rate.

3. A patient with a history of COPD and heart failure is admitted to the intensive care unit (ICU) with acute respiratory failure. The patient has a long history of obstructive lung disease and frequent pneumonia. At baseline, his Pa_{CO_2} is 65 mm Hg. As you evaluate your intubated, ventilated patient, you obtain arterial blood gas with F_{IO_2} of 0.5; it shows: Pa_{O_2} 85, Pa_{CO_2} 70, pH 7.30. The patient is being ventilated with volume ventilation with tidal volume of 5 mL/kg and respiratory rate 14/min. At this time, what would you consider?
   A. Increase the tidal volume.
   B. Increase the respiratory rate.
   C. Decrease the F_{IO_2}.
   D. Administer bicarbonate.

Answers

1. **Answer D. Decrease the respiratory rate**
   Rationale: The patient likely has dynamic hyperinflation because of severe expiratory resistance and insufficient time for exhalation with a respiratory rate of 24. By reducing the rate, expiratory time will increase, allowing the EELV to be lower. This will reduce the alveolar pressure at end inhalation, which may improve alveolar ventilation (remember, high alveolar pressure may produce dead space by compressing the alveolar capillaries—see Chapter 4 for review). An increase in tidal volume or respiratory rate, which might seem to be appropriate for a rising Pa_{CO_2}, may paradoxically make Pa_{CO_2} worse by leading to even greater hyperinflation and alveolar pressure. Similarly, increasing the applied PEEP, if it goes above the PEEPi, may also worsen hyperinflation. Finally, the present O_2 saturation is adequate, and further increases in F_{IO_2} may worsen hypercapnia by worsening $\dot{V}/\dot{Q}$ mismatch and the Haldane effect.

2. **Answer A. Assess PEEPi**

   Rationale: The patient is failing to trigger the ventilator likely because of the presence of PEEPi, which places a load on the inspiratory muscles. In the presence of PEEPi, the muscles must generate a pressure equal to the PEEPi plus the set trigger threshold to activate the ventilator. One must measure PEEPi and then set applied PEEP at about 80% of PEEPi to reduce the work of breathing. Although sedating the patient may prevent the dyssynchrony by eliminating spontaneous breathing efforts, we always try to minimize sedation, which can lead to delirium and other complications. Increasing tidal volume may worsen dynamic hyperinflation and PEEPi as will providing a higher respiratory rate.

3. **Answer C. Decrease the F_{IO_2}**

   Rationale: The patient's $Paco_2$ is near his baseline level of chronic hypercapnia. Using a $Paco_2$ target that is at or near the baseline level is appropriate to facilitate ultimate weaning from mechanical ventilation and extubation, as long as the kidneys can compensate for the respiratory acidosis. The arterial blood gas is consistent with an acute on chronic respiratory acidosis and a pH of 7.30 should not pose any major risk to the patient. Bicarbonate is not a meaningful buffer for respiratory acid; a proton that binds to bicarbonate becomes carbonic acid, which dissociates to CO_2 and H_2O. Because the CO_2 cannot be removed unless alveolar ventilation is increased, it will accumulate, increase the degree of hypercapnia, and force the chemical reaction in the opposite direction. Increasing the respiratory rate and/or tidal volume may lead to dynamic hyperinflation with worsening gas exchange. Reducing the F_{IO_2} is appropriate because the Pao_2 is higher than needed and may be contributing to the elevated $Paco_2$ by worsening $\dot{V}/\dot{Q}$ mismatch.

Suggested Readings

Panu SR, Dziactzko MA, Gajic O. How much oxygen? Oxygen titration goals during mechanical ventilation. *Am J Respir Crit Care Med.* 2016;193:4-5.

Ranieri VM, Giuliani R, Cinnella G, Pesce C, Brienza N, Ippolito EL, et al. Physiological effects of positive end-expiratory pressure in patients with obstructive pulmonary disease during acute ventilatory failure and controlled mechanical ventilation. *Am Rev Respr Dis.* 1993;147:5-13.

Ranieri VM, Mascia L, Tetruzzelli V, Bruno F, Brienza A, Guiliani R. Inspiratory effort and measurement of dynamic intrinsic PEEP in COPD patients: Effects of ventilator triggering systems. *Intensive Care Med.* 1995;21:896-903.

Mechanical Ventilation for Acute Asthma Exacerbation

Elias Baedorf Kassis

LEARNING OBJECTIVES

- Explain the basic mechanisms of the pathophysiology of asthma.
- Detail the typical clinical picture of life-threatening asthma.
- Describe the pharmacology of the treatment of asthma.
- Explain the use of noninvasive ventilation in acute asthma.
- Explore the concept of dynamic hyperinflation in acute asthma and its impact on plateau pressure measurements with mechanical ventilation.
- Describe the ventilator strategies used for patients with acute respiratory failure with asthma.
- Explore the role of extracorporeal membrane oxygenation (ECMO) in patients with acute respiratory failure with asthma.

INTRODUCTION

The frequency of intubation for asthma exacerbations has thankfully decreased dramatically in recent times. This is primarily due to improved outpatient control of asthma with home use of inhaled beta-agonists, antimuscarinics, steroids, leukotriene receptor agonists, and antibody therapy directed at inflammatory cytokines, particularly for patients with significant eosinophilia, as well as asthma action plans for patients, all of which have decreased the severity and incidence of asthma exacerbations. Although the incidence of patients presenting with status asthmaticus has notably decreased, these types of admissions still occur regularly (particularly in underserved populations with less access to healthcare), and it is imperative that we know how to approach the care for these patients. Severe asthma exacerbations may be life-threatening and result in significant morbidity and mortality if caught too late or improperly treated.

This chapter briefly discusses asthma exacerbations, the medications that form the backbone for severe exacerbations, and the ventilation strategies.

BRIEF BACKGROUND ON ASTHMA

Although this chapter is not a review of asthma, it is worth quickly discussing why asthma exacerbations can lead to severe illness. Asthma is a common condition impacting the airways of the lungs, with a particular effect on the smaller distal bronchioles. Patients with asthma develop inflammation, increased mucus production, and airway smooth muscle contraction, resulting in the narrowing of the airways. This narrowing causes high airway resistance, which leads to impaired flow. As you can imagine, not being able to fully exhale due to slow flow can lead to dyspnea, impaired clearance of CO_2, impaired oxygenation, and breath stacking with dynamic hyperinflation, which can lead to lung injury and hemodynamic compromise; interestingly, most of the dyspnea associated with severe obstructive lung disease is experienced breathing in not out. This probably relates to the fact that inspiration is more active than exhalation and the consequences of dynamic hyperinflation (including reduced compliance of the respiratory system, shortening of the inspiratory muscles, and the development of intrinsic positive end-expiratory pressure [PEEP]). Patients with acute bronchospasm also complain of "chest tightness," which is felt to arise from airway receptors stimulated by bronchoconstriction. As we discuss in this chapter, the primary goal for mechanical ventilation of patients with severe asthma exacerbations is to provide safe levels of gas exchange and ventilation while minimizing the harmful impact of dynamic hyperinflation and giving the patient time for the asthma exacerbation to respond to anti-inflammatory and bronchodilator therapy. It is important to note that mechanical ventilation for asthma is primarily supportive in patients with severe disease and that the "breaking" of the asthma attack is through treatment of asthma itself and elimination of any precipitants that can be identified as having triggered the attack.

PRESENTATION OF LIFE-THREATENING ASTHMA THAT MAY REQUIRE MECHANICAL VENTILATION

Although asthma exacerbations are still common, most are relatively minor and can be addressed at home or with a short visit to the hospital. It is important to identify the subset of patients in whom the exacerbation is more concerning and about whom you should be concerned for the development of possible deterioration and life-threatening event. Although there are no specific signs or predictive scores for this, there are several clinical and laboratory findings that should make you concerned that the patient could be presenting with a potentially life-threatening asthma exacerbation.

Patients with a less severe exacerbation are typically able to speak in full sentences without having to pause to take a breath (reflecting a good vital capacity and the absence of significant tachypnea); consequently, if a patient presents with an inability to talk secondary to the severity of dyspnea, this is a concerning finding. In addition, if patients become fatigued and develop altered mental status, this can be a sign of severe hypercarbia requiring mechanical support: Alternatively, if the $Paco_2$ is rising, it may be evidence of fatigue and should heighten your concern. When exacerbations become sufficiently severe, flow becomes so limited that patients may no longer even have wheezing on examination due to hyperinflation and poor movement of air (wheezes reflect vibration of airways due to turbulent flow; when flow is greatly reduced, there may be insufficient turbulence to generate the sound). Patients will often demonstrate accessory muscle use and intercostal retractions (the latter reflecting the very negative intrathoracic pressure being generated to overcome airway resistance and reduced respiratory system compliance at high lung volume). As the severity of dynamic hyperinflation worsens, intrathoracic pressure may become positive during exhalation to a degree that it will impair venous return, leading to bradycardia, dropping blood pressure, and, in severe cases, even cardiac arrest. Asthmatic patients often become very comfortable checking their own peak flow, and, if this drops below 20% of their predicted or personal best, this is another sign of a life-threatening exacerbation. The presence of any of these findings should make a clinician highly concerned about the patient and make the clinician consider the need for mechanical ventilatory support.

MEDICATIONS

Although this chapter is focused on mechanical ventilation for asthma exacerbations, we quickly touch on the medications available to treat the underlying problem with mechanical ventilation mostly providing enough time for these medications to work.

Inhaled beta-agonist medications represent the backbone of treatment (grade 1B evidence). Albuterol is the most commonly chosen short-acting inhaled agent and the first-line choice. Patients may prefer nebulizer, although metered-dose inhaler (MDI), particularly if used with a spacer, may be equivalent in most patients. When getting to the point of considering mechanical ventilation, however, nebulizers have the advantage of being able to provide continuous support; alternatively, they can be provided as "stacked" dosing, a term that denotes several doses are given in a row (roughly 10 to 15 mg/h dosing).

Inhaled short-acting muscarinic antagonists represent another pillar of treatment for severe acute exacerbations (grade 1B evidence). The typical medication used is ipratropium, which can be delivered via nebulizer, and often is given simultaneously with albuterol. Notably, combined beta-agonists and antimuscarinics is more effective than either in isolation, especially in severe exacerbations. Beta-agonists and antimuscarinics result in smooth muscle relaxation, but they may not relieve the underlying driver of the exacerbation and do nothing to reverse the inflammatory process that is key to poorly controlled asthma and asthma exacerbations.

The use of oral (PO) or intravenous (IV) steroids is supported by the best evidence in acute exacerbations (grade 1A evidence). Where the beta-agonist and antimuscarinic medications temporarily cause smooth muscle relaxation, steroids decrease the underlying inflammation that is ultimately the driver of the exacerbation. Steroids, however, are not immediately effective, and their use in combination with beta-agonists and antimuscarinics is generally required. Of note, a single best dose for steroids has not been identified in the literature; it is clear, however, that the earlier they are initiated, the better the outcomes. In patients with severe life-threatening illness who are at risk for mechanical ventilation, the usual course is IV Solu-Medrol with a dose of 60 to 80 mg Q12 to Q24 hours; some providers advocate for even higher doses upfront. Although many patients may already be receiving inhaled steroids, continuing these during an acute exacerbation when the patient is receiving PO or IV steroids is of unclear benefit.

The use of *magnesium sulfate* during an acute exacerbation is more controversial; there is some evidence for its efficacy, but relatively low-quality data (grade 2C evidence). Magnesium may have bronchodilator effects through inhibition of calcium into airway smooth muscle and, in general, has very minimal side effects and a good safety profile. It should be noted, however, that there is likely less benefit with routine use, and it should be reserved for severe asthma exacerbations. The typical dosing is to give 2 g of IV Mg over 20 minutes.

Most other medications have more limited supporting evidence and cannot be strongly recommended at this point. Ketamine has been used as a sedative adjunct owing to both its sedative effects without respiratory depression and potential bronchodilating effects. Unfortunately, it is important to recognize the poor quality of evidence for its use and that the limited data available suggesting meaningful benefit are mostly in the form of case reports. The typical dose is 0.5 to 1 mg/kg bolus followed by continuous infusion at 0.5 to 2 mg/kg/hour. It can be used to help improve comfort and tolerance of bilevel positive airway pressure (BiPAP) while hoping to provide the patient enough time to bridge to recovery with other standard pharmacologic interventions or it may be considered after intubation in patients who are difficult to ventilate, but the optimal application remains unknown.

Inhaled anesthetics, such as halothane, isoflurane, and sevoflurane, have bronchodilating effects and have also been considered for use during severe exacerbations requiring mechanical ventilation. Currently, there is limited use of these drugs clinically because of the need for an anesthesiologist to remain at bedside, the expense associated with the treatment, and the need for the correct equipment (anesthesia machine) to allow delivery in an intensive care unit (ICU) setting. In addition, inhaled anesthetics may result in side effects including hypotension, which may limit its use in some patients. Although these medications are intriguing, more research is needed before they can be considered routine.

In contrast to inhaled beta-agonists, the data supporting the use of *IV beta-agonists* are less clear. Importantly, the evidence suggests no benefit when these agents are added to inhaled beta-agonists (which most patients will already have been receiving). As such, the use of these preparations should primarily be reserved for patients who are unable to receive inhaled agents, or if there is a severe allergic reaction contributing to the asthma exacerbation (in which case epinephrine would be useful).

Helium-oxygen (more commonly referred to as *Heliox*) is a gas mixture that is available at set oxygen concentrations. Heliox has been thought to be of potential benefit because of the low density of helium that decreases airway resistance by transforming turbulent to laminar flow (**Figure 12-1**); see Chapter 2 for more complete explanation. It should be noted that asthma typically involves the small airways where flow is often already laminar and Heliox would, in theory, work better with larger airway obstruction. Although it is still frequently used for asthma exacerbations, there is no clear role for Heliox in acute asthma before intubation. It should be noted, however, that some data suggest that Heliox may improve the delivery of

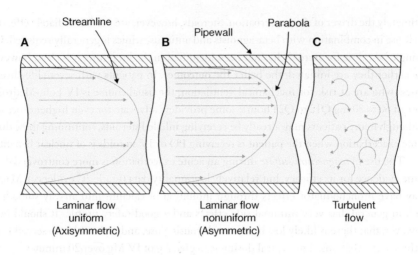

A. Reynolds number < 2000

B. Transient Reynolds number = 2000–4000

C. Turbulent Reynolds number > 4000

Figure 12-1: When gas flows through a tube, it can occur via either laminar flow (with linear movement) or turbulent flow (where flow eddies and does not consistently move in a single direction). The Reynolds number formula determines if a gas moving through a tube moves with linear or turbulent flow and is directly related to the density and velocity of the gas as well as the length of the tube and is inversely related to the viscosity of the gas. A lower Reynolds number would suggest laminar flow (<2000), and higher Reynolds number (>4000) is more likely to be associated with turbulent flow. As such, a lower density gas such as helium would thus have a lower Reynolds number and would result in more laminar flow. Enhanced laminar flow through airways results in lower airway resistance (and reduce work of breathing), which is why helium-oxygen (Heliox) has been postulated to be useful in asthma patients with severe exacerbations.

nebulized medications to deeper lung regions, which could provide some additional benefit; remember, however, Heliox is not considered part of the standard of care for status asthmaticus.

There are several other treatments that are important to highlight, although they are not recommended during acute exacerbations of asthma. Leukotriene receptor antagonists, although effective in chronic asthma, have no role in and there is no evidence for employing them for the treatment during acute exacerbations. Methylxanthines (including theophylline and aminophylline) were formerly considered part of the standard of care; however, there is no clear evidence for additional bronchodilating effect beyond beta-agonists and there are increased adverse events, including vomiting, arrhythmias, and palpitations, along with a narrow toxic to therapeutic range. Lastly, there is no clear evidence for antibiotics unless the exacerbation is clearly secondary to bacterial infection.

BILEVEL POSITIVE AIRWAY PRESSURE IN ASTHMA

The use of BiPAP in asthma is covered in more detail in Chapter 10, which comprehensively covers noninvasive ventilation and high-flow nasal cannula. In brief, there is unfortunately a paucity of evidence to define the role of the use of BiPAP in severe asthma exacerbations.

Despite the lack of evidence, however, BiPAP is still very commonly used during acute presentations and anecdotally has seemed to help bridge patients to recovery without requiring intubation (this has been seen in the clinical practice of the authors as well). BiPAP may theoretically provide benefit for patients by reopening airways collapsed from mucus plugging, improve obstruction, reduce the work of breathing by providing positive pressure to support inhalation and minimizing the work of breathing associated with intrinsic PEEP (see Chapter 7), and, consequently, improve patient comfort and ventilation. These benefits, although physiologically well founded, remain mostly theoretical at this time. In contrast, however, BiPAP might not be helpful (or even be harmful) in some patients by worsening the severity of hyperinflation secondary to the application of higher airway pressures; again, it is unclear in whom and when this harm would occur. The minimal evidence that we do have suggests a potential for improved spirometry and decreased admissions, and a recent large retrospective study (from over 50,000 patients) suggested lower odds of needing mechanical ventilation and lower mortality when using BiPAP, but this has not been tested prospectively. What do we make of this discussion? Despite the lack of definitive evidence, we suggest trying BiPAP in many patients with asthma exacerbations with close monitoring to determine whether they need to be intubated.

INTUBATION DURING ASTHMA EXACERBATION

It is important to recognize that while intubation may be necessary and lifesaving in patients with severe asthma exacerbations, the intubation itself may at times be challenging and result (hopefully only briefly) in decompensation of the patient after initiation of mechanical ventilation. This may occur for several reasons, which we briefly discuss.

The insertion of the endotracheal tube into reactive and sensitive airways may be associated with laryngospasm and worsened bronchoconstriction, which may worsen their obstruction. While many patients with severe asthma exacerbations demonstrate severe flow limitation, some are still relying on their muscles of expiration to augment expiratory flow and improve minute ventilation; with removal of these expiratory efforts, patients may have trouble augmenting their total ventilation as expiration shifts to being fully passive, resulting in higher P_{CO_2} and lower pH. Furthermore, these patients before intubation may have little physiologic reserve, with ramped-up adrenergic tone due to the effort required to breathe. Removal of this drive after intubation (with sedatives and paralytics, which are commonly used) may reduce adrenergic tone (and its effect on the cardiovascular system), and it is very common for intubation and sedation (in addition to the dynamic hyperinflation and intrinsic PEEP associated with asthma, as covered later in this chapter) to result in an acute drop in blood pressure. Consequently, hemodynamic decompensation should be expected in many patients, and preparation for this possibility should be made with a plan in place to address the resulting hypotension.

DYNAMIC HYPERINFLATION

The concept of dynamic hyperinflation (also addressed in Chapters 2 and 7) must be considered when preparing for the impact of severe asthma exacerbations on patients and the subsequent complications that may result. Dynamic hyperinflation (also sometimes referred to as *air trapping* or *breath stacking*, although this latter term has multiple meanings as are discussed in Chapter 18) occurs when an inspiration begins before the prior exhalation is completed

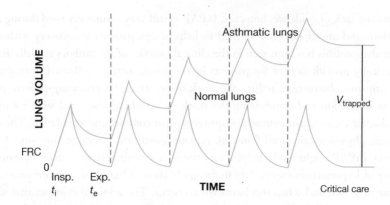

Figure 12-2: This schematic demonstrates lung volume as a function of time comparing a patient with normal lungs and a patient with asthma. The patient with asthma, despite the same initial delivered volume, does not have sufficient time for full exhalation before initiation of the next breath, causing the subsequent breath to be "stacked" on the prior. This results over time in an increase in total lung volumes, the "$V_{trapped}$" in the diagram. This trapped volume represents dynamic hyperinflation, which can lead to barotrauma, pneumothorax, lower lung compliance, impaired CO_2 clearance, and hemodynamic compromise. FRC, functional residual capacity.

(**Figure 12-2**). This means that the patient did not exhale back fully to their relaxation volume, with airway pressure equal to atmospheric pressure or 0, and that, at end expiration, there was still expiratory flow. Dynamic hyperinflation is associated with high levels of measured auto-PEEP (also called *intrinsic PEEP*—see Chapter 7). Recall that if there is residual expiratory flow at end expiration, there has to be a continued pressure gradient driving this flow, and this increased residual pressure within the lungs is the auto-PEEP (see Chapter 7 for more information on auto-PEEP).

The impact of dynamic hyperinflation may be distinct in a spontaneously breathing patient compared with a patient receiving mechanical ventilation. During spontaneous breathing, it becomes progressively more difficult for a patient to take an inspiratory effort as the intrathoracic volumes increase. The diaphragm becomes increasingly ineffective at contraction as it shortens at higher lung volume and the inspiratory effort required to generate inspiratory flow surges. This may lead to the patient tiring out and being unable to maintain sufficient tidal volume and respiratory rate to allow for adequate ventilation.

In mechanically ventilated patients, dynamic hyperinflation will result in increasing mean airway pressures with a different impact in pressure versus volume control settings (as discussed later). Hyperinflation as it worsens may cause direct barotrauma/volutrauma and pneumothorax if it becomes severe. The respiratory system becomes less compliant as end-inspiratory volume increases, which makes the lungs much stiffer than expected; reduced compliance of the lungs in an asthmatic should raise the question for clinicians about potential overdistension from dynamic hyperinflation. In addition, as intrathoracic pressures increase from dynamic hyperinflation, this can impair V̇/Q matching, resulting in increased dead space fraction and worsened CO_2 clearance (see Chapter 3 for more detailed explanation). Furthermore, the high pressures may impair venous return and reduce the cardiac output with hemodynamic effects as well, including bradycardia and hypotension, and, in severe cases, has resulted in cardiac arrest (see Chapter 4 for a discussion of the physiology of this phenomenon). As a reminder, the primary treatment to reduce dynamic hyperinflation is to reduce the airway resistance and lengthen the expiratory time to allow for adequate deflation time as we discuss.

Peak Versus Plateau Pressure Measurements During Asthma Exacerbation

When providing mechanical ventilation support for patients with status asthmaticus, it is very important to be comfortable measuring the peak and plateau pressures and to understand the implications of those measurements (see Chapter 2 for a review of the peak and plateau pressure) (**Figure 12-3**). It is very common for the peak pressures (which reflect both resistive and elastic forces) to be elevated during exacerbations, but in typical asthma exacerbations, the plateau pressure (which reflects only the elastic forces of the lung and chest wall) remains relatively low with a large pressure difference between the peak and plateau pressures. This large peak-plateau pressure gradient is secondary to the high airway resistance from bronchospasm, mucus plugging, and bronchoconstriction. In contrast, when the plateau pressure begins to increase, this may be evidence of worsened dynamic hyperinflation, causing lung overdistension. This overdistension might result in pneumothorax and additional lung injury.

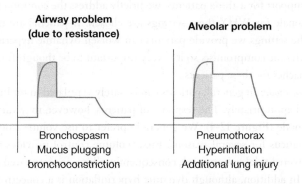

**Airway problem
(due to resistance)**

Alveolar problem

Bronchospasm
Mucus plugging
bronchoconstriction

Pneumothorax
Hyperinflation
Additional lung injury

Figure 12-3: It is important to recognize the difference between the peak pressure and the plateau pressure when monitoring patients with asthma exacerbations. It is common in asthmatic patients to have high airway resistance, resulting in high peak pressures secondary to bronchospasm, mucus plugging, and bronchoconstriction. If the pathology is primarily due to high airway resistance, however, the measured plateau pressure (measured during a breath-hold at end inspiration) will be relatively normal with a large difference in pressure between the peak and plateau measurements. This suggests that although the resistance of the airways is elevated, the underlying lung parenchyma is less impacted and has preserved compliance. In some patients with severe asthma, however, the peak pressure elevation is not JUST due to high airway resistance. Patients' lungs may become stiffer if they have additional lung injury (leading to altered surfactant), if they have developed a pneumothorax, or if they are suffering from dynamic hyperinflation, and in these cases, the plateau pressure (and the resulting driving pressure) will also be elevated more than expected. If this is found, then the clinician needs to be concerned about possible additional barotrauma/volutrauma, investigate why the high plateau pressures are occurring, and adjust the ventilator to counter this development.

MECHANICAL VENTILATION STRATEGIES

After intubation, the main goal for mechanical ventilation is to provide supportive care until the underlying asthma exacerbation has time to resolve sufficiently to allow patients to breathe independently. In a very basic sense, this involves the following goal: provide adequate and safe levels of gas exchange in a way that limits injury to the lungs. In the majority of patients with severe asthma exacerbations, the primary issue with gas exchange is CO_2 removal, with hypoxemia being less of a primary concern (although some patients may have both issues, especially when the asthma exacerbation has been triggered by an additional pulmonary insult such as pneumonia, or in particularly severe cases). Oxygenation goals should target Spo_2 and Pao_2 levels similar to patients with chronic obstructive lung disease (COPD) (oxygen saturation 89% to 92%); limiting overoxygenation may help prevent worsened ventilation-perfusion mismatch and hypercapnia (see Chapter 3 to review details on this process). As mentioned, the usual issue in patients with asthma is maintaining sufficient minute ventilation for safe levels of CO_2 clearance. Permissive hypercapnia (consciously using ventilator settings that allow the $Paco_2$ to be elevated) may be required and helpful in these settings, as it may allow for less intense mechanical ventilation and prevent subsequent injury by limiting the applied pressures and reducing the risk for barotrauma/volutrauma and pneumothorax. Although "safe" thresholds for pH and pco_2 are debatable and not well defined, patients often are able to tolerate a pH as low as 7.2, and in younger healthy patients, this tolerable level may be lower.

Although there is not a single best prescriptive approach to providing mechanical ventilation support for asthma patients, we briefly address the common settings that are used and the rationale for WHY these settings are chosen. If patients are not optimized on the ventilator, the settings we provide patients can worsen dynamic hyperinflation, lung injury, and hemodynamic compromise, so it is very important to be thoughtful, careful, and flexible in our approaches for these patients.

Ventilator mode: In general, patients can be safely ventilated in multiple modes if they are administered appropriately. The response of patients, however, may vary quite a bit depending on the mode (**Figure 12-4**). We generally prefer to use volume control in patients with status asthmaticus for several reasons. First, volume control provides more precise control over the delivered tidal volume and, consequently, allows for improved regulation of minute ventilation. In addition, although dynamic hyperinflation is a concern in any mode, the response to pressure control and volume control modes with respect to dynamic hyperinflation is quite distinct. In volume control, as total intrathoracic volume and pressure increases with each delivered tidal volume (which remain constant), the peak pressure, the plateau pressure, and the driving pressure increase as dynamic hyperinflation worsens, indicating the increased stiffness of the lungs at higher total intrathoracic volume. Consequently, in volume control, it is important to monitor the peak and plateau pressures to ensure that they are within acceptable and safe limits. In pressure control, the applied pressure remains constant, with each breath with increasing auto-PEEP over subsequent breaths actually reducing the driving pressure and reducing the delivered tidal volumes. Although pressure control might allow "safer" control of the pressure that is applied, the reduction in tidal volumes may not allow for as consistent minute ventilation and CO_2 clearance.

Respiratory Rate

Initial settings should aim for as low a respiratory rate as is tolerated empirically by the patient in terms of CO_2 clearance (remember that we can tolerate fairly significant hypercapnia as

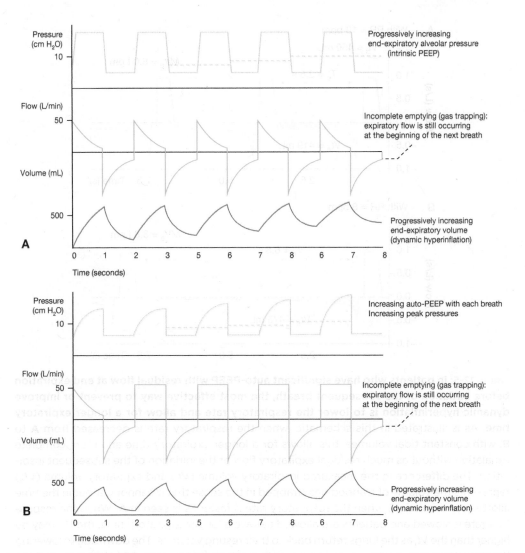

Figure 12-4: The response to dynamic hyperinflation is distinct depending on whether a patient is being managed with pressure control (A) or volume control (B)—in both situations, we depict applied PEEP by the ventilator. In pressure control (A), the applied pressure during inspiration is held constant with each delivered breath, resulting in minimal change in the inspiratory pressure. As dynamic hyperinflation leads to incomplete emptying with each breath, the intrinsic PEEP leads to progressively higher measured or total PEEP, resulting in a lower driving pressure. In the volume channel, however, the total lung volume at end inspiration remains the same, but with incomplete emptying, the tidal volumes get smaller in size and the end-expiratory thoracic volume increases. Pressure control may prevent high peak pressures but may make control over total minute ventilation more challenging. In contrast, volume control (B) shows the tidal volumes remaining constant as dynamic hyperinflation worsens. This leads to both an increase in the peak pressures and end-expiratory pressure (the measured PEEP). Although it may be easier to control the minute ventilation in these patients, they may be at higher risk for barotrauma/volutrauma with the increasing pressure associated with worsening dynamic hyperinflation. PEEP, positive end-expiratory pressure.

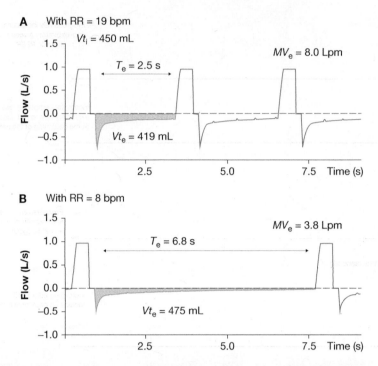

Figure 12-5: In patients who have significant auto-PEEP with residual flow at end expiration before initiation of the subsequent breath, the most effective way to prevent or improve dynamic hyperinflation is to lower the respiratory rate and allow for a longer expiratory time. As is illustrated in this schematic, when the respiratory rate is decreased from **A** to **B**, with constant tidal volumes, this allows for a longer expiratory time and more complete exhalation without as much residual expiratory flow at the initiation of the subsequent inspiration. The difference in the measured inspiratory volume (Vt_i) and expiratory volume (Vt_e) represents the volume of trapped gas (trapped in the sense that it cannot get out in the time allotted for exhalation) when the respiratory rate is faster as is seen in **A**. When the respiratory rate is slowed and patients are allowed to have a longer expiratory time, the Vt_e may be higher than the Vt_i as the lungs return back to their resting volumes. The downside to lowering the respiratory rate is a lower minute ventilation, which may worsen CO_2 clearance, and the decision to change the rate is often a balance between the severity of hypercapnia and the desire to protect the lungs against further injury from overdistension. PEEP, positive end-expiratory pressure. (From Junhasavasdikul D, Telias I, Grieco DL, Chen L, Gutierrez CM, Piraino T, Brochard L. Expiratory flow limitation during mechanical ventilation. *Chest*. 2018;154(4): 948-962. doi: 10.1016/j.chest.2018.01.046. Epub 2018 Feb 9. PMID: 29432712.)

long as the kidney can compensate for the respiratory acidosis by secreting acid from the distal tubule and the Pco₂ is not so high that it alters the patient's level of awareness). This will allow for the longest possible exhalation time, reduce the severity of auto-PEEP, and reduce the subsequent dynamic hyperinflation (**Figure 12-5**). Typical initial respiratory rate is roughly 10 to 12 bpm; although, if hypercapnia is not an issue, this can be titrated lower in some cases.

Tidal Volume

A safe initial default is to use typical lung-protective tidal volumes in the 6 to 8 mL/kg range. There are no data to define the optimal range in asthma patients, but this represents a likely safe initial goal and then titration can occur thereafter as needed for the individual patient.

Some patients with higher compliance may be able to tolerate marginally larger volumes, but it is important to remember that as the volumes increase, it takes longer for full exhalation to occur, so increasing the volumes too high can worsen auto-PEEP and dynamic hyperinflation. Indeed, smaller tidal volumes are generally preferred in severe asthma cases to limit volutrauma and lung injury. Recall that minute ventilation is the product of respiratory rate and tidal volume and that both of these variables can impact dynamic hyperinflation, requiring a delicate balance during clinical care.

Inspiratory Time and Flow

In order to maximize the expiratory time, the set inspiratory time can be reduced in some patients to allow for more rapid delivery of the breath and more time (within a set respiratory rate) for exhalation to occur. This will result in increased inspiratory flow (remember, tidal volume divided by inspiratory time equals inspiratory flow—if inspiratory time is reduced and tidal volume is held constant, inspiratory flow must increase), however, which will result in increased peak pressures for any given airway resistance; in some cases, this will limit how much adjustment is possible with the inspiratory time and flow.

Positive End-Expiratory Pressure

In general, there is minimal benefit from higher levels of set PEEP in patients with status asthmaticus. When patients are fully passive (meaning no spontaneous efforts), PEEP is typically set to lower levels to reduce the total applied pressures. As patients begin to breathe spontaneously, the PEEP may, in some cases, need to be slightly increased to "match" their measured auto-PEEP and make it easier for them to initiate (and have the ventilator sense) an inspiratory effort. The classic teaching is to set the PEEP to roughly 80% of the total measured PEEP; like many other teachings, however, this is not based on quality evidence, and the PEEP setting should be titrated to the individual patient based on gas exchange and patient comfort.

Fio$_2$

As is typical for any mechanically ventilated patient, the Fio$_2$ should be as low as tolerated to provide adequate O$_2$ saturations and appropriate Pao$_2$ and Paco$_2$. In patients with hypercapnia, this is particularly important because hyperoxia can worsen CO$_2$ retention (in a similar manner to COPD) by worsening ventilation-perfusion mismatch (see Chapter 3).

Pressure Limits

To limit the negative impact of dynamic hyperinflation, typical "lung-protective" settings and parameters should be maintained. Although the plateau pressure limit of 30 cm H$_2$O is not a data-driven value, it is generally a good target to utilize when determining the safety of mechanical ventilation in asthmatics. Similarly, the goal driving pressure cutoff of 15 cm H$_2$O is also an appropriate target. If either of these are above the goal, it raises concern for dynamic hyperinflation, resulting in overdistension and lung injury and may increase the risk for the development of pneumothorax.

EXTRACORPOREAL MEMBRANE OXYGENATION

So what should we do if we have optimized the ventilator, but our patient is demonstrating evidence of barotrauma with high peak and plateau pressures or pneumothorax, or that we are still unable to provide adequate or safe ventilation? In this case, we should consider the

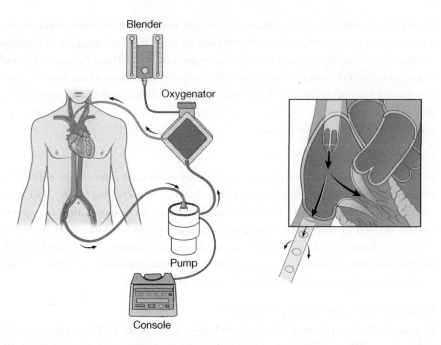

Figure 12-6: Schematic showing how the ECMO circuit functions. This demonstrates a two-site cannulation approach with cannulation of the internal jugular (IJ) and the femoral veins. Single-site cannulation (in the right IJ with a specialty catheter) or central cannulation directly into the heart is less commonly used. Deoxygenated venous blood is removed from the patient by the drainage cannula (typically in the femoral). A centrifugal pump creates flow through the "artificial lung" where the blood is oxygenated and carbon dioxide is removed. This oxygenated blood is then returned to the patient's venous system and pumped systemically via the patient's native cardiac function. ECMO may be very effective in severe cases of asthma by allowing lung rest, thereby preventing further lung injury while the underlying asthma exacerbation is given time to resolve. ECMO, extracorporeal membrane oxygenation.

initiation of extracorporeal membrane oxygenation (ECMO) or extracorporeal CO_2 removal (ECCOR). We do not delve too far into ECMO and ECCOR, but, briefly, these systems allow for gas exchange (O_2 and/or CO_2 regulation), independent from the lungs (**Figure 12-6**). In patients with asthma, ECMO will allow for full lung rest, preventing the propagation of further lung injury until the patient's airway resistance improves (see Figure 12-6). Although there is limited evidence for its use in patients with status asthmaticus, there is clear clinical benefit in selected patients. ECMO in asthma is one of the more satisfying and noncontroversial applications because the required course of ECMO is typically much shorter than when it is employed in acute respiratory distress syndrome (ARDS), which may lead to better clinical outcomes as recovery from the primary respiratory problem is more assured.

In particular, you should be considering the use of ECMO, or the transfer to an ECMO-capable center if (1) you are having persistent issues with adequate ventilation (meaning the $Paco_2$ remains very high on arterial blood gas [ABG] measurements), (2) there are negative effects due to the severity of hypercapnia (such as hemodynamic compromise), or (3) there is evidence of lung injury (such as pneumothorax) or risk for lung injury (high peak and plateau pressures). When the decision is made to initiate ECMO, ultra-lung rest settings may be applied with very slow respiratory rate at 5 breaths/min, reduced inspiratory flow to limit peak pressures, and very small tidal volumes and long expiratory times to limit dynamic hyperinflation. As patients begin to improve, the measured resistance will decrease, and patients can be slowly weaned from mechanical ventilation and decannulated and removed from ECMO.

SUMMARY

The management of severe asthma exacerbations and status asthmaticus involves a combination of bronchodilators and anti-inflammatory medication, an initial trial of BiPAP if the patient is sufficiently stable, and a low threshold for intubation and mechanical ventilation in patients who are failing to respond to therapy. Once the patient is intubated and mechanically ventilated, the goal should be to provide adequate gas exchange with permissive hypercapnia as needed, protecting the lungs from injury while allowing time for the underlying asthma exacerbation to break. Careful control of the respiratory rate, the tidal volumes, and the PEEP is required to prevent dynamic hyperinflation, thereby reducing the risk of barotrauma and pneumothorax in these patients. If despite these strategies, either the gas exchange remains dangerously impaired or there is evidence of ventilatory-induced lung injury, ECMO may be needed in some cases to rest the lungs and allow time for resolution of the exacerbation.

KEY POINTS

- Recognition of severe life-threatening asthma exacerbations is of critical importance, in particular looking for evidence of difficulty speaking, significant tachypnea, significant accessory muscle use, altered mental status, hypercapnia, or hemodynamic instability.
- Medications including beta-agonists, antimuscarinics, and steroids have the best data for use in acute exacerbations, whereas additional agents such as magnesium, ketamine, or inhaled sedation may be considered on an individual basis.
- The primary goal of using BiPAP or invasive ventilation is to give the patient time for the medications to work and the exacerbation to "break," while preventing the patient from injuring their own lungs or developing hemodynamic compromise.
- BiPAP has limited prospective data for its use, but can be considered in many patients with acute exacerbations because of the physiologic rationale for benefit.
- Dynamic hyperinflation is the primary cause of lung injury and hemodynamic compromise in severe asthma, and ventilation strategies should be targeted at limiting this potential harm.
- During mechanical ventilation, there is no established "best" practice; however, the goal should be to prevent dynamic hyperinflation by balancing tidal volume and respiratory rate and tolerating permissive hypercapnia.
- If conventional mechanical ventilation is unable to keep patients safe while waiting for the exacerbation to "break," then support with ECMO should be considered to allow the lungs to rest without further injury until the exacerbation improves.

STUDY QUESTIONS AND ANSWERS

Questions

1. A patient intubated for asthma is mechanically ventilated with volume control and now has peak pressures that have increased from 28 to 36 cm H_2O with the plateau pressure remaining the same. What does this change in value suggest?
   A. The patient is showing evidence of dynamic hyperinflation.
   B. The patient developed a pneumothorax.
   C. The patient's airway resistance is increasing.
   D. The patient is developing a superimposed pneumonia.
   E. All of the above.

2. A patient with asthma mechanically ventilated on volume control develops increased peak pressures without any other changes to the ventilator. When the plateau pressure is checked, it is also noted that this has increased as well. Which of the following clinical causes would you be concerned about?
   A. Pneumothorax
   B. Barotrauma
   C. Dynamic hyperinflation
   D. Pneumonia
   E. All of the above

3. A 36-year-old otherwise healthy patient with asthma who is deeply sedated is being mechanically ventilated on volume control without any spontaneous breathing with 400-mL tidal volumes, respiratory rate of 24 breaths/min, FIO_2 40%, and PEEP 8 cm H_2O. The compliance is measured, and the lungs appear stiff at 25 mL/cm H_2O. An ABG demonstrates pH 7.28, PCO_2 72 mm Hg, and PaO_2 75 mm Hg. An expiratory breath-hold is performed, and a total PEEP of 14 cm H_2O is measured. The nurse notes that the patient's blood pressure has been slowly dropping over the last 20 minutes and they have had to go up on her IV vasopressors. What is the next best step?
   A. Increase the respiratory rate.
   B. Increase the tidal volume.
   C. Increase the PEEP.
   D. Decrease the respiratory rate.
   E. Decrease the tidal volume.

4. A 42-year-old man with long-standing asthma is intubated after presenting with status asthmaticus and failing a brief trial of BiPAP. Several hours after intubation, the team notes that the patient has decreased breath sounds over the right lung. The peak pressure has also increased to 56 cm H_2O and the plateau is 34 cm H_2O, despite trials to optimize the tidal volume (currently with tidal volumes set to 5 mL/kg) and respiratory rate (currently set to 12 breaths/min). The $PaCO_2$ remains elevated at 96 mm Hg with pH 7.05. A chest radiograph reveals a new right pneumothorax. What should be the next consideration for the patient in addition to placing a chest tube?
   A. Continuing current ventilator settings.
   B. Increasing respiratory rate to increased minute ventilation.
   C. Adding inhaled anesthetic agents.
   D. Referring to ECMO center or calling for local ECMO consult.
   E. All of the above.

Answers

1. **Answer C. The patient's airway resistance is increasing**

   Rationale: The patient likely has had an increase in airway resistance, causing the increase in peak pressure without any change in the plateau pressure. A large difference between the peak and plateau pressures suggests a change in airway resistance. The resistance is calculated as the pressure difference between peak and plateau divided by the flow, demonstrating how the increased pressure difference would be suggestive of increased resistance. The other answer choices are incorrect as these would only result in both an increase in peak pressures and plateau pressure (see Chapter 2).

2. **Answer E. All of the above**

   Rationale: Each of the options listed can cause lower compliance (increased stiffness) of the lungs.

3. **Answer D. Decrease the respiratory rate**

   Rationale: The patient is showing concerning findings for dynamic hyperinflation and breath stacking, with low compliance, high levels of auto-PEEP, and hemodynamic effects. Although the patient is already suffering from a respiratory acidosis, the dynamic hyperinflation itself may be further worsening CO_2 clearance with a further worsening of the dead space fraction as well. Consequently, you might worry about lowering the respiratory rate and causing a decrease in minute ventilation, which could further worsen the P_{CO_2}. The negative impact of dynamic hyperinflation, however, is the biggest immediate concern, and we will have to tolerate permissive hypercapnia in order to protect the lungs. A respiratory rate of 24 may be faster than the patient can tolerate, resulting in incomplete exhalation before the next delivered breath; this will cause dynamic hyperinflation. Lowering the respiratory rate will allow for longer expiratory time and gives the best chance to improve the dynamic hyperinflation. Choice A, Increase the respiratory rate, is wrong as the patient is already showing dynamic hyperinflation, which would only worsen with a higher breathing rate. Choice B, Increase the tidal volume, is wrong as the larger volumes, although increasing minute ventilation, may further worsen the hyperinflation. Choice C, Increase the PEEP, is wrong; while this may be needed at some point when the patient is spontaneously breathing, to help with triggering the ventilator as the patient's asthma is improving, the best current strategy is to reduce the auto-PEEP by decreasing the respiratory rate. Choice E, Decrease the tidal volume, may be needed and is not wrong per se, but it is not the next step that should be made in the care of this patient. Decreasing the tidal volume may be needed if the compliance remains low and you are concerned about causing barotrauma. The first step, however, should be to lower the respiratory rate.

4. **Answer D. Referring to ECMO center or calling for local ECMO consult**

   Rationale: This patient is demonstrating a failure of the current ventilator settings. Despite small tidal volume (5 mL/kg) and low respiratory rate (12 breath/min), the patient still developed a pneumothorax and has very high plateau pressures, which may result in further barotrauma. In addition, the patient is still not achieving adequate ventilation. Consequently, this is a patient who would likely benefit from ECMO evaluation, which could allow for ultraprotective ventilation strategies. Choice A, Continuing current ventilator settings, is

(continued)

STUDY QUESTIONS AND ANSWERS *(continued)*

incorrect as these settings are not providing adequate gas exchange and are still resulting in barotrauma. Choice B, Increasing the respiratory rate, is incorrect as this could worsen dynamic hyperinflation, which is likely the primary cause of the pneumothorax. Choice C, Adding inhaled anesthetics, is incorrect. While these medications may be considered, their use is not presently standard of care, and the severity of the impaired gas exchange and the existing barotrauma would make ECMO a better next step.

Suggested Readings

Althoff MD, Holguin F, Yang F, et al. Noninvasive ventilation use in critically ill patients with acute asthma exacerbations. *Am J Respir Crit Care Med*. 2020;202(11):1520-1530. doi:10.1164/rccm.201910-2021OC.

Kirkland SW, Vandenberghe C, Voaklander B, Nikel T, Campbell S, Rowe BH. Combined inhaled beta-agonist and anticholinergic agents for emergency management in adults with asthma. *Cochrane Database Syst Rev*. 2017;1(1):CD001284. doi:10.1002/14651858.CD001284.pub2.

Acute Respiratory Distress Syndrome

Elias Baedorf Kassis • Jakub Glowala

LEARNING OBJECTIVES

- List the Berlin criteria for the diagnosis of acute respiratory distress syndrome (ARDS).
- Identify the major pulmonary and extrapulmonary causes of ARDS.
- Identify the unifying histopathologic and radiologic features across various causes of ARDS.
- Identify the therapeutic goals in support of patients with ARDS.
- Explain the mechanisms by which ARDS makes lungs vulnerable to further damage.
- Link therapeutic interventions with the mechanisms by which they minimize lung damage in ARDS.
- Describe emerging concepts in the fields of acute lung injury (ALI) and ARDS.

INTRODUCTION TO ACUTE RESPIRATORY DISTRESS SYNDROME

The acute respiratory distress syndrome (ARDS) is a syndrome culminating in severe hypoxic respiratory failure. It represents a constellation of signs and symptoms that appear to converge into the clinical picture known as *ARDS* but almost certainly represents the culmination of a variety of underlying diseases and pathophysiologic mechanisms. This is evidenced by the expansive differential diagnosis for causes of ARDS ranging from infection, trauma, pancreatitis, transfusion-associated lung injury, to many more, which we discuss in detail later in this chapter. Our increasing understanding of the complexity of the pathophysiology of ARDS and the associated overlapping phenotypes has also given rise to increased investigation of more complex monitoring tools, treatments, and reconceptualization of the concept of "lung protection" as we manage the ventilator.

Ultimately, ARDS is a consequence of an underlying disease process that triggers injury and inflammation in the lungs. This inflammatory syndrome causes the lungs to become extremely sensitive to biomechanical stressors. Although investigations are ongoing to find ways to directly modulate this inflammatory cascade, significant strides have been made in designing ventilator strategies to minimize biomechanical stress while maintaining adequate respiratory support and oxygenation concurrently with treatment of the underlying disease process. Though morbidity and mortality from ARDS are still significant, progress is evidenced by steadily improving outcomes owing to careful attention to the mechanistic guidelines, which are discussed later in this chapter.

DIAGNOSTIC CRITERIA

The latest diagnostic criteria for ARDS, the 2012 Berlin criteria, are summarized in **Table 13-1**. Briefly, they categorize ARDS as acute onset of hypoxemia within a week of a clinical insult

TABLE 13-1 Berlin Criteria for the Diagnosis of Acute Respiratory Distress Syndrome

Respiratory symptoms must have begun within 1 week of a known clinical insult OR the patient must have new or worsening symptoms during the past week.

Bilateral opacities consistent with pulmonary edema must be present on a chest radiograph or computed tomography (CT) scan.
These opacities must not be fully explained by pleural effusions, lobar collapse, lung collapse, or pulmonary nodules.

A moderate-severe impairment of oxygenation must be present, as defined by the ratio of arterial oxygen tension to fraction of inspired oxygen (Pa_{O_2}/F_{IO_2}). The severity of the hypoxemia defines the severity of the ARDS:
- Mild ARDS: The Pa_{O_2}/F_{IO_2} is >200 mm Hg, but ≤300 mm Hg, on ventilator settings that include positive end-expiratory pressure (PEEP) or continuous positive airway pressure (CPAP) ≥5 cm H_2O.
- Moderate ARDS: The Pa_{O_2}/F_{IO_2} is >100 mm Hg, but ≤200 mm Hg, on ventilator settings that include PEEP ≥5 cm H_2O.
- Severe ARDS: The Pa_{O_2}/F_{IO_2} is ≤ 100 mm Hg on ventilator setting that includes PEEP ≥ 5 cm H_2O.

Derived from ARDS Definition Task Force; Ranieri VM, Rubenfeld GD, Thompson BT, et al. Acute respiratory distress syndrome: the Berlin Definition. *JAMA.* 2012;307(23):2526-2533.

known to cause ARDS with bilateral opacities on radiographic imaging that leads to respiratory failure necessitating mechanical ventilation with at least 5 cm H_2O positive end-expiratory pressure (PEEP). After excluding cardiogenic pulmonary edema, lung nodules, pleural effusions or atelectasis of the lung as the primary cause of this hypoxemia, and bilateral imaging abnormalities, the diagnosis is made by the ratio of the partial pressure of oxygen (Pao_2) to the fraction of inspired oxygen (Fio_2) (the Pao_2/Fio_2 ratio), with ARDS being defined as a value less than 300 mm Hg. Further stratification of the severity of ARDS can be made based on the Pao_2/Fio_2 range. It is worth noting that many patients with focal pneumonia, chronic obstructive pulmonary disease (COPD), asthma exacerbations, and other acute cardiopulmonary conditions will have a P/F ratio less than 300 but are not considered to have ARDS because they do not meet the other clinical criteria necessary for the diagnosis.

RADIOLOGIC FINDINGS

As the diagnosis of ARDS requires suggestive radiographic imaging, we briefly review the characteristic findings. Chest x-rays (CXRs) are generally sufficient for the diagnosis, but given the need to exclude other potential causes of hypoxemic respiratory failure, computed tomography (CT) can be used interchangeably in the hospital setting. On plain films of the chest, the most common findings are diffuse alveolar opacities in bilateral lung fields. Although any bilateral distribution can meet ARDS criteria, the opacities can often be found particularly in the dependent regions of the lung (see **Figure 13-1**). CT findings correspond similarly with widespread opacities that can range from ground-glass appearance to consolidative depending on the timing and severity of the ARDS. Importantly, the definitions of ARDS do not specify what types and pattern of opacities are required for a diagnosis of ARDS so long as they are bilateral and not explained by nodules, edema, pleural effusions, or collapse alone.

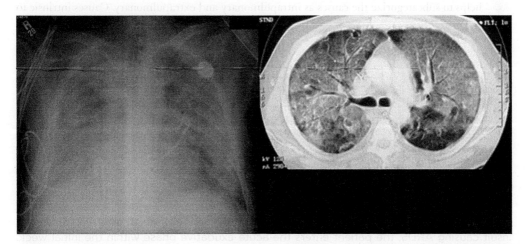

Figure 13-1: **ARDS imaging**. Imaging examples of ARDS with the requisite bilateral opacities. On chest x-ray alone, it may be challenging in all patients to exclude cardiogenic pulmonary edema or nodules. Chest computed tomography can also be used, which may improve diagnostic accuracy in some patients. Multiple different patterns and distributions of disease can be seen in ARDS with either homogenous or heterogeneous distribution, and opacities ranging from ground glass to denser consolidation. ARDS, acute respiratory distress syndrome.

PATHOPHYSIOLOGY

Ultimately, all patients with ARDS suffer from hypoxemic respiratory failure; the pathophysiologic cause of hypoxemia is intrapulmonary shunt. In some patients, and particularly as the severity of the condition worsens, clearance of CO_2 may also be impaired, resulting in additional hypercarbic respiratory failure as well. It should come as no surprise that this impairment in gas exchange correlates with histologic findings of alveolar dysfunction and injury.

ARDS typically proceeds through a series of three phases: an exudative, organizing, and fibrotic phase (**Figure 13-2**). The acute stage is characterized by exudation in the first 12 to 24 hours and can generally last through the initial week, but may be longer in some types of ARDS, particularly if there is ongoing injury. In this stage, the lung tends to have significant inflammation, and this may be the period in which it is most vulnerable. Toward the end of the first week and into the second week after initial injury, the subacute phase begins, which is characterized by the formation of granulation tissue and expansion of fibroblasts and myofibroblasts as the prior injury begins to organize. After this phase begins the chronic stage or fibrotic phase of the disease, which typically begins at weeks 3 to 4 after the initial injury. After roughly 2 to 4 weeks, the fibrotic stage is complete with the formation of granulation tissue, scarring, and fibrosis. The more severe and longer duration the ARDS, the worse this fibrosis tends to be in this final stage. More localized and heterogeneous damage can also be seen in some patients. Importantly, these three stages can be modified through proper treatment, and improvement may occur before significant fibrosis develops; the goal of ventilation strategies is to avoid ongoing lung injury and evolution to the fibrotic phase and allow for lung healing and recovery.

CAUSES OF ACUTE RESPIRATORY DISTRESS SYNDROME

ARDS carries an expansive differential diagnosis; to approach the etiologies systematically, it helps to subcategorize the causes as intrapulmonary and extrapulmonary. Causes intrinsic to

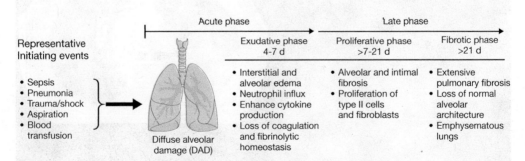

Figure 13-2: Pathology of ARDS and course of progression through stages. After the initial insult causing ARDS, the patient enters the acute exudative phase within the initial week. As the underlying diffuse alveolar damage begins to organize and heal, the patient enters the proliferative phase typically within the first 3 weeks. If patients' lung injury is severe, patients may then enter the late phase (fibrotic phase) after the initial 2 to 4 weeks of illness. The goal of lung-protective ventilation and treatment of patients with ARDS is to divert the path of recovery away from fibrosis toward healing, although this is not always possible depending on the severity of the presenting ARDS. ARDS, acute respiratory distress syndrome.

TABLE 13-2 Causes of Acute Respiratory Distress Syndrome	
Direct Lung Injury	**Indirect Lung Injury**
Pneumonia (bacteria, virus, fungi, parasites)	Sepsis and septic shock
Aspiration of gastric content	Multiple trauma
Air or fat emboli	Acute pancreatitis
Toxic inhalation	Massive transfusion
Near drowning	Transfusion-related acute lung injury
Lung contusion	Drug toxicity
Reperfusion after lung transplantation or thrombectomy	Neurogenic pulmonary edema
	Cardiopulmonary bypass

Aggravating common factors: fluid overload, hypervolemia, and increased intra-abdominal pressure.
Derived from Kollef MH, Schuster DP. The acute respiratory distress syndrome. *N Engl J Med*. 1995;332(1):27-37.

the lungs include pneumonia, aspiration, transfusion-related acute lung injury (TRALI), and post–lung transplant. Conceptually, the unifying theme in these causes of ARDS is a *localized* hyperinflammatory reaction to either infection, caustic chemicals, or foreign antigens. Extrapulmonary causes of ARDS are even broader and include any *systemic* hyperinflammatory reactions, including sepsis, drugs and alcohol, severe trauma, and massive transfusion. A more expansive list of causes is summarized in **Table 13-2**, but it is worth emphasizing that these various causes likely represent different pathophysiologic mechanisms that converge to produce a similar phenotype, or syndrome, known as *ARDS*.

CLINICAL OUTCOMES

The wide variability in both histopathologic and radiographic findings also mirrors the divergent outcomes experienced by patients with ARDS. Depending on the severity of the ARDS, mortality has ranged from 27% to 45%, though improvements mostly in ventilator management have seen that the number slowly decline year to year up until the COVID pandemic. Mortality, interestingly, is not usually due to respiratory failure; rather, most succumb to sepsis, ventilator-associated pneumonia, or multiorgan failure. There is evidence that systemic inflammation associated with lung injury contributes to multisystem organ failure in these patients. Ventilating patients in ways that minimize lung injury, consequently, may reduce mortality.

Patients may experience debilitating depression, post-traumatic stress disorder, and declines in functional capacity. There is increasing evidence that the ways in which we manage the ventilator, analgesia, and sedation in these individuals may contribute to the emotional and behavioral complications noted after recovery from respiratory failure.

LUNG INJURY IN ACUTE RESPIRATORY DISTRESS SYNDROME

The principal goal of therapy during mechanical ventilation for patients with ARDS, considering the lack of disease-modifying medications, is supportive care that minimizes additional injury to the lungs. The lungs of a patient with ARDS are particularly vulnerable to further injury due to the severe inflammatory response, reduction in lung compliance, and the need for high levels of ventilator support. Injury to the lungs has been characterized as "ventilator-induced lung injury" (VILI), based on studies indicating that some approaches to mechanical ventilation are associated with higher mortality rates; we review ventilator management strategies that reduce this risk in the subsequent section, but a newer understanding of lung mechanics and ARDS pathophysiology suggests that "self-inflicted lung injury" (P-SILI), that is, injury due to the patient's own breathing efforts, may also be important. Ultimately, however, VILI and P-SILI likely cause injury through the same mechanical and inflammatory pathways as we discuss later in this chapter.

VENTILATOR-INDUCED LUNG INJURY

A common framework, which we utilize to review the mechanisms of lung injury, for thinking about VILI stems from the concept of the "baby lung" of ARDS. Owing to the overwhelming inflammatory response and microvascular injury to the alveoli-capillary interface, only a fraction of the lung is functionally available for gas exchange. This is due to both portions of the lung having dysfunctional alveolar-capillary interfaces and consolidation as well as collapse and derecruitment of regions of the lung from reduced surfactant activity. Depending on various interventions, such as positioning and PEEP titration, the baby lung can be expanded by recruiting additional lung units, or even completely different regions of the lung, to participate in gas exchange. The important takeaway from this concept, though, is that depending on the severity of the ARDS, we are ventilating a patient's "baby lung" and not the entirety of their actual lung parenchyma. With that in mind, there are various mechanisms by which mechanical ventilation can induce lung injury and why the baby lung is particularly vulnerable. VILI is the "classic" concept for understanding lung injury and involves the related, though distinct concepts of overdistension, termed *volutrauma*, injury from cyclic lung collapse/reopening known as *atelectrauma*, and the resulting biotrauma, which are discussed later (**Figure 13-3**).

Overdistension Injury

Broadly speaking, patients who are mechanically ventilated receive a specified volume of air, which results in a certain pressure, or air is pushed into the lung at specified pressure, resulting in a certain volume. Because patients with ARDS have such significantly reduced functional lung, even "normal" volumes of air can excessively distend alveoli, causing volutrauma or damage due to excess volume. This form of injury can be conceptualized by discussing lung strain. **Strain** refers to the relative volumetric deformation of an area of lung relative to its resting volume. Inflating any area of the lung out of proportion to its resting volume can, therefore, cause strain and volutrauma. If the volumes are excessive, or even if they are appropriate for usual circumstances, the decreased compliance of the lungs (stiffness) can lead to significant pressure delivery to the lungs. The injury secondary to these high pressures is known as *barotrauma*, but as should be self-evident, barotrauma and volutrauma are inherently linked, albeit separate concepts (remember: compliance = change in volume/change in pressure). Conceptually, barotrauma is caused by excess **stress**, or change in pressure, across the lung (ie, transmural pressure or pressure in the alveolus minus the pressure in the pleural space—note: high pressure in the lung when there is a similarly high pressure in the pleural space, as occurs when you scuba dive, does not cause lung injury).

Strain can refer to either the total stress applied over an entire breath (estimated by the end-inspiratory pressure) or the cyclical stress applied by pressure changes over a series of

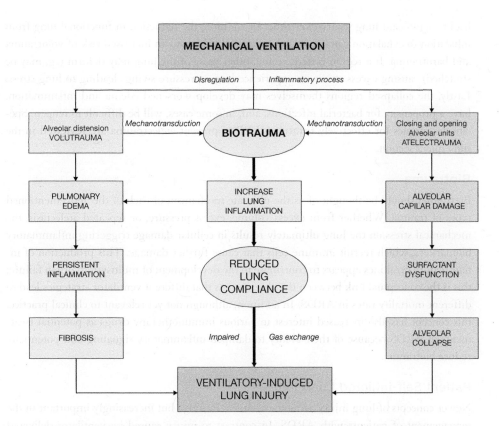

Figure 13-3: A conceptual schematic of ventilator-induced lung injury (VILI). Mechanical injury (both injury from overdistension and injury from collapse) is the primary type of injury caused by mechanical ventilation with secondary injury from inflammation (called *biotrauma*). Overdistension injury occurs from injurious volumes (known as *volutrauma*) and injurious pressure swings across the lungs. Injury from collapse is known as *atelectrauma* and occurs both from the collapse itself and the cyclic opening and closing of the alveoli and airways resulting in injurious shear stress. Mechanical injury worsens biotrauma, which, in turn, makes the lungs more sensitive to further mechanical injury. Much of the focus on "lung-protective ventilation" is on the limitation of mechanical trauma to prevent VILI and allow for improved recovery of the lungs during mechanical ventilation.

breaths (estimated by the driving pressure, which is further discussed later). Injury from overdistension (as we collectively refer to *volutrauma and barotrauma*) can occur if a patient is receiving too much volume relative to the size of their "baby lung." Overdistension can cause inflammatory damage to the already vulnerable lungs of patients with ARDS.

Atelectrauma

Atelectrauma should be understood as lung injury due to the collapse of the alveoli and airways during exhalation, with recurrent opening during the delivery of each new breath. If, during delivery of a breath, there is recruitment of a region of the lung but insufficient PEEP to maintain lung opening, then that area of the lung will collapse during exhalation. In the process of the lung reopening, very high levels of local shear stress cause local pressure injury along the airways and alveoli as they are "ripped" open. This recurring alveolar trauma can lead to significant lung injury over time. In addition, the reduction in functional lung from inhalation to exhalation can expose other regions of lung to an increased risk of volutrauma and barotrauma. If a region is derecruited, other parts of the lung may deform (eg, may be stretched) causing excess strain, or experience larger pressure swings leading to lung stress. Lastly, the collapsed regions themselves may develop worsened edema and inflammation, have a propensity for bacterial infections, and, in some cases, will be difficult to reopen. Specific techniques for effectively titrating PEEP to prevent atelectrauma are reviewed in the subsequent section.

Biotrauma

Biotrauma should be thought of as the ultimate mechanism of each of the abovementioned types of trauma. Whether from excess volume, excess pressure, or repeated atelectasis, the mechanical stress on the lung ultimately results in cellular damage triggering inflammatory biomarkers, which recruit immune cells that cause further damage. This production of inflammatory cytokines appears to contribute to the development of multisystem organ failure; this is the conceptual link between the observations that different ventilator strategies lead to different mortality rates in ARDS. In addition, although not yet relevant to clinical practice, this concept has also increased interest in various immunotherapy drugs as potential treatments in ARDS because of their ability to dampen inflammatory signaling and potentially reduce biotrauma.

Patient Self-Inflicted Lung Injury

Newer concepts of lung injury are somewhat less intuitive but increasingly important in the management of patients with ARDS. In contrast to injury caused by ventilator-delivered breaths, there is an emerging understanding of P-SILI. In these situations, the patient's own breathing efforts cause pressure and/or volume changes that can result in mechanical injury and biotrauma (**Figure 13-4**). The same basic concepts of volutrauma, barotrauma, and atelectrauma as the underlying mechanisms for lung injury with mechanical ventilation apply to P-SILI; the injury, however, is generated by the patient's own breathing efforts, which leads to a distinctive pattern owing to the unique effects of the diaphragm. Patients who are mechanically ventilated but triggering spontaneous breaths will have a combination of negative and positive pressure ventilation. Strong inspiratory efforts have been shown to produce much localized stress on lung tissue, particularly in the dependent regions of the lung, and in lung regions adjacent to the diaphragm. In addition, inspiratory efforts can create sufficiently strong transpulmonary pressure swings (pressure swings across the lung) to cause local overdistension or damage to the lung microvasculature causing local edema.

Lastly, asynchrony (which occurs when there is a discordance between the patient and ventilator), which is discussed in more detail in Chapter 18, can further worsen lung injury. Because asynchronies can occur at any point in the respiratory cycle, their effects can be variable. The simplest examples to understand are asynchronous inspiratory efforts that cause higher-than-intended tidal volumes or trigger premature stacked breaths that lead to some combination of volutrauma and barotrauma. Asynchronies can also cause atelectrauma similar to any inspiratory work done by the ventilator due to recruitment and derecruitment of the dependent lung regions.

While it might be tempting to think that we should remove all spontaneous breathing in patients with ARDS to avoid P-SILI, the typical **use of deeper sedation to remove these efforts**

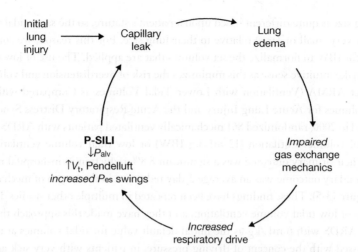

Initial
lung → Capillary → Lung
injury leak edema

P-SILI
↓P_{alv}
↑V_t, Pendelluft
increased P_{es} swings

*Impaired
gas exchange
mechanics*

*Increased
respiratory drive*

Figure 13-4: Schematic of patient self-inflicted lung injury (P-SILI). Mechanically the injury is similar to ventilator-induced lung injury (VILI), but simply generated through the patient's own breathing efforts. Mechanical injury occurs through overdistension of the lungs and injurious pressure swings across the lung from inspiratory efforts. Large inspiratory efforts cause a drop in alveolar pressure (P_{alv}), with large swings in pleural pressure as seen by large swings in esophageal pressure (P_{es}) causing large pressure swings across the lungs, large tidal volumes, and pendelluft (the movement of air between lung regions independent of bulk air movement in and out of the lungs, which can worsen lung stress). This causes worsened mechanical injury, capillary leak with resulting edema and impaired gas exchange, and worsened mechanics. This makes patients more susceptible to further injury and also can further increase the respiratory drive and further worsen the development of P-SILI.

may in some patients result in harm as well. Therefore, the determination of the "safety" of spontaneous breathing needs to be individualized for each patient, keeping in mind the length and severity of illness, the type of current ventilation employed, and the risks to the patient from increasing sedation.

LUNG-PROTECTIVE VENTILATION

With our understanding of the mechanisms of lung injury, we can turn to practical ways to ventilate and oxygenate patients with ARDS while maximally protecting the lungs from further damage. This is broadly termed *lung-protective ventilation* and consists of various ventilator considerations. The basics of ventilation are described in Section 2 of this book. We focus on pertinent parameters for lung-protective ventilation, the most basic of which is ventilator mode. Commonly used modes for patients with ARDS are volume (assist) control, pressure (assist) control, pressure-regulated volume control (PRVC), and airway pressure release ventilation (APRV). For more information on basic modes of ventilation, see Chapters 5 and 6, and for more information on advanced modes of ventilation, see Chapter 17. All of these modes can deliver lung-protective ventilation if properly used, which we elaborate on in the following sections.

Low-Volume Ventilation

Low tidal volume mechanical ventilation remains the most validated intervention and consists of minimizing tidal volumes to 4 to 8 mL/kg corrected for ideal body weight (IBW). Recall that lung size is quite different based upon a patient's stature, so the same tidal volume could be either very small or large relative to their lung size. For this reason, we correct the tidal volume for IBW to normalize the set volumes that are applied. The use of low tidal volumes should make intuitive sense as this minimizes the risk of overdistension and volutrauma. The ARDSnet ARMA (Ventilation with Lower Tidal Volumes as Compared with Traditional Tidal Volumes for Acute Lung Injury and the Acute Respiratory Distress Syndrome) study, published in 2000, randomized 861 mechanically ventilated patients with ARDS to traditional high tidal volume ventilation (12 mL/kg IBW) or low tidal volume ventilation (6 mL/kg IBW). Their primary outcome was a significant 8.8% reduction in in-hospital mortality, and their secondary outcome was an average 2-day reduction in the length of mechanical ventilation (**Figure 13-5**). These findings have been repeated in multiple other studies demonstrating the value of low tidal volume ventilation, and they have made this approach the standard of care for ARDS with 6 mL/kg as the initial default value for tidal volumes at many centers. As discussed with the concept of driving pressure, in patients with very sick and stiff lungs (low respiratory system compliance), the tidal volumes may need to be dropped to the 4 to 6 mL/kg range to prevent overdistension. Alternately in patients with preserved mechanics, that is, normal compliance, a higher range of volumes from 6 to 8 mL/kg may be safely tolerated.

Limitation of Plateau Pressure

As you recall from Chapter 2, the plateau pressure is the measurement of airway pressure during an occlusion at the end of inspiration. A plateau pressure measurement allows for a close estimation of the pressure within the alveoli (in contrast with peak pressure, which informs us about both the resistance of the airways and compliance of the lung) and can be used to determine the total pressure applied to the respiratory system from the combination of the volume delivered for the breath and the applied PEEP. The ARDSnet ARMA study also indirectly suggested that a plateau pressure of 30 cm H_2O or less should be targeted. The study utilized this as a secondary intervention if it could be achieved with low lung volumes, but,

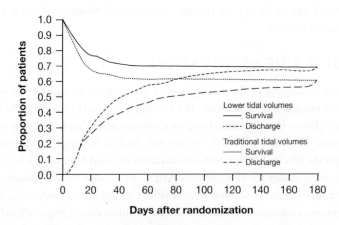

Figure 13-5: Kaplan-Meier curve from the 2000 ARMA trial consisting of 861 patients. This trial compared low tidal volume (6 mL/kg) versus traditional tidal volumes (12 mL/kg) and found significantly improved mortality and shorter duration of mechanical ventilation using low tidal volumes. (From Acute Respiratory Distress Syndrome Network; Brower RG, Matthay MA, Morris A, Schoenfeld D, Thompson BT, Wheeler A. Ventilation with lower tidal volumes as compared with traditional tidal volumes for acute lung injury and the acute respiratory distress syndrome. *N Engl J Med.* 2000;342(18):1301-1308. doi: 10.1056/NEJM200005043421801.)

unfortunately, the use of this cutoff value has not been independently investigated as a target. For this reason, targeting a plateau pressure of 30 cm H_2O or less is considered a consensus opinion at this time. Physiologically, this target is conceptually sound as the goal of using this value is to minimize the pressure and stress being applied directly to distend the lungs, and it could be a good indicator that the tidal volumes and PEEP are appropriate and safe. Conversely, end-inspiratory pressures have some limitations. They are a measurement of the total distending pressures for the respiratory system, so any other changes to the compliance of the system, such as excess body weight, stiffening of the rib cage, or any other restrictive physiology of the respiratory system, can falsely elevate end-inspiratory pressures without actually over distending the lungs. For more detail on this concept, see Chapter 18 and the discussion on esophageal manometry and transpulmonary pressure.

Driving Pressure

A related but distinct parameter that has been shown to potentially benefit patients with ARDS is the driving pressure. Driving pressure is calculated as the difference between the plateau pressure and PEEP and reflects the stress applied to the respiratory system and lungs during each inspiration; delivered pressure results in lung expansion (**Figure 13-6**). Conceptually, driving pressure provides a measurement that normalizes the delivered tidal volume relative to the size of the "baby lung" and the compliance. Put another way, the same delivered tidal volume (eg, 6 mL/kg) either can result in overdistension with high driving pressure in a patient with stiff lungs and multiple lung units that are collapsed and not receiving gas during

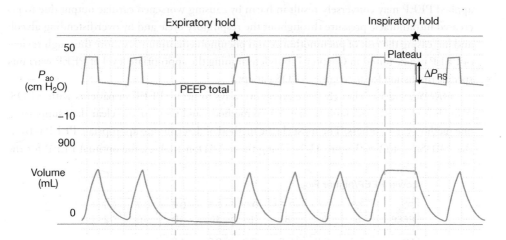

Figure 13-6: Driving pressure schematic. Driving pressure ΔP_{RS} is calculated first by identification of the plateau pressure. This pressure is obtained during an inspiratory breath-hold when there is no flow, and the measured airway pressure (the plateau pressure) provides a close estimate of the pressures in the alveoli. Patients then undergo an expiratory breath-hold as well to similarly measure the airway pressures when there is no flow to provide an estimate of the alveolar pressures at end expiration (the total positive end-expiratory pressure [PEEP]). In practice however, the set PEEP is often substituted in the calculation for the measured total PEEP when calculating driving pressure as this was the value that has been utilized in retrospective analysis on mortality. The driving pressure is then calculated as the difference between the plateau pressure and the PEEP. This pressure represents the cyclic pressure change during each breath and is secondary to both the size of the tidal volume delivered and the stiffness (compliance) of the lungs. P_{ao} represents the airway pressure.

the inspiration or be applied with safe driving pressure in a patient with normal (higher compliance) lungs. Importantly, retrospective data suggest that the benefit from lung-protective ventilation strategies is mediated primarily by the resulting lower driving pressure and that reduction in tidal volumes provides particular benefit in patients with stiffer lungs.

Functionally, this provides a direct marker to use clinically to assist in titration of PEEP and tidal volume. Based upon these retrospective data, a cutoff of 14 to 15 cm H_2O or less for driving pressure has been considered a reasonable safety threshold to utilize. For a given tidal volume, PEEP adjustments may result in changes in driving pressure, with lung collapse at inappropriately low levels of PEEP (leaving fewer lung units to receive the tidal volume) and overdistension at inappropriately high levels of PEEP, both causing increased "stiffness" of the lung (compliance of the lung falls at higher lung volume) and high driving pressures. Typically in early ARDS, there is a PEEP level at which collapse and overdistension are minimized and the driving pressure is lowest. Indeed, "best PEEP" measurements often directly or indirectly utilize driving pressure to assess the optimal PEEP. In addition, driving pressure may be decreased by lowering tidal volumes, and, as discussed earlier, driving pressures can help determine whether tidal volumes should be titrated to lower levels to prevent overdistension.

Positive End-Expiratory Pressure Titration

PEEP is the next parameter to consider for lung-protective ventilation. PEEP, to review, is the pressure maintained in the airways during expiration. Through prevention of atelectasis and derecruitment of the lung, PEEP improves oxygenation. In addition, by prevention of lung collapse at end expiration, PEEP can decrease VILI due to atelectrauma. Overly high levels of applied PEEP may conversely result in harm by causing worsened cardiac output due to increased intrathoracic pressure throughout the respiratory cycle and by overdistending alveoli and increasing the risk of pneumothorax and pneumomediastinum. A more thorough review of PEEP can be found in Chapter 7, but determining the appropriate level of PEEP warrants specific discussion for managing ARDS patients.

ARDSnet tables: Though there are many ways to titrate PEEP in patients with ARDS, many hospital centers default to one or two methods, and there are no clear data supporting one method versus others. The most classic method of determining appropriate PEEP is from the ARDSnet studies (**Figure 13-7**). Using these ARDSnet tables, the optimal PEEP for the

Lower PEEP/higher F_{IO_2}

F_{IO_2}	0.3	0.4	0.5	0.5	0.5	0.6	0.7	0.7
PEEP	5	5	8	8	10	10	10	12

F_{IO_2}	0.7	0.8	0.9	0.9	0.9	1.0
PEEP	14	14	14	16	18	18-24

Higher PEEP/higher F_{IO_2}

F_{IO_2}	0.3	0.3	0.3	0.3	0.3	0.4	0.4	0.5
PEEP	5	8	10	12	14	14	16	16

F_{IO_2}	0.5	0.5-0.8	0.8	0.9	1.0	1.0
PEEP	18	20	22	22	22	24

Figure 13-7: ARDSnet tables. It is not clear at this time if one table is superior to the other. The low PEEP table is used more often for clinical care, however, as many hospitals are less comfortable with the higher PEEP strategies suggested by the high PEEP table.

required F_{IO_2} can be easily determined at the bedside. As a patient requires more or less F_{IO_2} support, the ARDSnet tables would guide you on how to titrate the PEEP based on the sliding scales. Note that there have been two tables utilized for different ARDSnet studies: a low PEEP and a high PEEP table. While the high PEEP table has been used in several trials, the low PEEP table is far more commonly utilized for clinical care.

Physiologic PEEP titration: A more individual-tailored approach is to titrate the PEEP and determine the effect on lung mechanics through physiologic approaches. Of note, there are several techniques that are commonly employed depending on your site of practice, and the best physiologic technique is often the one with which your clinicians are most comfortable.

A particularly common approach is the use of the **decremental PEEP titration.** While PEEP can be adjusted in either an ascending or a descending manner, a decremental approach is preferred because of the faster equilibration of the lung mechanics at each PEEP level and the decrease in time required for a full decremental PEEP study. During this study, PEEP levels are initially raised to higher levels and then incrementally decreased with measurements of compliance, driving pressure, Spo_2, and vital signs at each PEEP level, assigning the "best PEEP" to the level that optimizes the mechanics and oxygenation such that the PEEP is not too low (and there is collapse) and the PEEP is not too high (and there is overdistension). Other related titration methods test the pressure and volume characteristics of the entire lung, or by looking at what is called the *stress index*, both of which are significantly more advanced and beyond the scope of this book. These methods may be locally used within your intensive care unit (ICU) but are far less common overall.

Lastly, there are even more specialized methods of titrating PEEP based on newer imaging modalities and using specialized pressure monitors. Esophageal manometry, which will be discussed in more detail in Chapter 18, allows one to titrate PEEP based on an estimate of the collapsing forces around the lungs from elevated pleural pressures: If the PEEP is set below the pleural pressure, there is an increased likelihood of derecruitment. CT imaging, bedside ultrasound, and electrical impedance tomography have all been suggested as possible methods of determining lung recruitment and for real-time monitoring of changes during titration of PEEP, which are beyond the scope of this book. Although they all have potential benefits and drawbacks to their use, none has yet been shown to be a reliable method of PEEP titration, and studies are ongoing to evaluate their value in regular clinical practice.

Permissive Hypercapnia

Permissive hypercapnia is the practice of tolerating ventilatory settings (specifically, low tidal volume leading to low minute ventilation) that result in hypercarbia and acidemia so long as oxygenation is appropriate. Acidemia as low as a pH of 7.2 is regularly tolerated in patients with ARDS as long as there are no direct negative sequelae. Permissive hypercapnia likely has benefit because it allows for lower tidal volumes and reduced the risk of volutrauma and makes it easier to achieve the various target parameters discussed earlier, even in patients with otherwise severe ARDS. There is also some speculation that there may be direct benefits of hypercarbia and acidemia in ARDS, though this mechanism is not completely clear yet, and it may simply be the decreased intensity of mechanical ventilation accompanying the hypercapnia that decreases injury. Of course, acute hypercapnia leads to respiratory acidosis, and a low pH will stimulate the respiratory controller, which may lead to dyspnea and spontaneous breathing efforts that can contribute to lung injury; patients may need analgesia and sedation until the pH improves with renal compensation.

Oxygenation Goals

Any discussion of hypoxic respiratory failure must discuss the role of F_{IO_2} in improving patient oxygenation. Given the long recovery times and need for prolonged mechanical ventilation, it warrants caution to avoid the potentially deleterious effects of overoxygenation. Lung-protective ventilation strategies allow patients to tolerate Pao_2 levels as low as 55 mm Hg without clear harm (although we typically aim for slightly higher values in the 65 to 75 mm Hg range to provide some degree of buffer should the patient worsen). Given known potential risks and lung toxicity associated with overoxygenation, F_{IO_2} should be increased to stabilize a patient while optimizing ventilator settings and then be weaned as readily as possible. Hyperoxia has been shown to promote free radical formation, dysregulate immune responses, and can worsen alveolar-capillary permeability, all of which can exacerbate the hyperinflammatory state of the lungs in ARDS and further injure the already damaged and vulnerable alveolar-capillary membrane. Absorption atelectasis may also be worsened by high levels of F_{IO_2}. Absorption atelectasis occurs when small pockets of trapped gas in the alveoli are reabsorbed, resulting in collapse; because blood in capillaries has a mixture of O_2, CO_2, and nitrogen dissolved in it, a pocket of gas in the lung with a very high Po_2 will have a high diffusion gradient for gas in the isolated pocket to move rapidly into the blood, thereby emptying that trapped pocket, which then collapses.

ESCALATING HYPOXEMIA STRATEGIES

Neuromuscular Blockade

Unfortunately, despite our best efforts at optimizing mechanical ventilation strategies, many patients continue to have severe hypoxemia requiring more aggressive interventions. One of the most initially promising ancillary treatments was neuromuscular blockade to induce paralysis. The ACURASYS (Neuromuscular Blockers in Early Acute Respiratory Distress Syndrome) study, published in 2010, showed a statistically significant improvement in 90-day mortality (hazard ratio 0.68) for patients with ARDS and a P/F ratio of less than 150 for those randomized to neuromuscular blockade with cisatracurium. This was challenged with the publication of the larger, multicenter ROSE (Early Neuromuscular Blockade in the Acute Respiratory Distress Syndrome) trial in 2019, showing no significant differences in mortality, ICU days, ventilator-dependent days, or any other secondary outcomes. Given the unclear benefits of routine paralysis for severe ARDS, these agents are generally reserved for patients exhibiting spontaneous respiratory activity or asynchrony that is felt to be worsening oxygenation, hemodynamic status, or could be sufficiently severe to induce P-SILI.

Despite the negative trial, paralytics are still routinely used by some centers; future studies, however, will be required to determine which patients are most at risk for self-injurious behavior and most likely to benefit from paralysis. These medications should not be used routinely in all patients with significant hypoxemia

Prone Positioning

Proning, though originally discussed as early as the 1970s, did not gain much popularity for routine clinical care until the publication of the PROSEVA (Prone Positioning in Severe Acute Respiratory Distress Syndrome) study in 2013, which showed an impressive 16.8% absolute reduction in 28-day mortality for patients randomized to proning. Despite these results, routine use of proning was not rapidly adopted. Thankfully, this has been changing over the past several years as education and experience with proning have improved.

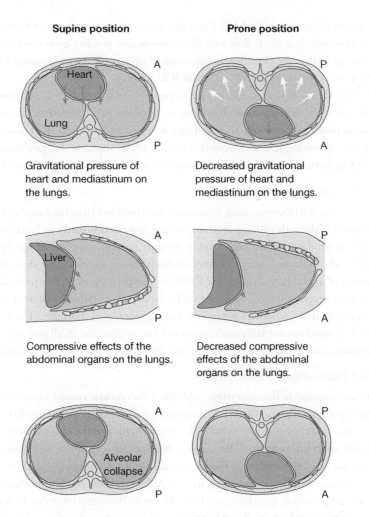

Supine position

Prone position

Gravitational pressure of heart and mediastinum on the lungs.

Decreased gravitational pressure of heart and mediastinum on the lungs.

Compressive effects of the abdominal organs on the lungs.

Decreased compressive effects of the abdominal organs on the lungs.

Expansion of the chest wall and overall less homogeneous chest wall compliance.

More homogeneous chest wall compliance due to restriction of anterior chest wall movement.

Figure 13-8: Proning provides benefit to patients in several ways. Prone position offloads the mediastinum, heart, and abdominal cavity of the lungs due to the change in position and the shape of the diaphragm, which can improve lung volumes and recruitment. There is also improved homogeneity of ventilation due to changes in chest wall compliance and improved matching of ventilation and perfusion, which may result in improved oxygenation as well. Note that A = anterior, P = posterior chest.

The prone position is felt to be beneficial for a few key reasons. For one, it offloads the weight of the heart and the mediastinum from the lungs and can improve recruitment of these areas of the lung, thereby improving the homogeneity of ventilation and decreasing the local stress distribution (**Figure 13-8**). Given the dysregulated ventilation/perfusion matching in the lungs of these patients, proning can also help aerate anterior areas of the lung that are now being perfused due to gravity, improving ventilation-perfusion matching and oxygenation. There is also some evidence to suggest that improved recruitment of lung in the prone position may reduce the risk of VILI and that the prone position makes it easier for patients to clear secretions. It is likely that with the expertise and practice gained over the COVID-19 pandemic, as well as the clear benefits in terms of patient outcomes, proning will continue to become more regularly practiced within all ICU settings.

Patients should be maintained in a prone position for at least 16 hours of every 24 hours period. Because most of these patients have tenuous respiratory and hemodynamic status, care must be taken to prone patients without dislodging access or endotracheal (ET) tubes. Should these patients decompensate, it is also important to be ready to supinate (lay patients on their backs) these patients in the event that cardiopulmonary resuscitation (CPR) protocols are required.

Recruitment Maneuvers

In patients with ARDS, some lung regions are collapsed but have the capacity to be reopened or "recruited." Methods of lung recruitment are described broadly as "recruitment maneuvers" but are similar in that a high level of pressure is applied for a prolonged period of time to reinflate the collapsed lung. Various methods exist ranging from short periods (up to 30 seconds) of applying high-pressure PEEP, to ramping up to higher pressures slowly and holding it for several minutes. Studies thus far have been variable, with some suggesting improved oxygenation and others potentially causing increased mortality. The best way to use these tools clinically is not fully understood yet, but routine use in all patients with ARDS is **not recommended** at this time and should only be performed by an expert clinician.

Inhaled Pulmonary Vasodilators

As patients continue to decompensate, additional therapeutic considerations include administration of pulmonary vasodilators. Commonly used agents are either inhaled nitric oxide or prostacyclins, and they work by inducing local vasodilation of the blood vessels adjacent to the alveoli that are being ventilated. Because medication delivery and vasodilation only occur in areas that are actively ventilating, this intervention can help improve matching of ventilation and perfusion and thus improve oxygenation. Although these medications can help stabilize a patient's oxygenation, they have not been shown to have any mortality benefits, and their effects may not be robust in all patients. They are better thought of as stabilizing agents (eg, they may allow you to reduce the Fio_2 and avoid the potential toxicity associated with high concentrations of inspired oxygen), and if patients do not improve, consideration of bridging to more advanced therapies should be quickly considered.

One major contraindication to keep in mind with inhaled vasodilators is that their use in any sort of cardiogenic edema can worsen pulmonary edema and should be avoided. This is due to the fundamental relationship between flow and resistance. Pulmonary vasoconstriction secondary to alveolar hypoxia increases resistance to blood flowing from the right side of the heart and, consequently, reduces flow to the left side of the heart. In patients with cardiogenic edema and heart failure, decreasing resistance of the pulmonary vasculature and increasing the flow of blood to the left side of the heart will only worsen filling pressures and lead to further increases in pulmonary capillary pressures. These vasodilated vessels are already prone to leakage due to the ARDS, and the vasodilators can further worsen pulmonary edema and hypoxic respiratory failure.

Extracorporeal Membrane Oxygenation

The final option available to patients with continuing decompensation despite all the abovementioned interventions is to bypass the lungs as a means of oxygenation and utilize extracorporeal membrane oxygenation (ECMO). It is always important to remember that ECMO is not without severe complications and risk and should only be thought of as a temporary life-sustaining measure if the patient is felt to have a chance of recovery.

Given that the primary pathology in ARDS is alveolar-capillary interface dysfunction, ECMO is generally only needed to assist with CO_2 removal and oxygenation of the blood. Assuming cardiac pump function is intact, most patients with ARDS only require veno-venous (VV) ECMO as opposed to veno-arterial ECMO, which supports the cardiovascular system and is not discussed further in this chapter. VV-ECMO can be started via various methods, but the general principle is to remove deoxygenated venous blood from the patient, provide oxygenation and CO_2 removal via the artificial lung, and then return the blood to the venous system. This oxygenated blood is then pumped via the patient's native circulatory system through the lungs, which are still mechanically ventilated (see Chapter 12, Figure 12-6). Given the extracorporeal oxygenation and CO_2 removal, highly restrictive lung-protective ventilation parameters (eg, very low tidal volume and inflation pressure) can be used to "rest" the lung and prevent further lung injury.

ECMO management is generally reserved for multidisciplinary specialist teams, and the decision to initiate cannulation is typically performed within tertiary care centers by high-level experts in the field. While ECMO can clearly be lifesaving in the right population of patients, the existing literature on ECMO has not clearly defined the best use in ARDS. In addition, there can be numerous complications associated with its use; consequently, it should only be used in the most critically ill patients who have a chance for lung recovery, or a previously described plan for lung transplant.

SUMMARY

ARDS is a poorly understood but highly morbid form of hypoxic respiratory failure. Although significant advancements in our understanding of the underlying pathophysiology have been made, they have also shown significant variability in phenotypes and prognosis. Despite this progress, all management is largely supportive, focusing on maintaining appropriate oxygenation while minimizing further damage to the lungs or worsening inflammation. *Lung-protective ventilation* refers to a series of respiratory interventions that have shown significant promise in improving outcomes and minimizing volutrauma, barotrauma, and atelectrauma. Further management is targeted at the presumed underlying etiology of ARDS and escalating strategies including proning, paralysis, pulmonary vasodilators, and ECMO, which can improve outcomes in select patient populations.

KEY POINTS

- ARDS is a syndrome of hypoxic respiratory failure defined by the 2012 Berlin criteria.
- Underlying triggers for ARDS are highly variable but can be broadly grouped into pulmonary and extrapulmonary causes.
- Lung injury in ARDS is caused by barotrauma, volutrauma, and atelectrauma and can also be caused by spontaneous inspiratory efforts (P-SILI).
- Evidence-based interventions in all patients with ARDS include low-volume ventilation (~6 mL/kg), maintaining low driving and plateau pressures, and titrating PEEP to maximize compliance of the lungs.
- Advanced oxygenation strategies include proning, paralysis, pulmonary vasodilators, and ECMO, which can be considered in select patients with sufficiently severe ARDS.

- Despite improvements in management, morbidity and mortality in ARDS remain high.
- Our understanding of the pathophysiology, prognosis, and mechanism of lung injury continues to expand. In the coming years, an enhanced understanding of the various ARDS phenotypes will likely modify clinical practice.

STUDY QUESTIONS AND ANSWERS

Questions

1. A 46-year-old woman with COVID pneumonia is admitted to the emergency department (ED) and intubated. She is noted to have bilateral lung opacities, no evidence of heart failure, and a Pao_2/Fio_2 ratio of 220 mm Hg on 100% Fio_2. Her PEEP is set empirically to 5 cm H_2O, and tidal volumes are at 9 mL/kg. Which of the following ventilation and management strategies should be considered in this patient (pick all that apply)?
   A. Tidal volume set to 6 mL/kg.
   B. Lower the Fio_2.
   C. Prone the patient.
   D. Initiate neuromuscular blockade (also known as *paralysis*).
   E. **A** and **B** are correct.

2. This same patient continues to worsen over the next 24 hours, now with a Pao_2/Fio_2 of 154 mm Hg on Fio_2 50%. Her driving pressure on current tidal volumes is noted to be 18 cm H_2O. PEEP is still only at 5 cm H_2O. What would be the next best intervention?
   A. Perform a "best PEEP" trial.
   B. Lower tidal volumes below 6 mL/kg.
   C. Raise the tidal volumes above 6 mL/kg.
   D. Increase the Fio_2.

3. After the abovementioned adjustment in PEEP to 12 cm H_2O, the patient now has a driving pressure of 15 cm H_2O, but unfortunately, the Pao_2/Fio_2 ratio has decreased further to 120 mm Hg despite an increase in Fio_2 to 80%. The patient is also noted to be dyssynchronous with the ventilator despite higher levels of sedation. Which would be the next best interventions to consider (pick all that apply)?
   A. Increase PEEP further.
   B. Increase the Fio_2 further.
   C. Prone the patient.
   D. Initiate neuromuscular blockade.
   E. Initiate ECMO.

4. Assuming an intubated patient with ARDS and IBW of 50 kg, which of the following patients are on inappropriate ventilator settings and why?
   A. RR: 12, V_t: 500, PEEP 5, Fio_2 30%, peak cm H_2O, plateau 20 cm H_2O
   B. RR: 12, V_t: 300, PEEP 10, Fio_2 30%, peak 35 cm H_2O, plateau 24 cm H_2O
   C. RR: 12, V_t: 300, PEEP 5, Fio_2 30%, peak 35 cm H_2O, plateau 25 cm H_2O
   D. RR: 12, V_t: 300, PEEP 18, Fio_2 50%, peak 35 cm H_2O, plateau 32 cm H_2O
   E. Both **C** and **D** are correct

Answers

1. **Answer E. Tidal volume set to 6 mL/kg and Lower the F_{IO_2}**

   Rationale: The initial tidal volume of 9 mL/kg may be too high for this patient, and a safe default initial setting is 6 mL/kg. The tidal volume can then be further adjusted as needed based upon the patient and the compliance of the lungs and ventilation needs. The patient is also receiving $F_{IO_2} = 1.0$, which is too high, especially considering the high Pao_2/F_{IO_2} ratio. This should be titrated down while monitoring the Pao_2 and Spo_2. **C** is not correct because the patient is not sick enough to warrant being placed in the prone position. This should be reserved for patients with a Pao_2/F_{IO_2} ratio of less than 150 mm Hg after initial stabilization and optimization. If needed, however, the evidence is very strong for its use in ARDS. **D** is not correct as paralytics should not be routinely used in patients with ARDS. The current evidence suggests that in a broad population of patients with moderate-severe ARDS (Pao_2/F_{IO_2} of <150), there was no difference in outcomes compared with the control. That being said, in patients who are severely hypoxemic and very dyssynchronous with the ventilator despite deep sedation, paralytics are still required in some patients but need to be applied carefully.

2. **Answer A. Perform a "best PEEP" trial**

   Rationale: The patient despite moderately severe ARDS is only on 5 cm H_2O of PEEP, which may be too low for this patient. This can cause both overly low oxygenation as seen by the lower Pao_2/F_{IO_2} ratio and worsened stiffness of the lungs as seen by the high driving pressure. In theory, titration of the PEEP through a "best PEEP" trial can address both of these issues. **B.** Lowering the tidal volumes may be eventually needed if the best PEEP maneuver is not sufficient to improve the mechanics and the driving pressure remains elevated, but this would not be the first step. **C.** Raising the tidal volumes could in theory improve oxygenation, but it would also worsen the overdistension of the lungs and result in worsened lung injury. **D.** Increasing the F_{IO_2} is not required at this point and would not help the underlying issue. Indeed, overly high F_{IO_2} (>0.6) may result in increased harm.

3. **Answer E. Initiate ECMO**

   Rationale: The patient is now increasingly hypoxemic with a Pao_2/F_{IO_2} less than 150 mm Hg. This means that the patient should be placed in prone position. The data from the PROSEVA trial in 2013 showed a substantial benefit in mortality in this group of patients, and this should be considered the "standard of care" in any ICU. Prone position should be maintained for at least 16 hours per day and continued until the patient shows evidence of durable recovery. In addition, while neuromuscular blockade should not be used in every patient with severe hypoxemia, it may still be needed in some patients in whom there is significant dyssynchrony, which could be worsening the severity of hypoxemia. In addition, it is often used in combination with proning to limit mishaps associated with turning the patient, especially when proning is initiated. **A** is incorrect as the PEEP has been optimized already and there would likely be a minimal benefit in further increasing. **B** is incorrect as well. While this may be needed eventually should the patient further worsen, the level of oxygenation remains adequate, and increasing the F_{IO_2} would not provide further benefit yet. **E** is incorrect as the patient does not yet meet the criteria for ECMO (is not sick enough) and other optimization should always be performed first.

(continued)

4. **Answer B. RR: 12, V_t : 300, PEEP 10, F_{IO_2} 30%, peak 35 cm H_2O , plateau 24 cm H_2O**

   Rationale: This is correct as all of the parameters provided are within the "optimal" goals.
   A is incorrect because V_t is too high. Patient is receiving 10 mL/kg. If inadequate alveolar
   ventilation is being reached with lower tidal volume, the RR should be increased to compensate. **C** is incorrect because the driving pressure is too high. A plateau of 25 cm H_2O and
   a PEEP of 5 cm H_2O result in a driving pressure or 20 cm H_2O , which is greater than the
   desired driving pressure of 15. PEEP should be either uptitrated to try and improve lung
   recruitment or V_t should be decreased to lower plateau pressures. **D** is incorrect because the
   plateau pressure is too high. Aim to keep plateau pressures below 30 cm H_2O . Patient is on
   high ventilator settings, so options may be limited, but possible options include lowering V_t
   to decrease the plateau or titrating the PEEP downward to see if perhaps overdistending
   the lung.

Suggested Readings

Acute Respiratory Distress Syndrome Network; Brower RG, Matthay MA, Morris A, Schoenfeld D,
   Thompson BT, Wheeler A. Ventilation with lower tidal volumes as compared with traditional
   tidal volumes for acute lung injury and the acute respiratory distress syndrome. *N Engl J Med*.
   2000;342(18):1301-1308. doi: 10.1056/NEJM200005043421801.

Guérin C, Reignier J, Richard JC, et al. Prone positioning in severe acute respiratory distress syndrome.
   NEJM. 2013;368(23):2159-2168. doi:10.1056/NEJMoa1214103

National Heart, Lung, and Blood Institute Acute Respiratory Distress Syndrome (ARDS) Clinical Trials
   Network, Wiedemann HP, Wheeler AP, et al. Comparison of two fluid-management strategies in
   acute lung injury. *NEJM*. 2006;354(24):2564-2575. doi:10.1056/NEJMoa062200

National Heart, Lung, and Blood Institute PETAL Clinical Trials Network; Moss M, Huang DT,
   Brower RG, et al. Early neuromuscular blockade in the acute respiratory distress syndrome. *N Engl J
   Med*. 2019;380(21):1997–2008. doi: 10.1056/NEJMoa1901686. Epub 2019 May 19.

Papazian L, Forel JM, Gacouin A, et al; ACURASYS Study Investigators. Neuromuscular blockers
   in early acute respiratory distress syndrome. *N Engl J Med*. 2010;363(12):1107–1116. doi: 10.1056/
   NEJMoa1005372.

Wilson JG, Calfee CS. ARDS subphenotypes: understanding a heterogeneous syndrome. *Crit Care*.
   2020;24(1):102. doi:10.1186/s13054-020-2778-x

Interstitial Lung Disease

Jeremy B. Richards • Kavitha C. Selvan

LEARNING OBJECTIVES

- Delineate the pathophysiology and basic classification of interstitial lung disease (ILD).
- Describe strategies for overcoming the challenges associated with the use of mechanical ventilation in patients with ILD.
- Discuss the alternatives to mechanical ventilation in patients with ILD, including the use of noninvasive positive pressure ventilation (NIPPV) and high-flow nasal cannula (HFNC).
- Review strategies that can be used to mitigate ventilator-induced lung injury in patients with ILD requiring mechanical ventilation, and describe the physiologic mechanisms that underlie these strategies.

INTRODUCTION TO INTERSTITIAL LUNG DISEASE

The management of interstitial lung disease (ILD) in the intensive care unit (ICU) poses a particular challenge to clinicians. Owing to the complex and progressive nature of the disease, patients with ILD frequently develop acute hypoxemic respiratory failure that leads to the need to consider intubation and the initiation of mechanical ventilation. In this chapter, we review the pathophysiology and classification of ILD in an effort to understand the principles guiding the application of mechanical ventilation in these patients. We then explore the challenges, practical considerations, and recommendations available for clinicians considering the use of mechanical ventilation in patients with ILD.

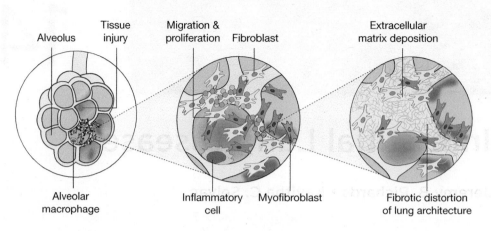

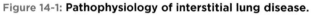

Figure 14-1: **Pathophysiology of interstitial lung disease.**

Pathophysiology

ILD is a heterogeneous group of lung diseases that leads to remodeling of the extracellular pulmonary matrix and distal airspaces and ultimately impairs respiratory mechanics and gas exchange. Remodeling is thought to be driven by aberrant wound healing in response to tissue injury that leads to progressive and irreversible deposition of collagen and extracellular matrix protein by differentiated fibroblasts (myofibroblasts) that have migrated to the interstitium (**Figure 14-1**). The mechanism by which fibroblasts differentiate into activated myofibroblasts is unclear, but it is thought to be the result of complex signaling pathways that occur between endothelial cells, activated immune cells, and injured alveolar epithelial cells. Bleomycin animal models of pulmonary fibrosis and other animal studies have demonstrated that surfactant dysfunction and alveolar epithelial cell apoptosis may play a key role early in this pathway.

Classification of Interstitial Lung Diseases

ILDs can be broadly classified as those with an identified etiology or idiopathic conditions (**Table 14-1**). It can be further classified by phenotype, characterized by either an inflammatory and/or fibrotic clinical and histopathologic presentation. Notably, there can be significant

TABLE 14-1	Classification of Interstitial Lung Diseases
Interstitial Lung Disease	
Known Etiology	**Idiopathic**
Exposure related	Idiopathic interstitial pneumonias (IIPs)
Connective tissue disease	Sarcoidosis
Infection	Langerhans cell histiocytosis (LCH)
Genetic (familial ILD)	Lymphangioleiomyomatosis (LAM)
	Eosinophilic pneumonia
	Pulmonary alveolar proteinosis (PAP)
	Unclassifiable ILD

ILD, interstitial lung disease.

overlap between these two phenotypes. Inflammatory ILDs present predominantly with ground-glass opacities on high-resolution computed tomography (HRCT) of the chest, called *nonspecific interstitial pneumonia* (NSIP) pattern. Fibrotic ILDs presents with irregular reticulations, traction bronchiectasis, and honeycombing, termed *usual interstitial pneumonia* (UIP) pattern (**Figure 14-2**). The most commonly encountered fibrotic ILD is idiopathic pulmonary fibrosis (IPF).

While some forms of fibrosis are partially reversible, others are irreversible, and a subset of patients with fibrotic ILD develop progressive deterioration in lung function, dyspnea, and quality of life that has coined the term *progressive fibrosing ILD* (PF-ILD). In general, fibrotic ILDs are associated with a significantly worse prognosis and lower survival rates than inflammatory ILDs.

Acute Exacerbations of Interstitial Lung Disease

Throughout the course of their disease, patients with ILD may develop acute worsening of their dyspnea. *Acute exacerbations of ILD* (AE-ILD) are defined as an acute, clinically significant respiratory decompensation that develops within less than 1 month without an obvious clinical cause, such as pulmonary edema, pulmonary embolism, or pneumothorax. AE-ILD occur at the highest frequency in patients with IPF and are associated with poor prognosis and increased mortality. Patients typically present with increased cough, sputum production, and severe hypoxemia that may lead to admission to an ICU and consideration of mechanical ventilation. Radiographically, AE-ILD present with diffuse ground-glass opacities with or without consolidations on HRCT chest, often superimposed over baseline fibrotic disease, and the extent of radiographic disease correlates with clinical outcomes. Physiologically, oxygenation worsens and fails to respond significantly to supplemental oxygen, consistent with shunt physiology. Exacerbations are frequently triggered by infection, microaspiration, and procedural intervention, but oftentimes, clinicians are unable to identify a clear trigger.

In addition, it has been suggested that IPF patients have the potential for sudden and rapid clinical decompensation driven by the concept of percolation, derived from the physics literature. With repeated stretching, such as that occurring with the application of tidal volume during mechanical ventilation, bands of fibrosis increase in number until they reach a critical density, coined the "percolation threshold" (**Figure 14-3**). After reaching the percolation threshold, isolated bands of fibrosis become connected and expand across the lung tissue, leading to a sudden and detectable decrease in lung elasticity and a fall in lung compliance. In patients with IPF or other fibrotic ILDs requiring mechanical ventilation, this phenomenon may ultimately preclude the ability to liberate from mechanical ventilation.

Treatment

There are a variety of treatments with varying efficacies available for ILD, based on the underlying etiology of pulmonary inflammation and/or fibrosis. Treatments range from avoidance of triggers in exposure-related ILDs, corticosteroids in patients with inflammatory ILDs, steroid-sparing immunosuppression in ILD associated with connective tissue disease, and antifibrotic agents in progressive fibrotic ILDs. In patients with severe disease or disease refractory to medical management, prognosis is generally poor and lung transplantation may be considered in select patients.

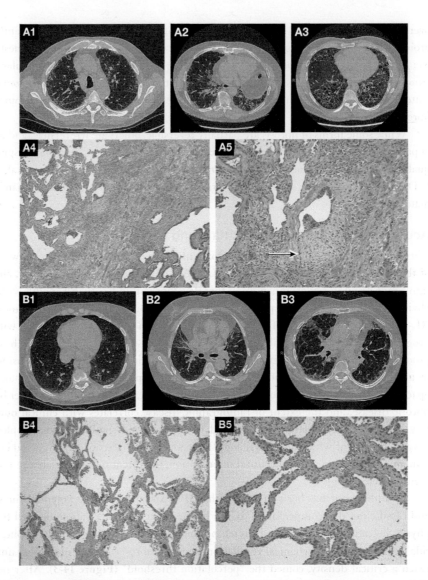

Figure 14-2: Interstitial lung disease phenotypes. A1-A3, Representative axial HRCT images of a UIP pattern with characteristic peripheral-predominant reticulations, honey-combing, and traction bronchiectasis. Note that the subsequent panels depict progression over time. **A4-A5,** Low- and high-power magnification of a representative section of UIP. **A4** (low power) depicts microscopic honeycombing in the bottom right-hand corner with subsequent partial destruction of alveolar lung architecture. **A5** (high power) demonstrates the pathognomonic fibroblastic foci (*arrow*) with myxoid stroma separating spindle cells. **B1-B3,** Representative axial HRCT images of an NSIP pattern with characteristic symmetric ground-glass opacities and fine reticulations. Note that the subsequent panels depict progression over time. **B4-B5,** Low- and high-power magnification of a representative section of NSIP. **B4** (low power) depicts mild interstitial thickening with characteristic preservation of alveolar architecture. **B5** (high power) demonstrates mild fibrosis and chronic inflammation, which together lead to interstitial thickening. HRCT, high-resolution computed tomography; NSIP, nonspecific interstitial pneumonia; UIP, usual interstitial pneumonia. (Images courtesy of Aliya Husain, MD.)

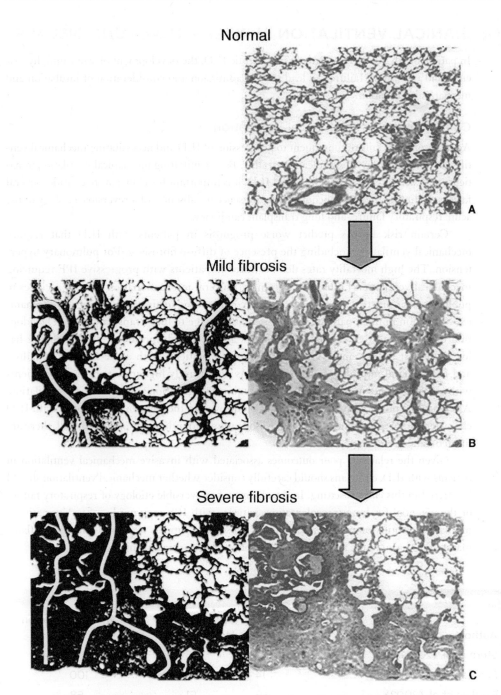

Figure 14-3: Percolation threshold. This figure taken from Bates et al. depicts the percolation threshold at a microscopic level. **A,** Normal lung tissue. **B,** Mild fibrosis with focal areas of fibrosis surrounded by normal lung tissue. **C,** Severe fibrosis with dense bands of fibrosis expanding across the entire section of lung tissue. It is postulated that this progression, from mild to severe lung fibrosis, occurs over time in patients with fibrosis who are subjected mechanical ventilation. (From Bates J, Davis G, Majumdar A, Butnor K, Suki B. Linking parenchymal disease progression to changes in lung mechanical function by percolation. *Am J Respir Crit Care Med.* 2007;176(6):617-623. Figure 3.)

MECHANICAL VENTILATION IN INTERSTITIAL LUNG DISEASE

In patients with AE-ILD or progressive fibrotic ILD, the development of worsening hypoxemia and respiratory failure can lead to ICU admission and consideration of intubation and mechanical ventilation.

Consideration of Mechanical Ventilation

Acute respiratory failure consequent to progression of ILD and necessitating mechanical ventilation is associated with significant mortality. Before initiating mechanical ventilation in patients with acute respiratory failure and ILD, it is important for clinicians to consider several factors, including the ILD phenotype, the presence (or absence) of a reversible etiology of the acute respiratory failure, and lung transplant candidacy.

Certain risk factors predict worse prognosis in patients with ILD that require mechanical ventilation, including the presence of diffuse fibrosis and/or pulmonary hypertension. The high mortality rates demonstrated in patients with progressive IPF requiring mechanical ventilation (**Table 14-2**) prompted several international respiratory societies to publish a joint practice guideline in 2011 recommending against intubation and mechanical ventilation in these patients, unless used as a bridge to lung transplantation. The adoption of lung-protective ventilation strategies and other advancements in critical care has led to modest improvement in mortality rates for patients with acute respiratory failure and ILD; overall mortality, however, remains significantly higher as compared to patients with other etiologies of pulmonary disease requiring intubation and mechanical ventilation. Alternatively, outcomes may be somewhat improved in the subgroup of patients with ILD characterized predominantly by cellular infiltration and inflammation, but overall, there are limited data on this topic.

Given the relatively poor outcomes associated with invasive mechanical ventilation in patients with ILD, clinicians should carefully consider whether mechanical ventilation should be offered in this clinical setting. In the absence of a reversible etiology of respiratory failure or the potential for lung transplantation, patients with IPF may not benefit. Alternatively, mechanical ventilation may be reasonable to consider in patients with predominantly inflammatory ILD, even in the absence of a reversible etiology or transplant eligibility.

TABLE 14-2 Outcomes in Fibrotic ILD Requiring Hospital Admission			
Author	**Study Size**	**In-Hospital Mortality (%)**	**Mechanical Ventilation Mortality (%)**
Stern et al. (2001)	23	96	96
Fumeaux et al. (2001)	14	100	100
Saydain et al. (2002)	38	61	68
Al-Hameed and Sharma (2004)	25	96	100
Rush et al. (2016)	17,770	–	49
Mooney et al. (2017)	22,350	–	56
Durheim et al. (2019)	6,665	31	55
Schrader et al. (2021)	411	35	49

ILD, interstitial lung disease.

Alternatives to Mechanical Ventilation

Given the poor prognosis associated with the use of intubation and invasive mechanical ventilation in ILD, there has been interest in investigating the role of noninvasive positive pressure ventilation (NIPPV). Studies have demonstrated that NIPPV in patients with acute respiratory distress syndrome (ARDS) allowed for the avoidance of intubation, which subsequently led to an improved overall mortality rate compared to patients who require mechanical ventilation, but there are limited data available on outcomes of NIPPV in ILD.

The mortality rate associated with the use of NIPPV in IPF is approximately half of that seen with invasive mechanical ventilation, and the use has more than doubled between 2006 and 2012, though mortality has not significantly declined with increased use. The use of NIPPV may be of particular value in patients with ILD who have an Acute Physiology and Chronic Health Evaluation (APACHE II) score less than 20 or acute respiratory failure secondary to pneumonia. In addition, there is increased survival with early use of NIPPV in patients with hypoxemia and suspected AE-ILD. However, the failure rate for NIPPV is high, and the need for continuous NIPPV seems to portend poor prognosis.

Despite the paucity of data available, many clinicians are now advocating for the use of NIPPV over invasive mechanical ventilation in the subset of ILD patients who have a fibrotic phenotype, but additional investigation is still needed. We recommend an individualized approach, with consideration of patients' overall goals of care, ILD phenotype, and etiology and/or reversibility of acute respiratory failure. Owing to the poor outcomes associated with the use of invasive mechanical ventilation in fibrotic ILD, we strongly recommend early initiation of NIPPV in conjunction with palliative care consultation in patients with fibrotic ILD with AE-ILD without a reversible etiology. Alternatively, in patients with a predominantly inflammatory ILD and/or an identified, reversible etiology of AE-ILD, it is reasonable to consider invasive mechanical ventilation as first-line therapy, given the relatively high failure rates of NIPPV reported in patients with ILD.

The application of heated, humidified air delivered via high-flow nasal cannula (HFNC) may also be considered in patients with ILD and acute respiratory failure. Although HFNC does not offer the mechanical ventilatory support or positive end-expiratory pressure (PEEP) provided by NIPPV, it is able to provide a high fraction of inspired oxygen (Fio_2) up to 1.0 and may be an ideal device choice in patients with predominantly hypoxemic respiratory failure, as opposed to hypercapnic. In addition to providing high levels Fio_2, HFNC is more comfortable and tolerable for patients than NIPPV and is safe to use in patients suffering from ICU delirium or encephalopathy. Though data suggest that application of HFNC does not reduce the need for endotracheal intubation, we recommend considering HFNC as a first-line alternative to mechanical ventilation in patients with fibrotic ILD and severe hypoxemia that are unlikely to benefit from mechanical ventilation.

Strategies for the Application of Mechanical Ventilation

At present, there are no specific consensus guidelines on the optimal strategy for mechanical ventilation in ILD. It is clear, however, that clinicians should seek to limit ventilator-induced lung injury (VILI), or acute lung injury caused or perpetuated by mechanical ventilation. Alveolar overdistension ("volutrauma") and injury from repeated alveolar collapse ("atelectrauma"), which occur with the application of mechanical ventilation, have been linked to increased morbidity and mortality in patients with ARDS. Patients with ILD are particularly susceptible to overdistension injuries (relatively normal regions of lung get a disproportionate fraction of the tidal volume given the very low compliance of the diseased regions); it is less clear whether individuals with pulmonary fibrosis suffer from the same extent of atelectrauma seen in patients with ARDS who have a deficiency of normal surfactant.

Lung-protective ventilation refers to the practice of applying low tidal volumes in order to limit plateau (airway) pressures to less than 28 to 30 cm H_2O. The use of tidal volumes of 6 mL/kg of predicted body weight has been definitively proven to reduce mortality in patients with ARDS when compared to high tidal volume strategies. There is consensus agreement that these same ventilatory strategies should be applied to patients with ILD despite the sparse available literature confirming this clinical practice. There are some data that demonstrate worse survival for ILD patients with higher plateau and mean airway pressures. With decreased lung compliance, further reduced in the setting of acutely worsening disease, even a low tidal volume strategy may be associated with higher plateau pressures than is deemed appropriate to avoid volutrauma in the relatively normal regions of lung.

Respiratory acidosis is a frequent complication of both progressive ILD and lung-protective strategies of mechanical ventilation and poses a significant challenge in the management of these patients. As a consequence of progressive interstitial and alveolar abnormalities, patients with ILD develop increased physiologic *dead space*, defined as areas of lung that continue to receive inhaled gas but do not receive blood flow (Q = 0). The increase in dead space ventilation is driven by increases in both anatomic dead space, secondary to the increased volume of the conducting airways (recall that airways are tethered open by surrounding lung tissue and the recoil forces of the lung are increased with interstitial inflammation and fibrosis), and alveolar dead space secondary to decreased perfusion to areas of involved lung (**Figure 14-4**).

Increased dead space fraction has been identified as an independent risk factor for death in patients with ARDS and, interestingly, has been reported as a defining feature of IPF. In contrast with other ILDs, patients with IPF do not seem to experience the normal reduction in dead space fraction associated with exercise.

The rising carbon dioxide levels that characterize clinically significant increased dead space ventilation in ILD are mitigated by increasing minute ventilation ($V_E = V_t \times f$; V_t = tidal volume, f = respiratory rate [RR]), which typically ranges from 4 to 6 L/min in healthy individuals. Patients with ILD may require a significantly higher minute ventilation in order to eliminate carbon dioxide in the setting of increased dead space ventilation ($V_E = V_A + V_d$) and to manage respiratory acidosis. For patients who are intubated and mechanically ventilated, it is recommended that the first step in augmenting minute ventilation in individuals with ILD is to increase RR, given the high pressures that would be needed to increase tidal volume in many cases.

As established in the landmark ARDSNet trial, incremental increases in RR up to 35 breaths/min should be made in order to achieve a pH of 7.30 to 7.45. In patients with severe ILD, the degree of respiratory acidosis that develops may overwhelm compensation achieved with the maximal recommended RR. In these scenarios, clinicians are faced with the dilemma of whether to further augment RR above 35 breaths/min, which could paradoxically worsen ventilation by leading to the development of intrinsic PEEP, which may worsen physiologic dead space (see Chapter 7), or to increase the tidal volume (to increase minute ventilation), which would violate lung-protective strategies.

There are several methods for monitoring respiratory acidosis, including the use of end-tidal carbon dioxide ($Etco_2$) monitors, serial measurements of the partial pressure of carbon dioxide on arterial blood gas (ABG) ($Paco_2$), or serial calculations of the dead space fraction (ratio of dead space ventilation to tidal volume, or V_d/V_t).

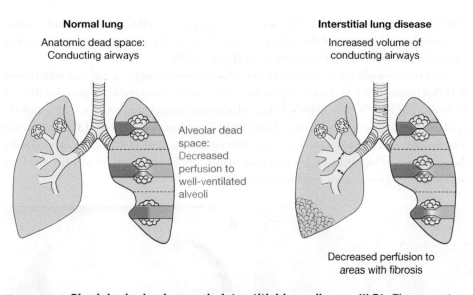

Normal lung

Anatomic dead space:
Conducting airways

Interstitial lung disease

Increased volume of
conducting airways

Alveolar dead
space:
Decreased
perfusion to
well-ventilated
alveoli

Decreased perfusion to
areas with fibrosis

Figure 14-4: **Physiologic dead space in interstitial lung disease (ILD).** There are two main sources of dead space in the lung: anatomic and alveolar. In the normal lung, anatomic dead space comes from the conducting airways, made up of the nose, pharynx, larynx, trachea, bronchi, and bronchioles, and is ~150 mL. Alveolar dead space is created by areas of the lung that are well ventilated, but poorly perfused (West Lung Zone 1). In patients with ILD (*right*), there is increased volume of the conducting airways and decreased perfusion to areas with fibrosis, leading to an increase in both anatomic and alveolar dead space.

Another consideration in the application of mechanical ventilation is the titration of PEEP, which is applied to mitigate atelectrauma and improve lung compliance by recruiting collapsed alveoli. Recall that the functional residual capacity is reduced in ILD owing to the enhanced recoil forces and the risk of alveolar collapse is increased as a result. It is unclear, however, whether atelectrauma exerts a significant effect on fibrotic areas of lung, as these areas may be irreversibly collapsed.

Collapse induration, a hallmark feature of IPF, occurs as a consequence of surfactant dysfunction and subsequent overgrowth of alveolar epithelium in the alveolar space. In the absence of functional surfactant, alveolar epithelial cells are subjected to repetitive mechanical stress, which subsequently leads to cell hyperplasia and further increased surface tension. Together, these lead to alveolar collapse that may ultimately be unrecruitable. Bleomycin models of pulmonary fibrosis have demonstrated that in early phases of fibrosis before the onset of collapse induration, the application of PEEP leads to successful alveolar recruitment and improved lung compliance; however, after the onset of collapse induration, PEEP leads to worsening lung compliance, suggesting that PEEP, in this setting, is contributing to alveolar overdistension in relatively normal levels of lung.

The heterogeneity of involvement in ILD is likely responsible for these findings and leads to overdistension of relatively preserved alveoli, with little to no recruitment of collapsed alveoli. Recently, the idea of the "squishy ball lung" has been proposed to explain the lung injury and subsequent loss of lung compliance caused by high PEEP in fibrotic ILD. They postulate that in affected areas, the lung acts like a stress ball encased in an inelastic net ("squishy ball").

With the application of high PEEP, elastic lung tissue protrudes through the net and becomes increasingly rigid because of the high pressures generated by positive pressure ventilation. Tissue damage and VILI subsequently occur (**Figure 14-5**).

It is recommended that clinicians target a "lung resting strategy" in patients with fibrotic ILD that titrates PEEP to the lowest possible value to achieve acceptable oxygenation (Pao_2 > 50-60 mm Hg, Spo_2 > 88%-90%) with the goal of minimizing plateau pressures. Although the available data suggest against the use of high PEEP in patients with fibrotic ILD, it is less clear whether the same harm is seen in patients with inflammatory ILD. Clinicians may consider the application of higher PEEP levels, similar to those applied in ARDS, in patients who have predominantly ground-glass opacities on imaging.

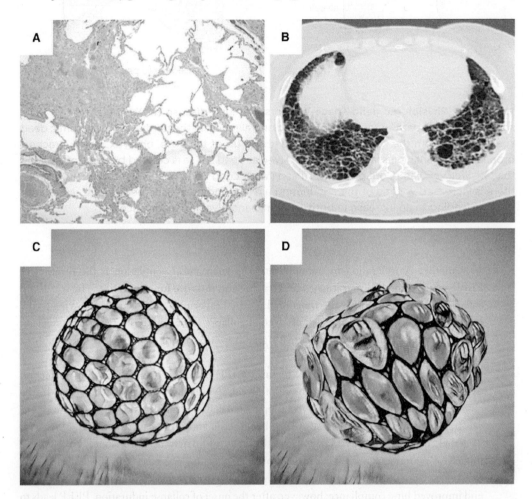

Figure 14-5: Squishy ball lung. A, Histologic usual interstitial pneumonia (UIP) pattern seen in fibrotic interstitial lung disease (ILD). **B,** High-resolution computed tomography (CT) image of UIP pattern. **C,** Visual depiction of the "squishy ball lung" depicting inelastic bands of fibrosis (*black net*) around normal elastic lung (clear) at rest. **D,** When internal pressure is applied, such as that exerted during mechanical ventilation, normal lung extrudes through the fibrotic bands and is subjected to overdistension injury. (From Marchioni A, Tonelli R, Rossi G, et al. Ventilatory support and mechanical properties of the fibrotic lung acting as a "squishy ball." *Ann Intensive Care.* 2020;10(1):13. Figure 2.)

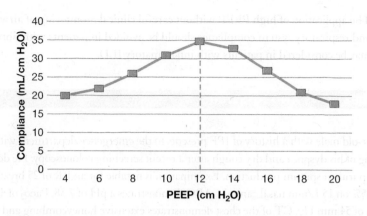

Figure 14-6: "Best PEEP" trial. In this figure, markers represent changes in respiratory system compliance ($C_{RS} = V_t/(P_{plat} - PEEP)$) with incremental changes in PEEP. The optimal, or "best" PEEP, indicated by the *dashed line*, corresponds to the highest compliance. PEEP, positive end-expiratory pressure.

"Best PEEP" trials, in which clinicians titrate PEEP to optimize driving pressure (DP = Pplat − PEEP) and, therefore, compliance, can be easily performed at the bedside and provide insight as to when overdistension occurs in individual patients (**Figure 14-6**). Notably, the optimal or "best" PEEP level is dependent on the delivered tidal volume and must be re-calculated if changes to tidal volume are made.

Liberation From Mechanical Ventilation

Assessing readiness for liberation from mechanical ventilation in patients with ILD can pose a particular challenge to clinicians owing to the underlying derangements in respiratory physiology these patients develop. At baseline, patients with ILD may breathe at faster rates and take relatively small tidal volumes because of their increased dead space and reduced lung compliance. As such, standard indices used to predict success in liberation, such as rapid shallow breathing index (RSBI) less than 105 breaths/min/mL, minute ventilation less than 10 L/min, or the integrative compliance, rate, oxygenation, and pressure (CROP) index greater 13 mL/breath/min, often suggest failure. At present, there is no available literature regarding ventilator liberation protocols for ILD, but we recommend a multifaceted assessment that accounts for improvement and/or resolution of the etiology of acute respiratory failure and adequate respiratory muscle strength when considering liberation.

KEY POINTS

- ILD is a heterogeneous group of lung diseases, and, clinically, patients can present with fibrotic or inflammatory disease.
- Patients with ILD are prone to AE-ILD that can lead to severe hypoxemia and the need to consider mechanical ventilation.
- The application of mechanical ventilation in ILD is challenging, and outcomes in patients with fibrotic ILD who require intubation and invasive mechanical ventilation are poor despite recent advances in critical care medicine.
- In all patients with ILD, low tidal volume ventilation and rapid RRs are recommended, given increased dead space ventilation and reduced lung compliance.

- The application of high PEEP without careful clinical monitoring of airway pressures and respiratory system compliance should be avoided in patients with fibrotic ILD but may be considered in patients with inflammatory ILD.

STUDY QUESTIONS AND ANSWERS

Questions

1. A 65-year-old male with a history of IPF presents to the emergency department with acute worsening of his dyspnea and dry cough after a recent screening colonoscopy. He denies fevers, chills, or purulent sputum production. Examination is notable for an RR of 25 breaths/min and SpO_2 of 85% on 15 L/min nasal cannula. ABG demonstrates a pH of 7.38, $PaCO_2$ of 45 mm Hg, and PaO_2 of 54 mm Hg. CT of the chest demonstrates extensive honeycombing and traction bronchiectasis that has progressed since a prior study performed 1 year ago. He is admitted to the ICU for higher level of care. Which of the following is most appropriate at this time?
   A. Continue low-flow nasal cannula.
   B. Administer NIPPV.
   C. Administer HFNC.
   D. Proceed to endotracheal intubation and mechanical ventilation.

2. A 73-year-old female with connective tissue disease–associated ILD (CTD-ILD) on rituximab presents to the emergency department with fevers, chills, and purulent sputum production. Examination is notable for a RR of 34 breaths/min and SpO_2 of 88% on nonrebreather mask. A chest x-ray is obtained and shows a new right middle lobe infiltrate, and sputum culture grows *Staphylococcus aureus*. The patient is intubated and admitted to the ICU. She is on volume control-assist control mode with the following initial settings: V_t 350 mL (6 mL/kg ideal birth weight [IBW]), RR 20 breaths/min, FiO_2 1.0, PEEP 8 cm H_2O. Plateau pressure is 30 cm H_2O. Initial ABG demonstrates a pH of 7.28, $PaCO_2$ of 60 mm Hg, and a PaO_2 of 80 mm Hg. Which of the following changes should be made?
   A. Increase V_t to 8 mL/kg IBW.
   B. Decrease V_t to 5 mL/kg IBW.
   C. Increase RR to 30 breaths/min.
   D. Increase PEEP to 10 cm H_2O.

3. You are evaluating a patient in the ICU who was intubated 12 hours ago for acute hypoxemic respiratory failure secondary to an exacerbation of their underlying fibrotic ILD. They are currently saturating 94% on volume control-assist control mode with the following settings: V_t 300 mL (6 mL/kg IBW), RR 20 breaths/min, FiO_2 0.6, PEEP 8 cm H_2O. You decide to perform a bedside PEEP titration and record the following values:

PEEP (cm H_2O)	Plateau pressure (cm H_2O)	PO_2 (mm Hg)
8	28	45
10	28	60
12	32	80

Which of the following is the "best" PEEP?
   A. 8 cm H_2O.
   B. 10 cm H_2O.
   C. 12 cm H_2O.

Answers

1. **Answer is C. Administer HFNC**

   Rationale: This patient with fibrotic ILD is presenting with an AE-ILD, likely triggered by sedation administered during his recent colonoscopy. He may benefit from the application of HFNC (Choice **C**) at this time. His blood gas demonstrates hypoxemic respiratory failure that is not responding to low-flow nasal cannula (Choice **A** is incorrect), and he does not have hypercapnia, which suggests that he does not require NIPPV at this time (Choice **B** is incorrect). Imaging does not suggest a reversible etiology for his exacerbation, such as a pneumonia or pulmonary embolism. As such, invasive mechanical ventilation (Choice **D** is incorrect) would not be advisable at this time.

2. **Answer is C. Increase RR to 30 breaths/min**

   Rationale: This patient presents with acute respiratory failure secondary to a community-acquired *S. aureus* pneumonia. Her initial ABG shows a significant respiratory acidosis that should be managed by an increase in minute ventilation. This can be achieved by increasing tidal volume (V_t) or RR. However, this patient is currently receiving the recommended lung-protective V_t of 6 mL/kg, and further increases to the V_t would violate the goal plateau pressure of less than 28 to 30 cm H_2O (Choice A is incorrect). Increasing the RR to 30 breaths/min (Choice **C**), however, would augment minute ventilation without violating lung-protective strategies. Decreasing V_t to 5 mL/kg IBW would decrease the minute ventilation and lead to worsening respiratory acidosis (Choice **B** is incorrect). Increasing PEEP to 10 cm H_2O would not be helpful (Choice **D** is incorrect) as the patient is currently saturating appropriately with the current amount of PEEP.

3. **Answer is B. 10 cm H_2O**

   Rationale: The "best PEEP" is 10 cm H_2O (Choice **B** is correct). The goal of PEEP application in fibrotic ILD is to provide the lowest amount of PEEP possible to achieve adequate oxygenation, while minimizing plateau pressures. With 8 cm H_2O of PEEP, plateau pressures are acceptable, but oxygenation is below the goal of 50 to 60 mm Hg (Choice **A** is incorrect). With 12 cm H_2O of PEEP, oxygenation is acceptable, but plateau pressure is above the goal of 28 to 30 cm H_2O (Choice **C** is incorrect).

Suggested Readings

Acute Respiratory Distress Syndrome Network, Brower RG, Matthay MA, et al. Ventilation with lower tidal volumes as compared with traditional tidal volumes for acute lung injury and the acute respiratory distress syndrome. *NEJM*. 2000;342(18):1301-1308.

Akira M, Kozuka T, Yamamoto S, Sakatani M. Computed tomography findings in acute exacerbation of idiopathic pulmonary fibrosis. *Am J Respir Crit Care Med*. 2008;178:372-378.

Al-Hameed FM, Sharma S. Outcome of patients admitted to the intensive care unit for acute exacerbation of idiopathic pulmonary fibrosis. *Can Respir J*. 2004;11:117-122.

Aliberti S, Messinesi G, Gamberini S, et al. Non-invasive mechanical ventilation in patients with diffuse interstitial lung diseases. *BMC Pulm Med*. 2014;14:194.

Amato MB, Barbas CS, Medeiros DM, et al. Effect of a protective-ventilation strategy on mortality in the acute respiratory distress syndrome. *NEJM*. 1998;338(6):347-354.

Antonelli M, Conti G, Esquinas A, et al. A multiple-center survey on the use in clinical practice of noninvasive ventilation as a first-line intervention for acute respiratory distress syndrome. *Crit Care Med*. 2007;35(1):18-25.

Bagnato G, Harari S. Cellular interactions in the pathogenesis of interstitial lung diseases. *Eur Respir Rev.* 2015;24:102-114.

Bates JH, Davis GS, Majumdar A, Butnor KJ, Suki B. Linking parenchymal disease progression to changes in lung mechanical function by percolation. *Am J Respir Crit Care Med.* 2007;176(6):617-623.

Baydur A. Mechanical ventilation in interstitial lung disease: which patients are likely to benefit? *Chest.* 2008;133(5):1062-1063.

Churg A, Muller NL. Cellular vs fibrosing interstitial pneumonias and prognosis: a practical classification of the idiopathic interstitial pneumonias and pathologically/radiologically similar conditions. *Chest.* 2006;130:1566-1570.

Durheim MT, Judy J, Bender S, et al. In-hospital mortality in patients with idiopathic pulmonary fibrosis: a US cohort study. *Lung.* 2019;197(6):699-707.

Fernandez-Perez ER, Yilmaz M, Jenad H, et al. Ventilator settings and outcome of respiratory failure in chronic interstitial lung disease. *Chest.* 2008;133(5):1113-1119.

Fujimoto K, Taniguchi H, Johkoh T, et al. Acute exacerbation of idiopathic pulmonary fibrosis: high-resolution CT scores predict mortality. *Eur Radiol.* 2012;22:83-92.

Fumeaux T, Rothmeier C, Jolliet P. Outcome of mechanical ventilation for acute respiratory failure in patients with pulmonary fibrosis. *Intensive Care Med.* 2001;27:1868-1874.

Glasser SW, Hardie WD, Hagood JS. Pathogenesis of interstitial lung disease in children and adults. *Pediatr Allergy Immunol Pulmonol.* 2010;23(1):9-14.

Grasselli G, Vergnano B, Pozzi MR, et al. Interstitial pneumonia with autoimmune features: an additional risk factor for ARDS? *Ann Intensive Care.* 2017;7(1):98.

Gungor G, Tatar D, Salturk C, et al. Why do patients with interstitial lung diseases fail in the ICU? A 2-center cohort study. *Respir Care.* 2013;58(3):525-531.

Huapaya JA, Wilfong EM, Harden CT, Brower RG, Danoff SK. Risk factors for mortality and mortality rates in interstitial lung disease patients in the intensive care unit. *Eur Respir Rev.* 2018;27(150):180061.

Judge EP, Fabre A, Adamali HI, Egan JJ. Acute exacerbations and pulmonary hypertension in advanced idiopathic pulmonary fibrosis. *Eur Respir J.* 2012;40:93-100.

Kim DS, Park JH, Park BK, Lee JS, Nicholson AG, Colby T. Acute exacerbation of idiopathic pulmonary fibrosis: frequency and clinical features. *Eur Respir J.* 2006;27:143-150.

Kishaba T, Tamaki H, Shimaoka Y, Fukuyama H, Yamashiro S. Staging of acute exacerbation in patients with idiopathic pulmonary fibrosis. *Lung.* 2014;192:141-149.

Kondoh Y, Taniguchi H, Katsuta T, et al. Risk factors of acute exacerbation of idiopathic pulmonary fibrosis. *Sarcoidosis Vasc Diffuse Lung Dis.* 2010;27:103-110.

Leuschner G, Behr J. Acute exacerbation in interstitial lung disease. *Front Med (Lausanne).* 2017;4:176.

Ley B, Collard HR. Epidemiology of idiopathic pulmonary fibrosis. *Clin Epidemiol.* 2013;5:483-492.

Lutz D, Gazdhar A, Lopez-Rodriguez E, et al. Alveolar derecruitment and collapse induration as crucial mechanisms in lung injury and fibrosis. *Am J Respir Cell Mol Biol.* 2015;52(2):232-243.

Marchioni A, Tonelli R, Rossi G, et al. Ventilatory support and mechanical properties of the fibrotic lung acting as a "squishy ball." *Ann Intensive Care.* 2020;10:13.

McKown AC, Semler MW, Rice TW. Best PEEP trials are dependent on tidal volume. *Crit Care.* 2018;22:115.

Miyazaki Y, Tateishi T, Akashi T, Ohtani Y, Inase N, Yoshizawa Y. Clinical predictors and histologic appearance of acute exacerbations in chronic hypersensitivity pneumonitis. *Chest.* 2008;134(6):1265-1270.

Mooney JJ, Raimundo K, Chang E, Broder MS. Mechanical ventilation in idiopathic pulmonary fibrosis: a nationwide analysis of ventilator use, outcomes, and resource burden. *BMC Pulm Med.* 2017;17(1):84.

Nemec SF, Eisenberg RL, Bankier AA. Noninfectious inflammatory lung disease: imaging considerations and clues to differential diagnosis. *AJR Am J Roentgenol.* 2013;201:278-294.

Nuckton TJ, Alonso JA, Kallet RH, et al. Pulmonary dead-space fraction as a risk factor for death in the acute respiratory distress syndrome. *N Engl J Med*. 2002;346:1281-1286.

Ohshimo S, Ishikawa N, Horimasu Y, et al. Baseline KL-6 predicts increased risk for acute exacerbation of idiopathic pulmonary fibrosis. *Respir Med*. 2014;108:1031-1039.

Olson AL, Huie TJ, Groshong SD, et al. Acute exacerbations of fibrotic hypersensitivity pneumonitis: a case series. *Chest*. 2008;134(4):844-850.

Park IN, Kim DS, Shim TS, et al. Acute exacerbation of interstitial pneumonia other than idiopathic pulmonary fibrosis. *Chest*. 2007;132(1):214-220.

Plantier L, Cazes A, Dinh-Xuan AT, Bancal C, Marchand-Adam S, Crestani B. Physiology of the lung in idiopathic pulmonary fibrosis. *Eur Respir Rev*. 2018;27:170062.

Raghu G, Collard HR, Egan JJ, et al. An official ATS/ERS/JRS/ALAT statement: idiopathic pulmonary fibrosis: evidence-based guidelines for diagnosis and management. *Am J Respir Crit Care Med*. 2011;183:788-824.

Raghu G, Rochwerg B, Zhang Y, et al. An official ATS/ERS/JRS/ALAT clinical practice guideline: treatment of idiopathic pulmonary fibrosis. An update of the 2011 clinical practice guideline. *Am J Respir Crit Care Med*. 2015;192(2):e3-e19.

Riha RL, Duhig EE, Clarke BE, Steele RH, Slaughter RE, Zimmerman PV. Survival of patients with biopsy-proven usual interstitial pneumonia and nonspecific interstitial pneumonia. *Eur Respir J*. 2002;19:1114-1118.

Rush B, Wiskar K, Berger L, Griesdale D. The use of mechanical ventilation in patients with idiopathic pulmonary fibrosis in the United States: a nationwide retrospective cohort analysis. *Respir Med*. 2016;111:72-76.

Saydain G, Islam A, Afessa B, Ryu JH, Scott JP, Peters SG. Outcome of patients with idiopathic pulmonary fibrosis admitted to the intensive care unit. *Am J Respir Crit Care Med*. 2002;166:839-842.

Schrader M, Sathananthan M, Jeganathan N. Patients with idiopathic pulmonary fibrosis admitted to the ICU with acute respiratory failure: a reevaluation of the risk factors and outcomes. *J Intensive Care Med*. 2021 ;37:342-351. doi:10.1177/0885066621989244. Epub ahead of print.

Shweish O, Dronavalli G. Indications for lung transplant referral and listing. *J Thorac Dis*. 2019;11(suppl 14):S1708-S1720.

Song JW, Hong SB, Lim CM, Koh Y, Kim DS. Acute exacerbation of idiopathic pulmonary fibrosis: incidence, risk factors and outcome. *Eur Respir J*. 2011;37(2):356-363.

Stern JB, Mal H, Groussard O, et al. Prognosis of patients with advanced idiopathic pulmonary fibrosis requiring mechanical ventilation for acute respiratory failure. *Chest*. 2001;120:213-219.

Suda T, Kaida Y, Nakamura Y, et al. Acute exacerbation of interstitial pneumonia associated with collagen vascular diseases. *Respir Med*. 2009;103(6):846-853.

Tachikawa R, Tomii K, Ueda H, et al. Clinical features and outcome of acute exacerbation of interstitial pneumonia: collagen vascular diseases-related versus idiopathic. *Respiration*. 2012;83(1):20-27.

Vourlekis JS, Schwarz MI, Cherniack RM, et al. The effect of pulmonary fibrosis on survival in patients with hypersensitivity pneumonitis. *Am J Med*. 2004;116:662-668.

Weill D. Lung transplantation: indications and contraindications. *J Thorac Dis*. 2018;10(7):4574-4587.

Wong AW, Ryerson CJ, Guler SA. Progression of fibrosing interstitial lung disease. *Respir Res*. 2020;21:32.

Yokoyama T, Kondoh Y, Taniguchi H, et al. Noninvasive ventilation in acute exacerbation of idiopathic pulmonary fibrosis. *Intern Med*. 2010;49(15):1509-1514.

Yokoyama T, Tsushima K, Yamamoto H, Koizumi T, Kubo K. Potential benefits of early continuous positive pressure ventilation in patients with rapidly progressive interstitial pneumonia. *Respirology*. 2012;17:315-321.

Zafrani L, Lemiale V, Lapidus N, Lorillon G, Schlemmer B, Azoulay E. Acute respiratory failure in critically ill patients with interstitial lung disease. *PLoS ONE*. 2014;9:e104897.

Complications of Mechanical Ventilation

Elias Baedorf Kassis

LEARNING OBJECTIVES

- Delineate the risks and benefits associated with the decision to initiate mechanical ventilation.
- Describe the risks associated with intubation.
- Discuss the complications associated with short-term mechanical ventilation.
- Outline the longer term complications that occur secondary to prolonged mechanical ventilation.

INTRODUCTION

Although mechanical ventilation is necessary to stabilize critically ill patients, deliver oxygen and remove carbon dioxide in patients unable to breathe independently, and provide support for the respiratory system in patients with fragile lungs who are challenged by an acute pulmonary disease, it is important to understand that mechanical ventilation may also be the source of complications and harm in patients, even when optimally applied. Mechanical ventilation is associated, unfortunately, with many potential problems and side effects, either directly or indirectly related to the ventilator. These side effects include injury to the lung from improper mechanical ventilation settings, injury from the patient's own breathing activity while being ventilated, the development of muscle weakness and injury related to disuse of respiratory muscles (diaphragm and peripheral skeletal muscles), and additional complications associated with prolonged ventilation (eg, pressure ulcers, ventilator-associated pneumonias [VAPs], delirium, prolonged hospitalization, and the need for a tracheostomy tube).

There is often little choice in the decision to intubate and mechanically ventilate patients when they are developing acute respiratory failure, or need intubation for an important procedure or operation. Awareness of these risks, however, may help guide management of the patient during intubation and enable you to limit the degree of risk and complications as much as possible. In addition, there may be some cases in which the decision to intubate is more nuanced and less straightforward; in these settings, the potential complications need to be weighed against the possible benefits from mechanical ventilation. Delaying intubation too long has been associated with worsened outcomes in patients, whereas intubating a patient too early might result in unnecessary intubations and increased patient complications from the intubation and mechanical ventilation. Although it is not possible to avoid intubation in all circumstances, it is imperative to understand the numerous complications and issues associated with mechanical ventilation (**Figure 15-1**).

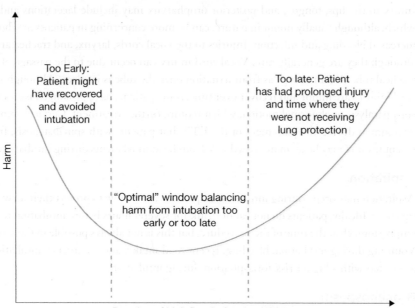

Figure 15-1: **Understanding the "sweet spot" in the decision to intubate and initiate mechanical ventilation**. Delaying intubation too long may result in worsened patient outcomes, while in contrast, intubating patients too soon may result in some patients getting mechanical ventilation who otherwise would have improved without it and are exposed to the additional duration, sedation, and complications associated with mechanical ventilation.

COMPLICATIONS FROM INTUBATION

Although many of the complications that are discussed in this chapter are secondary to mechanical ventilation and the prolonged hospitalization that may be associated with this therapy, the intubation procedure itself also carries a unique set of risks. Intubation is usually routine and safe, especially when done for an elective procedure or operation, but there are a number of important risks associated with intubation itself that are important to understand and discuss. Thankfully, most complications are minor (such as sore throat), whereas major complications from intubation are relatively rare, but there is an increased risk for complications when the procedure is done urgently or emergently.

Oropharyngeal Injuries

Although dental injuries may be considered a fairly minor complication from intubation, they are very common and represent the most frequent cause of malpractice claims. Poor baseline dentition and difficult intubations are associated with an increased risk of injury. Sore throat is another common (but minor) side effect of intubation and is relatively benign in nature and course. Typically, sore throat is present for the initial 48 hours after extubation and then subsequently resolves. If the sore throat persists, it may be evidence of a more serious soft-tissue injury and may require further investigation and diagnostic evaluation, such as imaging or direct visualization.

Soft-Tissue and Structural Injuries

Soft-tissue and structural injuries from intubation may range from minor to severe in nature. Injury to the lips, tongue, and posterior oropharynx may include lacerations and bleeding, which, although usually minor in nature, can be more concerning in patients in whom there is increased bleeding and infection. Injuries to the vocal cords, larynx, and trachea are possible, although they are generally rare. Vocal cord injury can occur due to the passage of the endotracheal tube (ETT) as well as from irritation once the tube is in place. Although most vocal cord injuries are minor and recover over time, some patients have prolonged issues with vocal cord paralysis or abnormal motion, which require further treatment. Cervical spine injury is uncommon during the placement of the ETT, but patients with spinal stenosis, fracture, or recent trauma may be at an increased risk from head movements during intubation.

Aspiration

Aspiration may occur during intubation as patients are unable to protect their airways during this time. Ideally, patients do not eat or drink for several hours before intubation to ensure an empty stomach at the time of the procedure, but this is not always possible in the acute setting. Vomiting during intubation, bleeding, recent food intake, and emergency intubations are all associated with a higher risk for aspiration during intubation.

Bronchospasm

Bronchospasm and laryngospasm may occur after intubation secondary to the irritation of the ETT within the trachea. This is particularly common in patients with baseline airway hyperreactivity, asthma, and chronic obstructive pulmonary disease (COPD), although they can occur in other patients as well. Typically, this manifests as a sudden increase in peak pressure during the inspiratory phase of mechanical ventilation, high measured airway resistance, difficulty delivering the desired tidal volume, or apparent patient discomfort.

Esophageal Intubation

With direct laryngoscopy or video laryngoscopy, the frequency of esophageal intubation should be low; however, it still has been estimated to account for up to 6% of airway complications. The use of capnography, which measures exhaled CO_2 levels, and the confirmation of bilateral breath sounds after intubation should be used in all patients to confirm correct placement.

HYPOXEMIA AND HYPERCARBIA

Hypoxemia and hypercarbia can be considered a complication of both intubation and mechanical ventilation. It is common for patients to acutely develop worsened hypoxemia after intubation, and this may occur secondary to decreased ventilation, lung collapse, or worsened ventilation-perfusion matching immediately after intubation. Because rapid sequence intubation techniques typically employ paralytics, the loss of muscle tone in the chest wall can have adverse consequences on the distribution of ventilation. While these gas exchange disturbances are particularly common in more critically ill patients who are intubated specifically for respiratory failure, it may occur in other seemingly lower risk patients as well. In particular, patients with obesity, pregnancy, or underlying pulmonary and cardiovascular pathologies are especially vulnerable to this period of hypoxemia postintubation.

Patients may similarly develop worsened hypercapnia after intubation. This can typically be addressed by increasing the minute ventilation (raising tidal volumes and/or respiratory rate) but may be persistent, particularly in patients with COPD and asthma exacerbations (see Chapters 11 and 12 for more details) who are at risk for dynamic hyperinflation, particularly with increased respiratory rate, and in patients with high dead space fraction who have high ventilation requirements (such as acute respiratory distress syndrome [ARDS], see Chapter 13).

Worsened hypoxemia and hypercapnia may also develop over the course of mechanical ventilation. In some cases, this may be a consequence of mechanical ventilation, particularly if secondary to ventilator-induced lung injury (VILI) (see later in this chapter), VAPs, or incorrect ventilator settings. Often, the worsening hypoxemia and hypercapnia, however, may just be secondary to the progression of the underlying disease that necessitated intubation.

HEMODYNAMIC COMPLICATIONS

As discussed in Chapters 4 and 7, the application of positive pressure and the resulting increase in intrathoracic pressures with initiation of mechanical ventilation can have significant hemodynamic effects, which, at times, may lead to large and dangerous decreases in blood pressure. This problem is accentuated when applying higher levels of positive end-expiratory pressure (PEEP) and in patients with high levels of auto-PEEP or dynamic hyperinflation in whom intrathoracic pressures are further increased. The risk of a decrease in cardiac output is particularly notable in patients with low intravascular volume and pulmonary vascular disease or right heart dysfunction. Hypotension can also occur in other patients secondary to the use of sedative medications, which reduce the high adrenergic tone associated with the respiratory distress before intubation; the anesthetics used for induction, which may cause vasodilation, further contribute to the problem. Hypotension is a common response found in up to 50% of critically ill patients undergoing intubation and, in severe cases, can lead to cardiac arrest. As such, planning ahead for expected hypotension is important when proceeding to intubation.

Patients often receive a small bolus of pressor medications (which raise the blood pressure) during induction, and a continuous infusion should be planned for before intubation to avoid dangerous and prolonged drops in the blood pressure.

Other hemodynamic side effects include hypertensive episodes and arrhythmias, both of which are less common than hypotension. Hypertension may be precipitated by intubation and is usually a sign of a large sympathetic nervous system discharge, indicative of inadequate sedation needed to blunt the pain/discomfort associated with intubation. Arrhythmias, particularly bradycardia, may be accompanied by hypotension, especially in patients with high vagal tone or predisposition to slow heart rate. In addition, hypoxemia during intubation can worsen the degree of bradycardia in some cases. Tachyarrhythmias are less common and tend to occur in patients with baseline cardiac dysfunction.

DEVELOPMENT OF LUNG INJURY DURING MECHANICAL VENTILATION

Ventilator-Induced Lung Injury

VILI represents several types of injury that can be incurred by a patient's lungs consequent to the mechanical ventilation. Although some degree of VILI may not be completely avoidable, particularly in patients with severely diseased lungs, understanding the potential mechanisms by which VILI is thought to arise may allow a clinician to limit this additional injury. The concept of VILI is also touched upon in Chapter 14 where we discuss mechanical ventilation for ARDS; VILI, however, is a potential complication associated with any lung disease or reason for intubation (including for surgery) if the ventilator is not properly utilized.

Lung injury from overdistension is secondary to both the pressures applied to the lungs and the physical deformation that results from the volumes that the lung achieves, and it is largely predicated on the finding that most lung diseases are heterogeneous; not all lung units are affected to the same degree in most pulmonary processes, which leads to variable compliance within the lung and, consequently, different effects of a given inspiratory pressure on the distribution of gas during lung inflation on varying lung units. The injury from pressure (also known as *barotrauma*) and the injury from physical deformation (also known as *volutrauma*) are intimately related to each other via the concept of compliance described in Chapter 2. Lung stress correlates with the pressure being applied to the lungs, and lung strain is a manifestation of the volume of deformation; for the purposes of our discussion, however, these concepts can be considered together as the mechanical injury that occurs secondary to overdistension.

Imagine a balloon that is overinflated to the point of failure; the lungs can similarly be injured by overdistension. Limiting overdistension is primarily achieved via control over delivered tidal volumes, peak pressures, end-inspiratory pressures during an inspiratory breath-hold (also known as the *plateau pressure*—see Chapter 2), and the pressure that is needed to ensure the delivery of the desired volume (also known as the *driving pressure*, which is calculated as the plateau pressure minus the end-expiratory pressure). These values are easily monitored at the bedside to determine the safety of the current ventilator settings and thereby limit additional injury (**Figure 15-2**). Chapter 13 discusses the concepts of lung-protective ventilation strategies in further detail, but the overlying goal of these strategies is to prevent overdistension and further VILI.

Lung injury can also occur secondary to collapse or atelectasis of regions of the lungs and the repetitive opening and collapse of lung units during mechanical ventilation. This injury

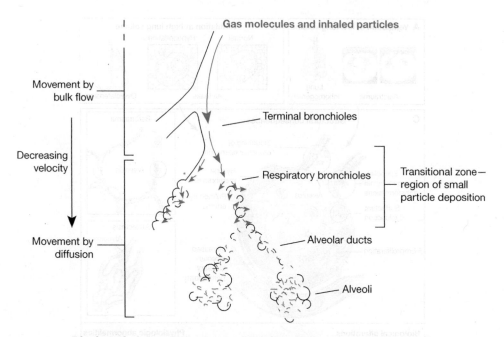

Figure 15-2: Display of plateau pressure and driving pressure.

from the repetitive collapse and opening on each breath is termed *atelectrauma* (from the cyclic atelectasis that occurs). Atelectrauma occurs secondary to high levels of shear stress along the tissue interface as they are repetitively ripped open and then allowed to collapse again. As discussed in Chapter 7, the application of PEEP serves in part to increase the end-expiratory lung volume and thereby prevent the collapse at end expiration and the consequent degree of atelectrauma.

The combination of mechanical trauma from overdistension and cyclic collapse results in a local and systemic inflammatory response, which is called *biotrauma*. In addition, biotrauma may be precipitated by other local and systemic pathologies in the body, which may further worsen the lungs response to mechanical trauma. Although some degree of inflammation may be needed for proper healing, the response may be injurious and contribute to the development of fibrosis and scarring (**Figure 15-3**).

Role of the Patient in Lung Injury Complications From Mechanical Ventilation

More recently, the understanding of injury during mechanical ventilation has evolved, and increasing attention has been focused on the potential for lung injury caused by a patient's own breathing activity. This concept has been termed *patient self-induced lung injury* (P-SILI). Although this can be considered a possible complication in patients receiving mechanical ventilation if the ventilation parameters are set incorrectly, appropriate application of mechanical ventilation and the use of sedation and other adjunctive treatments can also protect patients again from developing P-SILI.

In patients without significant lung injury, spontaneous breathing is preferred during mechanical ventilation. Spontaneous breathing with pressure support assistance in these patients improves ventilation-perfusion matching; prevents lung collapse, particularly in

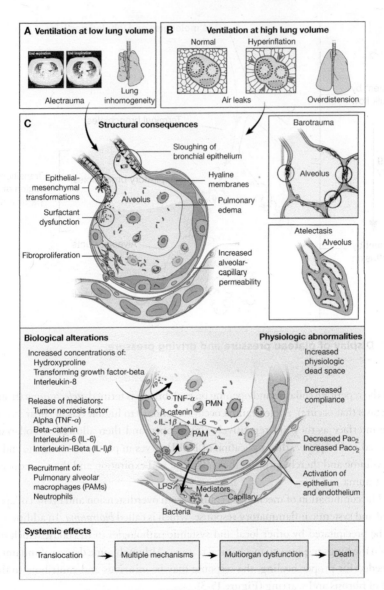

Figure 15-3: **Overview of the types of ventilator-induced lung injury (VILI). A**, Lung collapse at end expiration and overdistension at end inspiration occur secondary to lung heterogeneity. **B**, Ventilation at high lung volumes results in overdistension injury. **C**, VILI can occur secondary to both lung overdistension and collapse and the resulting inflammation that occurs from this repetitive sequence. Collapse of the lungs at low lung volumes and low levels of positive end-expiratory pressure (PEEP) results in cyclic opening and closing of the alveoli (atelectrauma), which causes shear stress injury, and is further amplified by lung heterogeneity, with some areas of lung exhibiting very low compliance while other regions may have normal compliance. With high levels of PEEP and large tidal volume, the lung can become overdistended, leading to trauma from both the applied pressures (barotrauma) and the physical deformation associated with the larger volumes (volutrauma). Volutrauma and barotrauma are inherently related but distinct. Both injuries from collapse and overdistension can create mechanical damage that further amplifies or causes resulting inflammation, which provides an additional type of injury (biotrauma). (Redrawn from Slutsky AS, Ranieri VM. Ventilator-induced lung injury. *N Engl J Med.* 2013 Nov 28;369(22):2126-2136.)

dependent lung regions; and helps prevent atrophy and weakness of the respiratory muscles, including the diaphragm. As the lung disease worsens, however, as occurs with ARDS, several factors associated with spontaneous breathing may result in lung injury. Spontaneous breathing can be associated with uncontrolled tidal volumes, which may be significantly larger than would otherwise be desired for sick injured lungs, leading to volutrauma. In concert with these larger tidal volumes, especially in patients with decreased compliance, the driving pressures may also be elevated to dangerous and injurious levels. Driving pressure may not initially make sense conceptually in spontaneously breathing patients; the "driving" pressure in this case is the combination of the patient's own inspiratory effort in addition to the applied pressure support that is required to expand the lungs during inspiration. As discussed earlier, the driving pressure is calculated as the difference between the plateau pressure (measured during an inspiratory occlusion) and the total PEEP level (measured during an expiratory occlusion). These measurements require some practice to acquire in spontaneously breathing patients, but quality data can be obtained to assure safe levels of lung stretch during spontaneous breathing.

Lung injury from spontaneous breathing can also be caused and magnified by the variable ventilation pattern of the lungs and the uneven movement of the diaphragm during contraction. The diaphragm is tethered in a more cranial position anteriorly and more caudal position posteriorly. This results in greater vertical movement locally of the posterior portion of the diaphragm relative to the anterior portion, which results in increased local posterior ventilation during normal spontaneous breathing. While this serves to improve ventilation-perfusion matching in healthy patients, the increased local diaphragm forces result in increased local stress on these relatively low compliance regions of lung in individuals in whom the posterior/dependent lung regions become consolidated and collapsed; the resulting large pressure swings may worsen injury and edema in these regions. The variable distribution of gas in the lung is also magnified in some patients by a phenomenon called *pendelluft*. This occurs when air moves from one lung region to another, independent of the bulk air movement in and out of the lungs, and can occur during lung inflation and deflation. During spontaneous breathing, air is "pulled" during inspiration from anterior/nondependent regions into the posterior/dependent regions, resulting in locally increased volumes from both the bulk air movement from outside the lungs and the air movement from within the lungs (the pendelluft phenomenon), which may result in local overdistension, particularly in the dependent lung regions (**Figure 15-4**).

There is increasing evidence that it is not only the applied lung volumes and pressure changes that may result in injury but also the degree of patient inspiratory effort associated with breathing. Patient effort has been given many names clinically and can be assessed partly via a bedside physical examination based upon a patient's degree of tachypnea, tidal volume, accessory muscle use, nasal fairing, intercostal retractions, and level of agitation. While these observations may be useful, they are difficult to standardize and may at times be misleading. More objective measurements of patient effort may be helpful to estimate when efforts are "safe" versus "injurious." The p0.1 is the pressure measured over the initial 100 msec of inspiratory effort against a closed airway (the inspiratory inlet of the ventilator is occluded during the prior exhalation). The greater the inspiratory effort, the larger the resulting pressure; this value may be useful in assessing the safety of spontaneous breathing in patients with ARDS (safe levels are considered to be between 0 and 4 cm H_2O) and to estimate whether patients will be successfully weaned from mechanical ventilation (with higher efforts associated with

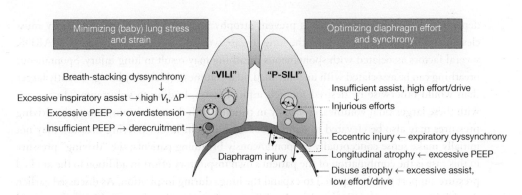

Figure 15-4: Patient self-induced lung injury. Self-induced lung injury results from injurious patient efforts during spontaneous breathing. This can occur particularly in early acute respiratory distress syndrome (ARDS) when the lung is inflamed or stiff, and vigorous patient respiratory efforts result in damaging pressure swings across the lungs. PEEP, positive end-expiratory pressure; P-SILI, patient self-induced lung injury; VILI, ventilator-induced lung injury (From Goligher EC, Jonkman AH, Dianti J, et al. Clinical strategies for implementing lung and diaphragm-protective ventilation: avoiding insufficient and excessive effort. *Intensive Care Med.* 2020 Dec;46(12):2314-2326.)

increased weaning failure; the presumption is that the higher effort, indicative of stimulation of the central controller component of the respiratory system, may represent worse underlying disease that has not yet resolved).

Dyssynchrony

Patient-ventilator dyssynchrony, which is covered in detail in Chapter 18, denotes circumstances in which the patient is making respiratory efforts that are not aligned with what the ventilator is trying to do, for example, the patient is trying to breathe in while the ventilator is in the expiratory phase, or the patient is assisting the ventilator in a way that may lead to lung injury. Dyssynchrony may cause a similar type of injury pattern as P-SILI secondary to strong patient respiratory efforts, large delivered volumes, and high-pressure swings across the lungs. Dyssynchrony has also been associated with worsened patient outcomes with prolonged intensive care unit (ICU) stay, increased duration of mechanical ventilation, and increased mortality. Patients with dyssynchrony may require increased sedative use, which (as covered later) may lead to sedative-specific complications, increased delirium, and prolongation of mechanical ventilation.

DIAPHRAGM AND SKELETAL MUSCLE INJURY

Diaphragm injury and weakness has been shown to occur rapidly in patients undergoing mechanical ventilation, a process known as *ventilator-induced diaphragmatic dysfunction* (VIDD). The diaphragm quickly atrophies with disuse as occurs when patients are deeply sedated or paralyzed and are fully passive with the ventilator performing all of the work of respiration. Atrophy may be more rapid in the setting of critical illness and is further exacerbated by the use of medications, such as steroids.

In addition, the diaphragm may be susceptible not only to atrophy but also to direct injury secondary to systemic inflammation and load-based injury (ie, struggling against moving the lungs with low compliance and/or high resistance) associated with spontaneous breathing efforts. This combination of atrophy and injury can lead to significant impairment of diaphragm function, which may require a prolonged period for recovery (**Figure 15-5**). This respiratory muscle impairment can lead to long-term morbidity, decreased functional status, difficulty with extubation, prolonged ventilation, and increased need for tracheostomy placement. Although this is an important complication about which you should be aware, it remains unclear how best to balance lung-protection ventilation strategies with diaphragm protection in all patients, as they may at times be at odds with each other—to prevent P-SILI and injury from dyssynchrony, we sedate the patient to prevent spontaneous breathing, which then may lead to the absence of neural stimulation of the diaphragm and consequent atrophy.

Skeletal muscle weakness and injury may also occur in patients undergoing mechanical ventilation. While the ventilator itself does not directly cause weakness and injury, the associated deep levels of sedation, use of paralytics in some patients, prolonged illness, and use of certain medications such as steroids in concert with minimal patient movement may cause skeletal muscle damage. Unfortunately, generalized weakness and myopathy are quite common and may lead to prolonged recovery and weakness. Prevention of this complication

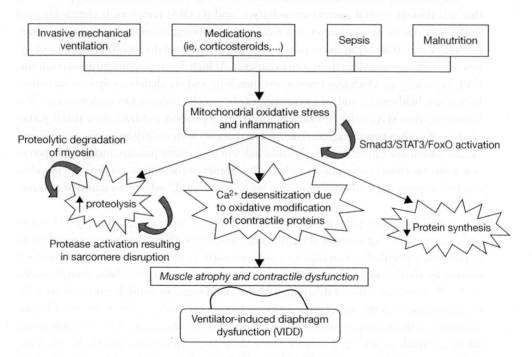

Figure 15-5: During mechanical ventilation, multiple factors contribute to diaphragm dysfunction (both atrophy and weakness). These include prolonged lack of use while in fully controlled modes of ventilation when patients are often passive over long durations, the medications that are used including paralytics and steroids, the lack of adequate nutrition, and the underlying disease and associated inflammation, which typically have systemic effects in these severely ill patients. Together, these factors can lead to profound diaphragm injury and weakness, which has been associated with worsened clinical outcomes. (From Peñuelas O, Keough E, López-Rodríguez L, et al. Ventilator-induced diaphragm dysfunction: Translational mechanisms lead to therapeutical alternatives in the critically ill. *Intensive Care Med Exp.* 2019 Jul 25;7(Suppl 1):48.)

includes early physical therapy and mobilization of the patient (even while intubated), minimization of sedation, paralytics and steroids, and adequate nutritional intake.

SEDATIVE USE

Intravenous sedation and analgesia are commonly required in order to allow the patient to tolerate mechanical ventilation. In particular, the standard best practice of "lung-protective ventilation" may inherently be uncomfortable for patients, providing lower tidal volumes than patients would typically desire and resulting in high Pco_2 levels and low pH levels, which can increase respiratory drive. In addition, mechanical ventilation can cause discomfort from the ETT, and many of the disease states that result in the need for mechanical ventilation are associated with increased pain (such as surgery, trauma, and pancreatitis). Patients often require high levels of sedatives and analgesics while on mechanical ventilation with consequent complications that may occur directly from the sedatives or as a secondary effect due to difficulty in weaning sedatives necessitating prolonged mechanical ventilation as the period of critical illness resolves.

Direct toxicity from sedatives includes the following: Propofol, which is a hypnotic drug that acts through central gamma-aminobutyric acid (GABA) receptors, is commonly used in the ICU due to its rapid onset and recovery, titratability, antiemetic and anticonvulsant properties, and its ability to use in patients with liver and renal disease. Bradycardia and hypotension are common side effects seen in patients. At high doses, propofol infusion syndrome (PRIS) can develop, which may cause severe metabolic acidosis, rhabdomyolysis, renal failure, liver injury, bradycardia, and, in severe cases, cardiovascular collapse. Dexmedetomidine (also known as *precedex*) is a sedative with less respiratory depression, a characteristic that is particularly useful when treating agitated delirium in patients with underlying respiratory disease. Dexmedetomidine can cause hemodynamic side effects in many patients, including hypotension with or without bradycardia or tachycardia. Abrupt discontinuation of dexmedetomidine can lead to physiologic changes associated with "withdrawal," which can manifest as severe hypertension.

Several benzodiazepines are commonly used to achieve sedation, including midazolam and lorazepam, during mechanical ventilation. These medications are sometimes used instead of propofol, particularly when clinicians are concerned about hemodynamics, or if there is a concern for the development of PRIS. Benzodiazepines, however, have been strongly associated with an increased risk of delirium, a complication found in multiple studies in critically ill patients; consequently, many critical care centers have moved away from the use of benzodiazepines in this patient population. Benzodiazepines may also accumulate in adipose tissue, which can result in prolonged sedation as the drug slowly recirculates into the blood. Withdrawal symptoms from cessation of benzodiazepines may be severe in some patients who have been treated for prolonged periods or who have been weaned too quickly. Opiates, including fentanyl and Dilaudid, are used in combination with sedatives, and prolonged use can result in chemical dependence and risk of withdrawal symptoms upon cessation (**Table 15-1**).

DELIRIUM

Although delirium is not unique to patients undergoing mechanical ventilation, the use of ventilators, the severe underlying illness leading to respiratory failure, and the medications, sedatives, and analgesics used throughout critical illness all can contribute to and worsen

TABLE 15-1 Use and Risk of Specific Sedatives

Drug	Mechanism of Action	Pharmacokinetics	Patient Care Considerations
Fentanyl	Mu opioid receptor agonist	Onset IV: immediate Duration IV: 0.5-1 h Half-life elimination IV: 2-4 h	Chest wall rigidity, accumulation in hepatic dysfunction, tachyphylaxis
Hydromorphone	Mu opioid receptor agonist	Onset IV: 5 min Duration IV: 3-4 h Half-life elimination IV: 2-3 h	Drug (rounding) errors, hypotension
Morphine	Mu opioid receptor agonist	Onset IV: 5-10 min Duration IV: 3-5 h Half-life elimination IV: 2-4 h	Hypotension, flushing, accumulation in renal dysfunction
Propofol	GABA agonist	Onset: 30 s Duration: 3-10 min, prolonged with prolonged use Half-life elimination: terminal 4-7 h, prolonged with prolonged use	Propofol-related infusion syndrome, triglyceridemia, pancreatitis, hypotension
Dexmedetomidine	Alpha-2 agonist	Onset: 15-30 min Duration: 60-120 min Half-life elimination: terminal 3 h	May be used in nonintubated patients; bradycardia, hypotension; analgesic-sparing effects
Midazolam	GABA agonist	Onset: 1-5 min Duration: <2 h Half-life elimination: 3-11 h	Delirium; prolonged sedation in patients with hepatic or renal dysfunction, obesity, or heart failure; active metabolites

GABA: gamma-aminobutyric acid; IV, intravenous. Modified from Mefford BM, Donaldson JC. Analgesia and sedation strategies in COVID-19 patients. *US Pharm.* 2021;47(3):HS-11-HS-16; Devlin JW, Skrobik Y, Gélinas C, et al. Clinical practice guidelines for the prevention and management of pain, agitation/sedation, delirium, immobility, and sleep disruption in adult patients in the ICU. *Crit Care Med.* 2018;46(9):e825-e873; Ammar MA, Sacha GL, Welch SC, et al. Sedation, analgesia, and paralysis in COVID-19 patients in the setting of drug shortages. *J Intensive Care Med.* 2021;36(2):157-174; Chanques G, Constantin JM, Devlin JW, et al. Analgesia and sedation in patients with ARDS. *Intensive Care Med.* 2020;46:2342-2356.

delirium. Delirium may manifest in a wide variety of confusional states ranging from somnolence to agitation and may have an enormous impact on patients, particularly in the elderly population. Delirium is associated with prolonged hospitalization, loss of functionality, and decreased ability to be sent home after the resolution of illness. Particularly notable is the impressive association between delirium and mortality, which is significantly increased even after adjusting for dementia and other potential confounders.

Delirium may persist for a prolonged period after the resolution of the initial illness and has been linked to accelerations in cognitive decline, particularly in patients with underlying baseline dementia. Delirium in patients undergoing mechanical ventilation may result in a longer duration of ventilation with an increased risk of other complications during this time; paradoxically, the treatment of delirium in mechanically ventilated patients may also prolong intubation and increase the total load of required sedatives.

VENTILATOR-ASSOCIATED PNEUMONIA

VAP is a common and sometimes severe complication from mechanical ventilation. It is associated with increased mortality, increased duration of mechanical ventilation, and prolonged stay within the ICU. VAPs are diagnosed in patients who have been undergoing mechanical ventilation for at least 48 hours. It is important to make the diagnosis of VAP because they are associated with more severe infections related to a specific set of pathogens.

VAPs are diagnosed when ventilated patients develop new symptoms, including fever, increased secretions, increased ventilator requirements, and worsened ventilatory mechanics in association with new infiltrates on chest imaging. VAPs occur probably secondary to the presence of the ETT, which inhibits some of the normal lung defenses against infection and can be a source of colonization for organisms; hence, the specific bacteria causing the new infection tend to be those that are endemic to the hospital and have established a home in the ETT. This combination of factors makes VAPs particularly dangerous because patients may become infected with multidrug-resistant nosocomial bacteria. The resistant and severe nature of these infections requires longer and more intensive courses of antibiotics, which can lead to further drug resistance.

OTHER INFECTIOUS RISKS

Patients receiving longer durations of mechanical ventilation are also at risk for additional nonpulmonary infectious complications. Many patients require central line placement during mechanical ventilation, and these lines can become infected, causing bacteremia and sepsis. Prolonged illness during mechanical ventilation may also be associated with urinary tract infections from Foley catheter placement, or *Clostridium difficile* colitis infections from the use of antibiotics. These infections may range from minor, to severe and life-threatening and can lead to hemodynamic collapse and severe septic shock.

TRACHEOSTOMY TUBE PLACEMENT

If patients are expected to require prolonged mechanical ventilation support, or are having difficulty weaning to extubation, tracheostomy placement may be needed. There are several (mostly theoretical) advantages to tracheostomy tubes compared with ETTs, including improved patient comfort (and decreased sedation needs), ease of suctioning, the ability for care to be performed outside the ICU and even outside the hospital after discharge, and the ability for patients to speak and eat food. While these advantages may seem to favor placement of tracheostomy tubes, the placement itself is a procedure that carries some risk and there are several possible disadvantages to tracheostomies as well. During placement, bleeding is a common issue, and there is a risk for possible trachea-innominate artery fistula formation. The stomal site itself can have persistent bleeding or infection issues, and the surgical site can provide a conduit to the mediastinum for infection. In addition, laryngeal injury is possible, and tracheal injury/stenosis can occur as well. Although the data are mixed (see later), tracheostomy may lead to

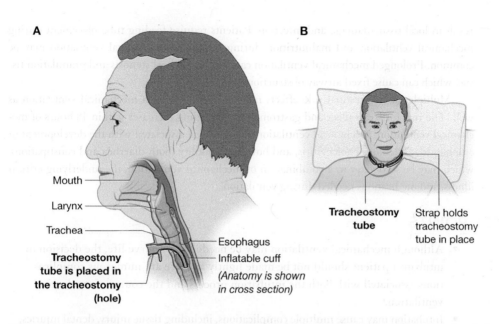

A

B

Mouth

Larynx

Trachea

Tracheostomy tube is placed in the tracheostomy (hole)

Esophagus

Inflatable cuff
(Anatomy is shown in cross section)

Tracheostomy tube

Strap holds tracheostomy tube in place

Figure 15-6: Anatomy of the upper airway and use of a tracheostomy tube. A, Lateral view showing the anatomy of the trachea and larynx relative to the position of the tracheostomy tube. **B,** The tracheostomy tube sits midline in the patient's neck, with straps holding the tube in place.

earlier extubation and cessation of mechanical ventilation in selected patients; psychologically, it is easier for an ICU team to "test" the ability of the patient to breathe on their own when a "failure" only necessitates reconnecting the tracheostomy tube to the ventilator in contrast to removing an orotracheal tube that then has to be replaced. Ultimately, the risks of tracheostomy must be balanced against the risks associated with prolonged orotracheal intubation.

A tracheostomy tube is placed either surgically or percutaneously usually after 1 to 3 weeks of intubation (**Figure 15-6**). There is no clear optimal timing for placement, and the decision to transition from an ETT to a tracheostomy tube is based upon the individual assessment of the patient's overall progress, expected ability to continue weaning from mechanical support, and the level of support required. Without clearly defined best timing, delayed tracheotomy tube placement is more common in patients who are unstable or remain on high levels of ventilator support.

A study in 2010 suggested a possible benefit from earlier tracheostomy placement (7 days vs 14 days) with a higher likelihood of weaning from the ventilator and discharge from the ICU within 28 days, as well as improved survival at 1 month. A larger follow-up study, however, comparing early versus late tracheostomy placement did not appear to result in any appreciable benefit from early tracheostomy placement; there was no benefit with respect to mortality or length of stay. Interestingly in this study, more than half of the patients randomized to late tracheostomy placement never actually required trach placement, which might suggest an advantage to delaying in many patients. In general, one considers tracheostomy at 14 to 21 days of intubation if it appears the patient will not be extubated imminently.

OTHER ASSOCIATED COMPLICATIONS

Prolonged mechanical ventilation with its associated sedation and reduced patient movement can result in pressure ulcer formation, even with proper positioning. Skin breakdown can result in local tissue damage and infection. Patients require feeding tube placement during mechanical ventilation and malnutrition during prolonged mechanical ventilation may be common. Prolonged mechanical ventilation can lead to tracheal stenosis and granulation tissue, which can cause fixed airway obstruction.

Multiple gastrointestinal side effects may be associated with mechanical ventilation as well. The risk for stress ulcer and gastrointestinal bleeding increases within 48 hours of mechanical ventilation. Mechanical ventilation has also been associated with the development of esophagitis, acalculous cholecystitis, and bowel dysmotility (both diarrhea and constipation), which may be secondary to a combination of mechanical ventilation, the underlying critical illness, and medications needed during ventilation.

KEY POINTS

- Although mechanical ventilation may be needed to preserve life, the decision to intubate a patient should not be made lightly as there are numerous complications associated with both the intubation process and the course of mechanical ventilation.
- Intubation may cause multiple complications, including tissue injury, dental injuries, aspiration, and bronchospasm.
- During intubation and over the course of mechanical ventilation for respiratory failure, patients are at risk for developing worsened hypoxemia and hypercarbia.
- During intubation and over the course of mechanical ventilation, hemodynamic complications are common and secondary to the use of sedatives and positive pressure.
- VILI can occur secondary to high lung volume, pressure, and localized atelectasis of the lungs.
- A patient's spontaneous breathing activity can result in injurious breathing patterns, for example, if they are generating large pressure swings during a breath, excessive respiratory efforts, or large tidal volume.
- Diaphragm and skeletal muscle injury may develop in association with prolonged ventilation secondary to disuse atrophy and direct muscle injury.
- High levels of sedatives may be required during mechanical ventilation; these may be difficult to wean, resulting ultimately in symptoms of drug withdrawal and a prolonged course of mechanical ventilation.
- Delirium is common in critically ill patients but is particularly prevalent in mechanically ventilated patients.
- VAP and other infections are commonly associated or caused by mechanical ventilation.
- If patients are having difficulty weaning to extubation, tracheostomy tube placement may be required.

STUDY QUESTIONS AND ANSWERS

Questions

1. What are the most frequent and the most serious risks from intubation?
   A. Sore throat
   B. Dental injury
   C. Hemodynamic compromise
   D. Bronchospasm
   E. All of the above

2. A patient with sepsis who is on low-dose vasopressors is intubated for worsening altered mental status. They are on 2 L nasal cannula at the time of intubation. They have not yet received any fluids and the patient has low urine output. What would be your biggest acute concern for the patient to occur with intubation?
   A. Worsened hypotension
   B. Bronchospasm
   C. Acute hypercarbia
   D. Acute hypoxemia

3. A patient with ARDS is having their sedation weaned after 2 days of intubation. They are exhibiting accessory muscle use and tachypnea, they are triggering breaths on the ventilator, and their oxygen saturation has worsened in the last hour since lightening sedation. What are you concerned about in this patient?
   A. Injury from overdistension (also known as barotrauma and volutrauma)
   B. Injury from biotrauma
   C. Injury from high respiratory drive and efforts
   D. Hemodynamic compromise
   E. All of the above

4. A patient has been requiring deep sedation for the last week because of their respiratory failure and ongoing severe dyssynchrony. What are the consequences and complications of their use in mechanically ventilated patients?
   A. Prolonged duration of intubation
   B. Worsened mortality
   C. Increased infections and ventilator-associated pneumonia
   D. Muscle and diaphragm myopathy
   E. All of the above

Answers

1. **Answer E. All of the above**
   Rationale: Sore throat and dental injuries are the most common side effects of intubation but are generally less serious in nature. More serious soft-tissue injuries and lacerations are less common but can occur and result in bleeding, scarring, or infections. Hemodynamic changes during intubation are common and can more rarely result in life-threatening decreases in blood pressure or cardiac arrest. Acute bronchospasm can occur particularly in patients with asthma or reactive airway disease. Hypoxemia and hypercapnia are also common during intubation.

(continued)

STUDY QUESTIONS AND ANSWERS   (continued)

2. **Answer A. Worsened hypotension**

    Rationale: Hypotension is common after intubation and during mechanical ventilation, and the causes may be multifactorial. The sedative and induction agents used during intubation and initiation of mechanical ventilation may directly cause vasodilation and decreased blood pressure. In acutely ill patients, the initiation of sedation may also remove the adrenergic tone that patients have had in response to their acute illness. Positive airway pressure from the ventilator may cause reduced venous return and decreased cardiac output, particularly in patients with right ventricular dysfunction, pulmonary vascular hypertension, and low intravascular volume.

3. **Answer E. All of the above**

    Rationale: VILI occurs when the applied ventilator settings cause injurious tidal volumes (called *volutrauma*), injurious total and cyclic pressures (called *barotrauma*), and injurious cyclic opening and collapse of the lungs (called *atelectrauma*). These mechanical injuries lead to inflammation and further injury (called *biotrauma*). Self-induced lung injury may similarly cause injury through injurious volumes, pressure swings, and atelectasis, but this injury is generated by a patient's own respiratory efforts, either in concert with the actions of the ventilator or independently from the ventilator support. Although the basic type of injury may be similar to mechanical injury leading to inflammation, the cause is distinctively different. The large intrathoracic swings in some patients may lead to hemodynamic changes as well.

4. **Answer E. All of the above**

    Rationale: Sedation is often required during mechanical ventilation to allow the patient to tolerate the ETT, uncomfortably low tidal volumes, and acidosis and to prevent dyssynchrony with the ventilator. Sedation may directly cause hemodynamic side effects, cause organ injury (including PRIS), may prolong the duration of mechanical ventilation, lead to tolerance and withdrawal, potentially worsen mortality, and increase the severity and duration of delirium.

Suggested Readings

Devlin JW, Skrobik Y, Gélinas C, et al. Clinical practice guidelines for the prevention and management of pain, agitation/sedation, delirium, immobility, and sleep disruption in adult patients in the ICU. *Crit Care Med.* 2018;46(9):e825-e873.

Gattinoni L, Protti A, Caironi P, Carlesso E. Ventilator-induced lung injury: the anatomical and physiological framework. *Crit Care Med.* 2010;38(10 Suppl):S539-S548.

Goligher EC, Dres M, Fan E, et al. Mechanical ventilation-induced diaphragm atrophy strongly impacts clinical outcomes. *Am J Respir Crit Care Med.* 2018;197(2):204-213.

MacIntyre NR, Epstein SK, Carson S, et al. Management of patients requiring prolonged mechanical ventilation: report of a NAMDRC consensus conference. *Chest.* 2005;128(6):3937-3954.

Schweickert WD, Hall J. ICU-acquired weakness. *Chest.* 2007;131(5):1541-1549.

Young D, Harrison DA, Cuthbertson BH, Rowan K; TracMan Collaborators. Effect of early vs late tracheostomy placement on survival in patients receiving mechanical ventilation: the TracMan randomized trial. *JAMA.* 2013;309(20):2121-2129.

Special Topics in Mechanical Ventilation

Esophageal Balloons and Pleural Pressure

Elias Baedorf Kassis • Jonah Rubin

LEARNING OBJECTIVES

- Understand the physiology and clinical applications of esophageal manometry.
- Understand the physiologic importance of transpulmonary pressure.
- Understand how to apply physiologic data and principles to ventilator management.

INTRODUCTION

Esophageal manometry, or the measurement of esophageal pressure, is an easily employed, minimally invasive technique to reliably estimate pleural pressure; it has several useful clinical applications that are reviewed in this chapter.

Much of our prior discussion about lung injury and mechanical ventilation has focused on monitoring and targeting treatment to the entire respiratory system; an important limitation of this discussion, however, has been the focus on monitoring only the **pressure at the airway opening (P_{ao})**, which is what a typical mechanical ventilator records and monitors. The P_{ao} measurement reflects the interaction of the patient's entire respiratory system, which includes both the lung and the chest wall; it may be challenging, however, to differentiate the relative contributions of lung and chest wall to P_{ao} using standard techniques. To discern the independent impact of the lung and chest wall on the respiratory system, we must first estimate the **pleural pressure (P_{pl})**, using esophageal manometry, to determine the chest wall mechanics, which may vary considerably depending on the patient's body habitus and disease. Estimation of the pleural pressure allows for calculation of the **transpulmonary pressure (P_L)**, the net pressure exerted across the lung, which is the most important measurement when considering the risk for ventilator-induced lung injury (VILI). As discussed further, pressure delivered by mechanical ventilation to the entire respiratory system may be significantly different from what is being felt by the lungs alone due to the impact of chest wall mechanics. Currently, esophageal manometry is the best way to estimate pleural pressure, derive transpulmonary pressure, and thereby quantify the potential size of individual lung units and the impact of various ventilator strategies.

In providing these physiologic data, esophageal manometry has transformed the current understanding of pulmonary pathophysiology. Nevertheless, although used extensively in research, it has not yet been widely adopted clinically. Still, even when not used in standard care, it is increasingly recognized as a powerful yet simple tool for the management of complex patients requiring individualized, physiologically based ventilator management, such as in obese patients and those with severe acute respiratory distress syndrome (ARDS).

BASIC CONCEPTS AND DEFINITIONS

Concept of Transmural Pressure

Before delving further into the principles and clinical applications of esophageal manometry, it is worth discussing a basic and fundamental concept that is critically important for a complete understanding of the physiology of the lungs. The "transmural pressure" is the pressure that is measured across the wall of a tube or balloon-like flexible structure. To explain this concept further, let us use the following example: A balloon is inflated, and the opening is tied off. The transmural pressure (P_{tm}) is the pressure measured across the balloon surface from the inside (P_i) to the outside (P_o) of the balloon ($P_{tm} = P_i - P_o$). After inflation, the P_i is the resulting pressure inside the balloon secondary to inflation and recoil forces of the balloon, and the P_o is atmospheric pressure (zero), so the transmural pressure equals the inside pressure. Now consider what happens to the P_i, the P_o, and the P_{tm} if the balloon is slowly submerged in water. In this case, as you might imagine, the P_o increases as the balloon is submerged deeper and the external force of the water around the balloon compresses it. The balloon's volume is reduced (remember, no air is coming out of the balloon!) as the P_o (from the pressure of the water) increases; as the volume inside the balloon decreases, there is a corresponding increase in the P_i (same gas content at a lower volume), but because the P_o has increased more than the corresponding increase in P_i (with a smaller balloon, the recoil force of the balloon is not as great), so the transmural pressure also decreases.

When the pressure outside the balloon exceeds the pressure inside the balloon, the transmural pressure becomes negative and the balloon collapses. This concept is of critical importance when considering the lung, as it is not the absolute pressure (the P_i) that determines the stress on the lung, but the transmural pressure or the pressure felt across the lung. As we discuss next, whereas the pressure inside the lung is easy to estimate using the ventilator, the pressure outside the lung (the pleural pressure) and the transmural pressure (or what we call *transpulmonary pressure*) are more complex.

Static Versus Dynamic Measurements

Briefly, another important concept to clarify in order to understand the measurements we elaborate in this chapter is the difference between static and dynamic measurements. As a reminder, the airway opening pressure (P_{ao}) (which stays at zero in spontaneously breathing patients who are not ventilated) in mechanically ventilated patients is the pressure that is measured or applied by the ventilator in the tubing outside of the patient. The P_{ao} represents an easily measured value and can be used to estimate the pressure within the alveoli (P_{alv}) when there is no air moving into or out of the lungs, that is, static conditions (remember a tube containing a fluid that is not moving, ie, static, has the same pressure at both ends; if the pressures were different, then flow would begin). At end inspiration and end expiration, if the clinician performs an occlusion (also known as *breath-hold*), a static column of gas is formed from the ventilator down the endotracheal tube, through the airways, and to the alveoli. Because there is no flow, the measured P_{ao} at this moment is equal to the P_{alv}. Of note, during dynamic states (when air is flowing in or out of the lungs), the P_{ao} and P_{alv} may be quite different because of the airway resistance.

When discussing transmural pressures, it may be initially confusing why we would use the P_{ao} to represent the pressure inside the lung in the calculation of the pressure across the lung. Indeed, ideally, we would use the P_{alv} measurement for dynamic transmural pressures, but this is not technically possible. Consequently, we use P_{ao} to estimate the P_{alv} at end inspiration and end expiration.

Estimation of Pleural Pressure Using Esophageal Manometry

Because pleural pressures cannot be directly measured, we rely upon estimations of pleural pressure using esophageal manometry. An esophageal balloon placed in the lower third of the esophagus allows us to assess the pressure within the thorax, which is functionally the same as the pleural space or the pleural pressure. Importantly, the pleural pressure is actually not constant or equal throughout the pleural space. More dependent regions have a higher pleural pressure from the weight of the less dependent structures (heart, lung, fluid), essentially squeezing the pleural space against the chest wall. This will further depend on the patient's position. In an upright patient, the highest pleural pressure will be at the lung bases, and the lowest, at the lung apices. In a supine patient, the highest pleural pressure will be the dorsum (both at the bases and apices), and the lowest pleural pressure will be at the ventral aspects of the pleural space (**Figure 16-1**).

This has been demonstrated nicely in both animal and human studies comparing direct measures of pleural pressure to measures via esophageal manometry. Although the absolute value of pleural pressure varied in different sites, these studies demonstrated that esophageal pressure measured by balloon in the mid-esophagus accurately reflects true pleural pressure at that same gravitational level.

In addition, despite this variability, several physiologic studies have demonstrated that an esophageal balloon, placed between the dependent and nondependent lung regions, provides reliable estimates of the average **effective** pleural pressure, which we can use to guide clinical care.

Chest Wall, Pleural Pressures, and Transpulmonary Pressure Measurements

Pleural pressure can be a confusing concept because the pleural space in a healthy individual is only a potential or virtual space containing a few cubic centimeters of fluid. The visceral and parietal pleura should be so closely apposed that no true, discernible space exists. Yet, the existence of this space connects the movement of chest wall expansion to the lung and facilitates "lung sliding" and inflation during inhalation. Pleural pressure varies throughout the thorax and increases in more dependent regions because of the weight of the lung compressing

Pleural pressure (P_{pl}) gradient

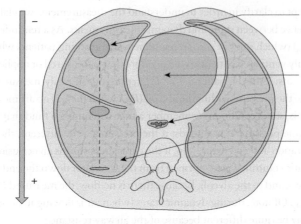

Open alveoli in nondependent areas as the alveolar pressure (P_{alv}) is greater than the P_{pl}

Heart and mediastinum

Esophageal balloon (P_{es})

Collapsed alveoli in dependent areas as the P_{alv} (same pressure as in nondependent areas) is less than P_{pl}

Figure 16-1: This schematic represents a cross section of the thoracic cavity in a patient lying supine with the orientation as would be typical in a computed tomography (CT) scan, with the right lung on the left side of the image and the left lung on the right side. The esophagus runs posterior to the mediastinum, which includes the heart, and the esophageal pressure is measured via the esophageal balloon (*yellow circle*). The esophageal pressure (P_{es}) provides a close estimate for the pleural pressure (P_{pl}) in the mid-thorax, providing a functional mean pleural pressure for clinical monitoring. Note, however, that the P_{pl} is not uniform within the thoracic cavity, with variability depending on the gravitational position. In this patient lying supine, the P_{pl} is lower in anterior nondependent regions of the thoracic cavity and becomes increasingly larger in posterior, dependent regions secondary to the weight of the lungs, mediastinal structures, and abdomen, which pushes on the diaphragm. The result of this variation in pleural pressure throughout the thorax is nonuniform alveolar distension during lung inflation despite the alveolar pressure (P_{alv}) being the same through the lungs, because the *transmural pressures will vary*. In anterior nondependent regions, the P_{alv} is greater than the P_{pl}, leading to open alveoli (*open blue circle*), whereas in posterior dependent regions of the lungs, the P_{pl} may be larger than the P_{alv}, leading to alveolar collapse (*collapsed blue circle*).

the pleural space against the chest wall, but generally ranges from approximately −3 to −5 cm H$_2$O in healthy individuals sitting upright at rest at the end of a relaxed exhalation (ie, at functional residual capacity or FRC). This negative pressure is created by the equal and opposite forces of the lung and the chest wall attempting to equilibrate in opposite directions. At end expiration, the elastic structure of the lung directs an inward "collapsing" vector of force, while simultaneously the chest wall expands outward. The degree of outward force from the chest wall and inward force from the lung determines both the relaxed total volume of the respiratory system (FRC) and the measured pleural pressure that serves as the interface between these structures, coupling one structure to the other. As an exercise, imagine what would occur with the removal of the lung from the chest: In this scenario, the elastic forces of the explanted lung cause further collapse, whereas the chest wall would expand outward, with both structures achieving new resting volumes (lower for the lungs, higher for the chest wall).

Thought Question 1

Can you imagine a clinical scenario in which the chest wall and the lungs become uncoupled from each other? What are the resulting clinical outcomes?

The pressure across the chest wall (trans-chest wall transmural pressure) is calculated as the pleural pressure (P_{pl}), which represents P_{inside}, minus the atmospheric pressure, which represents $P_{outside}$; thus, P_{tm} for the chest wall equals $P_{pl} - P_{atm}$. To isolate the pressures that the lung is exposed to, we measure the transmural pressure across the lung, also known as the *transpulmonary pressure* (P_L), which is calculated as the P_{ao} (which we measure during static conditions as earlier) minus the P_{pl} estimated by the esophageal pressures. These are demonstrated and described further in **Figure 16-2.**

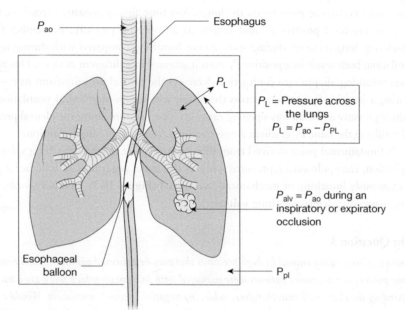

Figure 16-2: Individual pressures throughout the respiratory system. P_{ao} is the pressure measured at the airway opening. In nonintubated patients, this is equal to atmospheric pressure (P_{atm}). Note that regardless of whether or not someone is intubated, the P_{ao} equals the alveolar pressure (P_{alv}) under "static" conditions, that is, when there is no flow of gas into or out of the lung, for example, during breath-holds when there is no flow between the airway opening and the alveoli. In intubated patients undergoing positive pressure ventilation, P_{ao} is equal to the pressure applied by the ventilator. During exhalation, the P_{ao} equals the end-expiratory pressure, which may be zero or some higher number of the patient has auto-PEEP or if there is applied PEEP from the ventilator. At end inspiration during a breath-hold, the P_{ao} would be equal to the combined pressure required to distend the entire respiratory system, including both the lungs and the chest wall. As can be seen in the image, however, the P_{ao} at end inspiration, in order to inflate the lung, is exerting pressure not just on the lung but also, by extension, across the chest wall by changing the pleural pressure. Measurement of the pleural pressure, which is between the lung and the chest wall, helps differentiate the transpulmonary pressure from the trans-chest wall pressure. $P_{ao} - P_{pl}$ equals the transpulmonary pressure. The trans-chest wall pressure can also be calculated as $P_{pl} - P_{atm}$. The pressure in an appropriately placed esophageal balloon, also seen in this image, closely approximates the pressure in the pleural space. With P_{ao} measured by the ventilator, and P_{pl} measured by the balloon, transpulmonary pressure can be derived. These different pressures become important clinically when we are trying to determine the appropriate pressure to inflate the lung in patients with variable lung and chest wall compliance.

Thought Question 2

Imagine an elephant sitting on a patient's chest. What does this do to the pleural pressure? What do you think will happen to the lungs when the pleural pressure is greater than the airway pressure? Does this result in collapse or expansion of the lungs? Does this result in a negative or positive transpulmonary pressure? Can you think of any clinical scenarios that might illustrate the previous scenario (similar to but not involving an elephant)?

Any time pleural pressure exceeds airway pressure, this creates a **negative** P_L and inherently represents a collapsing pressure on the lungs. Any time airway pressure exceeds pleural pressure, this creates a **positive** P_L and represents an opening pressure. Remember this when considering lung inflation during spontaneous breathing compared with during mechanical ventilation; both result in a positive P_L even if attained in a different manner. During spontaneous breathing, diaphragm contraction decreases the pleural pressure from its resting state, creating a positive P_L gradient across the lungs, whereas in mechanical ventilation, applied positive pressure at the airway opening raises alveolar pressure above the pleural pressure, but still results in the same P_L gradient across the lungs, resulting in lung expansion.

A fundamental point derived from this concept is that for the same lung volume at end inspiration, transpulmonary pressure remains the same, regardless of whether a patient is spontaneously breathing or mechanically ventilated (**Figure 16-3**). In other words, transpulmonary pressure determines lung volume.

Thought Question 3

Barotrauma is a lung injury caused by high pressures that may be delivered via mechanical ventilation. During the polio epidemic, many patients were managed with iron lungs, which work via a vacuum effect expanding the chest wall and, therefore, achieving negative pressure ventilation. Would an iron lung be more protective against barotrauma, compared to positive pressure ventilation, or would it be the same?

IMPLICATIONS OF CHEST WALL PATHOLOGIES ON THE RESPIRATORY SYSTEM AND THE LUNGS

Certain conditions impact the pleural pressure in both otherwise healthy patients and critical illness. Obese patients tend to have positive pleural pressure generated by the weight of their chest wall (think the elephant sitting on the chest analogy in Thought Question 2). This positive pleural pressure is transmitted to the lungs and has a compressing effect, causing baseline atelectasis (in severe cases, reducing total lung capacity, FRC, and vital capacity). In ARDS, the weight of edematous consolidated lungs also increases pleural pressure, particularly in more dependent areas (lung bases when upright, dorsum when supine), as will other illness accompanying ARDS (such as pancreatitis, edema, and ascites, which increase intra-abdominal pressure pushing on the diaphragm, which is the inferior boundary of the thoracic cavity). In such a case, to expand the lung at all, either with spontaneous effort or via positive pressure ventilation, the positive pleural pressure exerted against the lungs must be overcome. Such conditions may be thought of as **basal pleural pressure elevation**. The problems all stem from an abnormally high end-expiratory pleural pressure.

Another condition that may affect the chest wall is **chest wall stiffness**, due to a wide range of diseases including neuromuscular disease, abdominal hypertension, chest wall edema, and critical illness. In such patients, pleural pressures may or may not be normal at end expiration depending

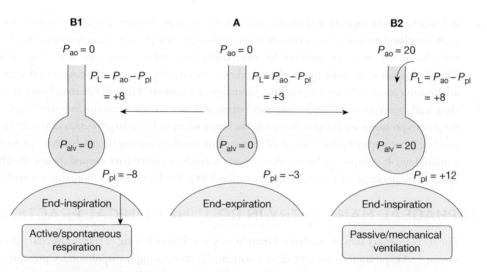

Figure 16-3: Pressure changes throughout the respiratory system during passive/mechanical and active/spontaneous respiration. A, Pressures throughout the respiratory system at rest at end exhalation are defined. Note that atmospheric pressure equals airway opening pressure and intra-alveolar pressure, as there is no flow at end exhalation (ie, static conditions are present; there cannot be a gradient). Pleural pressure is -3 cm H_2O, and transpulmonary pressure at end exhalation is $+3$ cm H_2O ($P_{ao} - P_{pl}$) representing the distending pressure needed to overcome the lung's innate recoil forces and maintain lung volume at functional residual capacity. **B1-B2**, Pressure changes found at end inhalation via active/spontaneous ventilation and passive/mechanical ventilation, respectively. In **B1**, for a patient breathing normally, inspiration is initiated by the muscles of respiration, predominantly the diaphragm. Diaphragmatic contraction expands the chest wall and results in more negative pleural pressure ($-3 \rightarrow -8$ cm H_2O). This change in pleural pressure is felt by the lung tissue as a pulling force, and the lung expands, creating negative intra-alveolar pressure ($0 \rightarrow -5$ cm H_2O). This creates a gradient between atmospheric pressure and the alveoli, drawing in air and increasing lung volume, until the gradient between P_{ao} and P_{alv} returns to 0, marking the end of inspiration. In this new steady state, note that pleural pressure has become more negative, which is necessary to maintain the lungs at this higher volume. Transpulmonary pressure became more positive, increasing from $+3$ to $+8$ mm Hg ($P_{ao} - P_{pl}$). In **B2**, for a patient undergoing mechanical ventilation, the process proceeds to produce similar pressure differentials between P_{ao} and P_{alv} but by a different mechanism. P_{ao} is increased, and this gets transmitted to the alveolus, creating flow and allowing the lung to expand until the pressure gradient resolves, such that $P_{ao} = P_{alv}$. In so doing, some pressure is exerted against the pleural space in order to expand the chest wall and overcome its elasticity as well, thereby increasing pleural pressure. At end expiration, we see that $P_{ao} = P_{alv} = 20$ mmHg. Pleural pressure has also increased and is now $+12$ cm H_2O, a function of the chest wall compliance. Note that the transpulmonary pressure is the same $+8$ cm H_2O ($P_{ao} - P_{pl} = 20 - 12 = 8$ cm H_2O) as the patient with spontaneous ventilation. In both scenarios, for the same patient, the tidal volume achieved would be the same, despite differences in P_{ao} and P_{pl}, because the transpulmonary pressure is equivalent. Numbers have been simplified to illustrate the concepts.

on the disease pathology. However, during inhalation in such a patient, the chest wall stiffness (reduced compliance) impairs or precludes full chest wall expansion; for any given change in alveolar pressure, one will get a smaller change in volume. In a spontaneously breathing patient, larger inspiratory muscle efforts are required to overcome the chest wall stiffness. This may result in lower total lung capacity and smaller tidal volume for a given inspiratory effort. In a mechanically ventilated patient, a larger portion of the applied positive pressure is dissipated by the chest wall; that is, the energy is "used up" by overcoming the reduced compliance of the chest wall. This dissipation of pressure by the chest wall may require larger applied pressures to deliver a tidal volume, even if the underlying lung parenchyma is normal. The reduced compliance of the chest wall causes an overall stiff respiratory system and may confuse clinicians into thinking that dangerous pressures are being delivered to the lungs when in fact a large portion of the applied pressure is not impacting the lungs at all (ie, the transmural pressure or transpulmonary pressure remains low). It is important to note that patients with **obesity often have normal chest wall stiffness,** but simply create elevated pleural pressure at FRC. We discuss this in more detail as well.

ESOPHAGEAL MANOMETRY IN ROUTINE CLINICAL PRACTICE

The three primary uses of esophageal manometry are (1) monitoring of transpulmonary pressure at end expiration to prevent derecruitment, (2) monitoring transpulmonary pressure at end inspiration to prevent overdistension, and (3) monitoring the change in transpulmonary pressure during each breath to assure safe levels of cyclic stress (desired pressure levels described in **Table 16-1**). Esophageal manometry can also be used for advanced monitoring of dyssynchrony (as is briefly covered in Chapter 21), to assess readiness for weaning, for measurement of work of breathing and other measures of patient effort, and for measurement of auto-positive end-expiratory pressure (PEEP). These more advanced applications of esophageal manometry are not touched upon in this chapter.

Preventing Lung Collapse in Acute Respiratory Distress Syndrome

As detailed earlier, certain clinical conditions lead to excessive end-expiratory positive pleural pressure (remember, in healthy individuals, pleural pressure is slightly negative at FRC). Examples include obesity, increased abdominal pressure, pleural effusions, pulmonary edema, and ARDS. This positive pleural pressure exerts a compressive force against the lungs (making the P_L negative at end expiration), predisposing to, or directly causing, collapse and atelectasis. These concepts provide the background for one of the easiest and most clinically helpful uses of esophageal manometry in mechanically ventilated patients undergoing positive pressure ventilation. If we can directly measure the increased "collapsing" pleural pressure, we may be able to directly counter this pressure by adjusting the applied pressure from the ventilator at the airway (the set PEEP).

At end expiration, if no pressure at all is applied by the ventilator ($P_{ao} = 0$, or PEEP = 0), then the positive pleural pressure can effectively collapse large portions of the lung (via a negative P_L), causing atelectasis, until the pressure in the system equilibrates. Note that in this case, even with high pleural pressures and very negative transpulmonary pressures, we will

TABLE 16-1 Goal Transpulmonary Pressure Levels for Safe Mechanical Ventilation	
	Target Transpulmonary Pressure
At end expiration (while adjusting PEEP)	0 cm H_2O (±2 cm H_2O)
At end inspiration (while measuring the plateau pressure)	<20 cm H_2O at all times Ideally ≤15 cm H_2O
Transpulmonary driving pressure	≤10-12 cm H_2O

PEEP, positive end-expiratory pressure.

not see full deflation of the lung due to gas trapping that occurs behind collapsed airways, and because of the vertical gravitational gradient of pleural pressure causing less collapse in nondependent regions.

For segments of the lung that do repeatedly collapse with expiration and reexpand with inspiration, the lung is vulnerable to atelectrauma, or injury from the shear forces generated by repeated collapse and reopening (as discussed in Chapters 13 and 15). Segments of the lung that remain collapsed are termed "derecruited." This means that the lung that might otherwise be able to participate in gas exchange is collapsed and receiving no ventilation, thereby leading to hypoxemia, hindering patient recovery, and potentially prolonging critical illness.

One of the main functions of PEEP is to prevent end-expiratory collapse of the lung that occurs secondary to both elevated pleural pressures and the inherent collapsing forces from surfactant depletion (see Chapters 2 and 13 for more detail on surfactant) and lung injury associated with many conditions of critical illness. As discussed in Chapters 7 and 13, there are many ways to estimate the "best" PEEP needed to prevent atelectasis and derecruitment. The use of esophageal manometry to assist in setting PEEP was a natural extrapolation, as the estimation of pleural pressure elevation would allow a corresponding targeted application of PEEP to counter these compressive pressures, target an end-expiratory transpulmonary pressure close to zero, and prevent collapse (while ensuring that end-inspiratory pressure is not excessive, as discussed later). PEEP can be increased or decreased to achieve this result **(Figure 16-4)**.

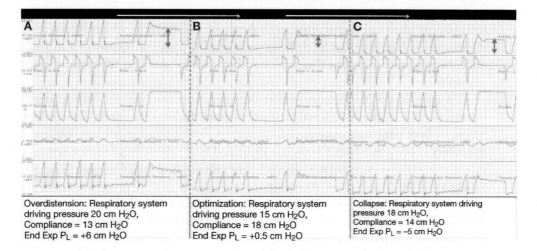

| Overdistension: Respiratory system driving pressure 20 cm H_2O, Compliance = 13 cm H_2O End Exp P_L = +6 cm H_2O | Optimization: Respiratory system driving pressure 15 cm H_2O, Compliance = 18 cm H_2O End Exp P_L = +0.5 cm H_2O | Collapse: Respiratory system driving pressure 18 cm H_2O, Compliance = 14 cm H_2O End Exp P_L = –5 cm H_2O |

Figure 16-4: PEEP titration to transpulmonary pressure. These panels demonstrate best PEEP selection using esophageal manometry for a patient with ARDS on volume control lung-protective ventilation at a tidal volume of 400 mL. Inspiratory and expiratory pauses are used to calculate the highest and lowest static transpulmonary pressures, respectively. For this patient, as seen in **A**, at a PEEP of 18 cm H_2O, plateau pressure is 38 cm H_2O, end-inspiratory P_L is 21 cm H_2O, and end-expiratory P_L is 6 cm H_2O. This high end-inspiratory and high end-expiratory transpulmonary pressure suggests that PEEP is excessively high and may be causing unnecessary overdistension and barotrauma/volutrauma. In **B**, at a PEEP of 12 cm H_2O, plateau pressure is 27 cm H_2O, end-inspiratory P_L is 12 cm H_2O, and end-expiratory P_L is 0.5 cm H_2O—both within the ideal ranges. In **C**, at a PEEP of 6 cm H_2O, end-inspiratory P_L was 10, and end-expiratory P_L is −5. This represents a compressive, closing force on the lung at end exhalation, likely causing atelectasis. ARDS, acute respiratory distress syndrome; PEEP, positive end-expiratory pressure.

In the initial EPvent clinical trial in 2008, this approach to PEEP titration yielded a higher applied PEEP compared to controls, improved oxygenation and compliance, improved survival in secondary analyses, and shortened time on mechanical ventilation. The subsequent multicenter EPvent2 study, although showing no overall benefit in all patients with moderate-severe ARDS, demonstrated in post hoc analysis a mortality benefit with PEEP titration using P_{es} in patients with lower Sequential Organ Failure Assessment (SOFA) and Acute Physiology and Chronic Health Evaluation (APACHE) scores (patients who are not dying of their other severe illness and with a greater chance for ARDS-specific benefit). In addition, there was improved mortality in patients whose P_L values were kept close to zero (-2 to $+2$ cm H_2O range), balancing atelectrauma injury at more negative P_L values and overdistension at higher P_L values. These data reaffirmed the target goal of titrating PEEP to maintain a P_L of close to zero.

Limiting Cyclical and Total Stress to Prevent Ventilator-Induced Lung Injury and Overdistension

The flip-side of ensuring that applied PEEP is sufficient to prevent derecruitment and atelectrauma is that excessive PEEP and the requisite tidal volumes that are delivered predispose to overdistension and lung stress (with cyclic and static stress outlined in Chapter 13 on ARDS when discussing driving pressure and plateau pressure measurements). If adequate PEEP is applied, it may be sufficient to overcome the recoil forces of the lung, thereby preventing lung collapse. Applying higher pressures or tidal volumes to the lung, however, can also cause barotrauma and volutrauma (see Chapters 13 and 15 for more information on lung injury). The challenge in setting PEEP and tidal volumes is to determine the ideal middle ground that minimizes both collapse and overdistension as much as possible.

Yet again, however, it becomes important to remember that, without esophageal manometry or other measures of pleural pressure, we cannot measure the impact of a ventilator setting on **lung** mechanics; without information on pleural pressure, we can only assess **respiratory system** mechanics. Choosing a PEEP and tidal volume based upon respiratory system values (P_{ao} on the ventilator) does not ensure the safety of lung distension due to the variability in the chest wall mechanics. In other words, the plateau pressure and driving pressure measured by P_{ao} inadequately take into account a patient's obesity, neuromuscular disease, severity of ARDS, or other factors affecting pleural pressure. Indeed, there are circumstances in which the P_{ao} pressures may be falsely reassuring or falsely concerning based upon the widely variable chest wall physiology that may not be measured. Using esophageal manometry, one can identify the true transpulmonary pressure and, therefore, the true total stress (end-inspiratory transpulmonary pressure) and cyclical stress (transpulmonary driving pressure) on the lung. Although the targets have not been extensively defined in the literature, in clinical practice, it is likely safest to target end-inspiratory transpulmonary pressures of roughly 15 cm H_2O or less (and never >20 cm H_2O) and targeting transpulmonary driving pressures of 10 to 12 cm H_2O or less (**Table 16-1**).

KEY POINTS

- Esophageal manometry is a readily available method to nearly directly measure transpulmonary pressure and guide individualized, physiology-based ventilator management.
- PEEP titrated to a near-zero end-expiratory transpulmonary pressure and end-inspiratory transpulmonary pressure below 20 cm H_2O can help maximize respiratory system compliance and minimize atelectasis and overdistension.

STUDY QUESTIONS AND ANSWERS

Thought Question Answers

1. A pneumothorax, or air in the pleural space, disrupts the apposition of the chest wall and the lung and decouples these two structures from each other. By eliminating this relationship, the chest wall can expand to a larger volume and the lung will collapse to a smaller volume until they achieve a new equilibrium.

2. An elephant sitting on a patient's chest will increase the positive pressure exerted on the lungs by the chest wall by increasing the pleural pressure. This positive pressure exerted on the lungs will create a *more negative* transpulmonary pressure and cause lung collapse. Any clinical scenario that increases pressure on the thorax or in the pleural space is akin to the elephant. This includes obesity, ascites, pleural effusions, and intra-abdominal hypertension.

3. Barotrauma predominantly depends on the transpulmonary pressure. As discussed extensively in the text, the transpulmonary pressure required to deliver a given tidal volume is the same whether delivered via positive pressure ventilation or negative pressure ventilation—such as spontaneous breathing or an iron lung. The solution for a patient on volume control with excessive transpulmonary pressures may be to reduce the tidal volume, if such a change does not adversely affect oxygenation or CO_2 removal, or to identify and correct other factors impairing the compliance of the respiratory system, such as derecruitment or suboptimal PEEP.

Multiple Choice Questions

1. For a tidal volume of 500 mL, in which of the following patients would you expect the transpulmonary pressure to be the *highest*?
   A. A patient with morbid obesity
   B. A patient with fibrotic lung disease
   C. A ventilator-dependent patient with amyotrophic lateral sclerosis (ALS)
   D. A patient with cirrhosis and ascites

2. A patient with morbid obesity and ARDS is admitted to the intensive care unit (ICU), intubated, and placed on volume control, lung-protective tidal volumes, a PEEP of 5, and an F_{IO_2} of 80%. Plateau pressure is 35 cm H_2O, and driving pressure is 17 cm H_2O. He is saturating 85%. You suspect the patient requires more PEEP. You place an esophageal balloon. Which of the following end-inspiratory and end-expiratory transpulmonary pressures do you most expect to see?
   A. End-expiratory: +17; end-inspiratory: +35
   B. End-expiratory: +5; end-inspiratory: +5
   C. End-expiratory: −7; end-inspiratory: −7
   D. End-expiratory: −7; end-inspiratory: +1

(continued)

3. You are testing to confirm appropriate placement of an esophageal balloon, and compress the chest during an end-expiratory pause, and see the following waveforms. You determine that the esophageal balloon is:

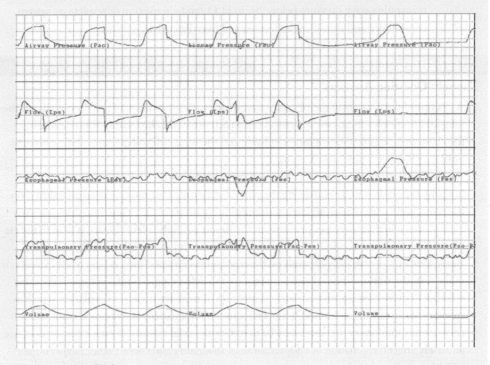

   A. Too shallow/high
   B. Correctly placed
   C. Deep/low
   D. None of the above

Multiple Choice Question Answers

1. **Answer B. A patient with fibrotic lung disease**

   Rationale: Only the patient with fibrotic lung disease has a disease process that reduces the compliance (or increases the elasticity) of the lungs, which means that more pressure must be exerted across the lungs—more transpulmonary pressure—to inflate the lung. A morbidly obese patient (Choice A) and a patient with abdominal ascites (Choice D) with normal lungs may require increased pressure at the airway opening (P_{ao}), but that is just to overcome the weight of the chest wall or the pressure from the abdominal contents on the thorax, but if measuring transpulmonary pressure with esophageal manometry, one would find a normal transpulmonary pressure. The patient with ALS has both normal lungs, and normal weight of the chest wall, and simply cannot ventilate themselves from neuromuscular impairment;

if undergoing mechanical ventilation, the patient would require a normal transpulmonary pressure to achieve an appropriate tidal volume, and also likely a normal P_{ao}.

2. **Answer D. End-expiratory: -7; end-inspiratory: $+1$**

Rationale: You suspect the patient requires more PEEP because they are derecruited from their obesity and ARDS. This patient likely has significantly high pleural pressure from both obesity (chest wall weight) and edematous lungs (lung weight). At end expiration, pressure inside the lungs (and P_{ao}) is at its lowest—in this case, at the PEEP set at only 5 cm H_2O. The excessively high pleural pressure is overwhelming, creating a *negative* transpulmonary pressure, exerting a *collapsing* force on the lung. Remember, $P_L = P_{ao} - P_{pl}$. If P_{ao} is relatively low, and P_{pl} is relatively high, P_L will be negative. Therefore, for this patient whom you suspect needs more PEEP, you expect the end-expiratory transpulmonary pressure to be *negative* (Choices A and B are incorrect). The end-inspiratory transpulmonary pressure may be high or low, depending on the severity of the ARDS on the patient's lung compliance. If the end-inspiratory pressure is high, this may limit options in managing this patient because increasing PEEP *may* increase end-inspiratory P_L. You may, perhaps seemingly paradoxically, decrease end-inspiratory P_L if, by increasing PEEP, more lung is recruited and lung compliance improves as well. Remember, however, when administering a tidal volume (this patient is on volume control), the end-inspiratory P_L must be greater than (and cannot be equal to) end-expiratory P_L (Choice C is incorrect).

3. **Answer B. Correctly placed**

Rationale: First, note the presence of cardiac oscillations on the esophageal pressure waveform. Next, note that, with a small chest compression, P_{ao} increases the same amount as P_{es}. This suggests that the esophageal balloon is correctly placed as you expect to see cardiac oscillations and an equal increase in airway and esophageal pressure with a chest push. Although this equal change in pressure can easily be determined visually, the change in airway pressure and change in esophageal pressure can also be directly measured. As the change in both should be the same, you can use the ratio of change to confirm. This ratio should be close to 1.0 with an acceptable range from 0.8 to 1.2. If there are no oscillations or if there is no equal change in pressure with chest pushes, the position needs to be adjusted.

Suggested Readings

Baedorf Kassis E, Talmor D. Clinical application of esophageal manometry: how I do it. *Crit Care.* 2021;25(1):6.

Beitler JR, Malhotra A, Thompson BT. Ventilator-induced lung injury. *Clin Chest Med.* 2016;37(4):633-646.

Beitler JR, Sarge T, Banner-Goodspeed VM, et al. Effect of titrating positive end-expiratory pressure (PEEP) with an esophageal pressure-guided strategy vs an empirical high peep-fio2 strategy on death and days free from mechanical ventilation among patients with acute respiratory distress syndrome: a randomized clinical trial. *JAMA.* 2019;321(9):846-857.

Pelosi P, Goldner M, McKibben A, et al. Recruitment and derecruitment during acute respiratory failure: an experimental study. *Am J Respir Crit Care Med*. 2001;164(1):122-130.

Talmor D, Sarge T, Malhotra A, et al. Mechanical ventilation guided by esophageal pressure in acute lung injury. *N Engl J Med*. 2008;359(20):2095-2104.

Yoshida T, Amato MBP, Grieco DL, et al. Esophageal manometry and regional transpulmonary pressure in lung injury. *Am J Respir Crit Care Med*. 2018;197(8):1018-1026.

Yoshida T, Brochard L. Esophageal pressure monitoring: why, when and how? *Curr Opin Crit Care*. 2018;24(3):216-222.

Advanced Modes of Ventilation

Elias Baedorf Kassis

LEARNING OBJECTIVES

- Explain the differences between pressure-regulated volume control (PRVC) and traditional volume and pressure control, and the potential benefits and downsides of this mode.
- Describe how airway pressure release ventilation (APRV) provides ventilator support, the patients in whom APRV might provide some benefit, and the potential downsides that limit its routine use.
- Describe the concept of "closed-loop" ventilation modes and several of the types of these advanced ventilator modes.
- Outline the potential use and limitations of neurally adjusted ventilator assist (NAVA).

INTRODUCTION

The majority of patients who are mechanically ventilated will only require traditional modes of mechanical ventilation with volume assist/control, pressure assist/control, and pressure-support ventilation (refer to Chapters 5 and 6 for a detailed description of these common ventilator modes and see **Figure 17-1**). Although these common modes are usually sufficient for the majority of patients, intensive care units (ICUs) are increasingly using uncommon or more advanced forms of ventilation as the local standard of care, and indeed, some patients may benefit from an expanded repertoire beyond the typical treatment modalities.

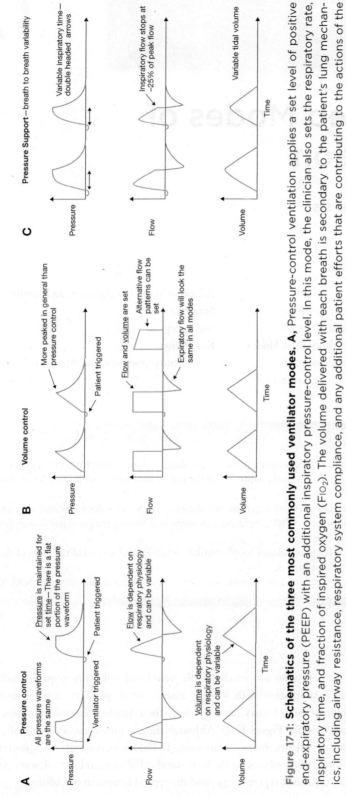

A Pressure control

Pressure

All pressure waveforms are the same

Pressure is maintained for set time—There is a flat portion of the pressure waveform

Ventilator triggered   Patient triggered

Flow

Flow is dependent on respiratory physiology and can be variable

Volume

Volume is dependent on respiratory physiology and can be variable

Time

B Volume control

Pressure

More peaked in general than pressure control

Patient triggered

Flow

Flow and volume are set

Alternative flow patterns can be set

Expiratory flow will look the same in all modes

Volume

Time

C Pressure Support—breath to breath variability

Pressure

Variable inspiratory time—double headed arrows

Flow

Inspiratory flow stops at ~25% of peak flow

Volume

Variable tidal volume

Time

Figure 17-1: Schematics of the three most commonly used ventilator modes. A, Pressure-control ventilation applies a set level of positive end-expiratory pressure (PEEP) with an additional inspiratory pressure-control level. In this mode, the clinician also sets the respiratory rate, inspiratory time, and fraction of inspired oxygen (FIO_2). The volume delivered with each breath is secondary to the patient's lung mechanics, including airway resistance, respiratory system compliance, and any additional patient efforts that are contributing to the actions of the ventilator. **B,** Volume-control ventilation applies a set flow pattern to achieve a specific tidal volume. Similar to pressure control, the clinician sets the inspiratory time, the respiratory rate, PEEP, and FIO_2. Unlike pressure-control ventilation, however, the resulting peak and plateau pressures (measured at end inspiration) are not controlled and are secondary to the patient's mechanics and resistance and the volume of gas delivered. **C,** Pressure support is the most commonly used ventilator mode providing assisted breathing for patients and relies upon the patient's ability to generate spontaneous efforts. In this mode, the clinician sets the PEEP level and pressure-support level in addition to the FIO_2.

While some of these "advanced" modes such as oscillatory ventilation and synchronized intermittent mandatory ventilation (also known as SIMV) are no longer used at all in adult populations owing to a lack of benefit or even harm (as was shown in two studies on oscillatory ventilation), other advanced and closed-loop ventilation modes are increasingly being utilized. With this in mind, a basic understanding of these less common or more advanced modes is important for healthcare providers working in the ICU to understand the risks, benefits, and correct application for each mode. This chapter describes several of these modes in detail, reviews the optimal patient for whom each mode may be appropriate, and outlines the potential complications for which one needs to be aware while using each mode.

AIRWAY PRESSURE RELEASE VENTILATION

Airway pressure release ventilation (APRV) inverts the typical time relationship between inhalation and exhalation by changing the "duty cycle" or proportion of each breath allotted for inspiration and expiration. Whereas usual mechanical ventilation modes provide support by applying pressure or volume to inflate the lungs for a relatively short time followed by a return to a set end-expiratory pressure during which exhalation occurs with passive recoil of the lungs (with an inspiratory-to-expiratory ratio [I/E] of 1/2 or 1/3), APRV inflates the lungs at a high pressure for a relatively long time and then provides intermittent release of this high applied pressure for very short intervals during which exhalation occurs; the I/E ratio is inverted with inhalation longer than exhalation. APRV applies an extreme version of what is known as "inverse ratio ventilation"—instead of I/E = 1/3 in conventional ventilation modes, we now see I/E = 3/1. Inverse ratio ventilation can be applied in any form of assist-control ventilation when the inspiratory time is set to be longer than the expiratory time.

The rationale for use of any form of inverse ratio ventilation is based upon the change in physiology that occurs when sick lungs have depleted surfactant stores, which results in an increase in surface tension in the alveolus and a predisposition for lung units to collapse. Notably, patients with sick lungs have a tendency to collapse/derecruit very quickly, while taking a *much* longer time to rerecruit. This is due to the inherent "viscoelastic" nature of the lungs (ie, the quality of the lungs reflects characteristics of both a liquid and solid when pressure is applied) and the time needed to overcome these properties of the lung parenchyma during inhalation when surface tension is particularly high, as occurs with deficient and/or abnormal surfactant. Inverse ratio ventilation applies prolonged inspiratory times (during which high pressure is maintained) to maximize recruitment during the inspiratory phase (while challenging the viscous lung component); in contrast, there are very short expiratory times (when low pressure, positive end-expiratory pressure [PEEP] is applied to the airway) to minimize the level of derecruitment during that time (which relates to the elastic properties of the lung). By minimizing the cycle of derecruitment (atelectasis) during exhalation and recruitment (opening the collapsed alveolus) during inhalation on each breath, we can minimize the lung injury termed *atelectrauma* in acute respiratory distress syndrome (ARDS) (see Chapter 13).

When employing APRV, the user sets a high pressure (P_{high}), a time (in seconds) for this pressure to be held (the T_{high}), a low pressure (P_{low}), and a very short duration or time for this low pressure to be maintained (the T_{low}). While inverse ratio ventilation in other control modes may shorten the expiratory duration, APRV typically shortens this release period even more dramatically in an attempt to limit the derecruitment that occurs as a consequence of the reduced compliance of the lung associated with diminished surfactant activity (**Figure 17-2**).

Notably, APRV can be used in both fully passive patients (without any additional inspiratory efforts) and patients who are spontaneously breathing. In passive patients, the pressure release generates

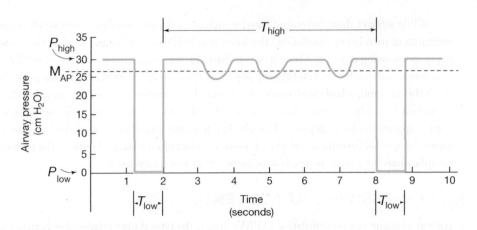

Figure 17-2: Schematic airway pressure waveform for airway pressure release ventilation (APRV). During ventilation with APRV, a high pressure (P_{high}) is held for a prolonged period (T_{high}), before a pressure is released to the low-pressure level (P_{low}), which is held for a very short amount of time (T_{low}) before pressure is increased back to the higher level once again. In patients who are fully passive, the tidal volumes are determined by the difference in pressure from the P_{high} and the P_{low} and the amount of auto-PEEP present during the pressure release. The respiratory rate in this case is dictated by the T_{high} and T_{low}. Patients can also be allowed to spontaneously breathe while in APRV at the high-pressure setting (somewhat like breathing while maintained at a constant pressure on continuous positive airway pressure [CPAP]), which may further augment ventilation. PEEP, positive end-expiratory pressure.

an intermittent exhaled tidal volume and the respiratory rate, and minute ventilation is determined by the duration of the inspiratory and expiratory phases. In addition, patients who make spontaneous efforts to breathe during the time the ventilator applies high and low pressures are able to do so via a mechanism similar to a continuous positive airway pressure (CPAP) mode superimposed on the sustained high and low pressures), and these spontaneous efforts may further augment recruitment and/or ventilation. This capability is particularly important in inverse ratio ventilation, which is not "natural" to normal respiratory physiology; other forms of inverse ratio ventilation, which do not allow these spontaneous respiratory efforts, require high levels of sedation for the patient.

APRV may be particularly helpful in patients whose lungs are "recruitable." Recruitability (see Chapter 13 for more information) is the determination of whether a patient's lungs (or potions of their lungs) have the ability to reexpand once they are collapsed. Stiff, fibrotic, chronically injured lungs likely will not reexpand when exposed to high pressures and are, therefore, not considered "recruitable." Indeed, in these patients, application of high pressures may only cause harm without any of the desired benefits because the relatively normal areas of lung will become overdistended and suffer volutrauma. In recruitable patients, in contrast, the use of APRV may support improved opening of the lungs by applying higher mean airway pressures with decreased time for derecruitment. The mode may improve hypoxemia in some patients, and experienced users can still apply "lung-protective" ventilation settings.

To ensure safety for the patient, a number of parameters should be monitored and adjusted in APRV, including (1) tight control over the P_{high} to assure pressures that are not overly high to prevent barotrauma and volutrauma; (2) performing expiratory breath-holds to measure the "total PEEP" (see Chapter 7 for more information on the total PEEP), in which APRV serves as the functional applied PEEP and will usually be significantly higher than the set P_{low} due to the short expiratory release time, which prevents the lung from returning to functional residual capacity before the next high-pressure segment is initiated by the ventilator; and (3) measurement of the "driving pressure" (see Chapter 14), which is calculated by subtracting the measured total PEEP from the P_{high} level. As monitored while in other ventilator modes, the driving pressure should be targeted with similar goals (generally ≤ 15 cm H_2O).

Unfortunately, APRV requires more experience and nuanced knowledge of ARDS compared to the typical ventilator modes to be applied correctly and safely. Incorrect application can lead to large driving pressure swings, derecruitment during expiratory release time, and large mean airway pressures, which could result in patient harm. In addition, there are minimal data at this time to direct the proper use of APRV. Despite the proposed physiologic benefits, the desired clinical benefit may not be feasible in many patients whose lungs are not recruitable or in whom the desired lung units that are sought to be protected and remain open are so stiff (with resulting very short time constants—low resistance and low compliance lung units) that they are still susceptible to collapse even during the very short pressure release times. As such, APRV should only be used by experienced clinicians in a very small subset of carefully selected patients, and the benefits may not be much greater than properly applied traditional ventilation modes.

PRESSURE-REGULATED VOLUME CONTROL

Pressure-regulated volume control (PRVC) is a hybrid partially closed-loop ventilator mode that utilizes aspects of both pressure-control ventilation and volume control in a single mode to target a set tidal volume while controlling applied pressure. This mode is commonly used in many ICUs as an alternative to standard volume control and indeed many clinicians may be using this mode instead of volume control without actually realizing it. Unfortunately, there is no standardized nomenclature to describe this mode, with different companies using a variety of acronyms and descriptions adding confusion to its use.

To understand PRVC, it is helpful to briefly rereview how volume-control and pressure-control modes operate. *Volume-control ventilation* determines an exact flow pattern over a set inspiratory time in order to specifically target and achieve the set tidal volume. The key aspect of this mode is the tight flow control that is maintained, which may cause dyspnea in patients who desire a different flow. In contrast, during *pressure-control ventilation*, rather than controlling the flow and tidal volume, a set pressure is applied over the inspiratory time; patients who wish a higher flow will receive it—as patients inspire more forcefully, pressure in the airway fall, which causes the ventilator to increase flow in an effort to achieve the predetermined pressure. Whatever tidal volume is achieved is not controlled or targeted in this mode, but is secondary to the resistance of airways, the stiffness of the lungs, and any additional patient efforts that may be additive to the applied pressure. For example, in pressure control, a patient with lungs that are less stiff (ie, more compliant) will receive a higher tidal volume in comparison to a patient with stiffer lungs for the same set pressure-control level.

PRVC utilizes aspects of both modes in a hybridized approach. With each individual breath while in PRVC, the ventilator applies a *pressure-controlled breath* without targeting a specific flow or flow pattern as would be done in volume control. With each breath, the ventilator then determines whether the achieved tidal volume was less than, greater than, or at the target tidal volume goal. By comparing the achieved and the target tidal volume with each breath, the ventilator then applies varying pressure on a breath-to-breath basis to achieve the target tidal volume goal. If the prior breath resulted in too large a volume, the next breath will have a reduced level of pressure control (providing less support for the inspiration and presumably achieving a smaller volume), and if the prior breath was too small, the subsequent breath will be given a higher level of pressure control (providing more support to the patient and resulting in a larger tidal volume) (see **Figure 17-3** for more details). Again, although this

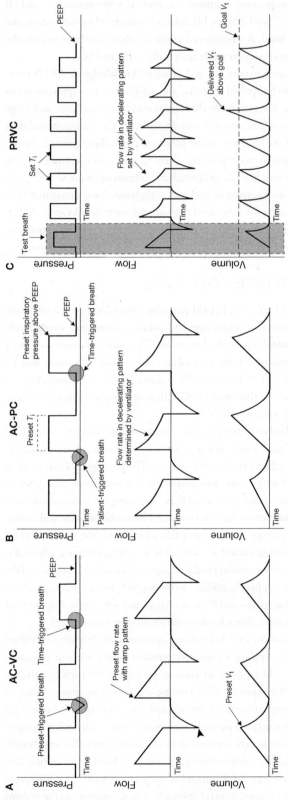

Figure 17-3: Comparison of volume-control, pressure-control, and pressure-regulated volume control (PRVC). A, Volume control allows for assisted and controlled breaths (ie, initiated by the ventilator), which utilize a set flow rate and pattern to deliver a precise target tidal volume. The resulting pressure generated during a breath is not controlled by the ventilator and is variable depending on the patient's spontaneous breathing, airway resistance, and respiratory system compliance. Note in the panel how a spontaneously initiated breath results in the same flow pattern and volumes as the subsequent passive breath. **B,** Pressure control sets a specific pressure, which remains constant during every breath delivery. Flow and volumes can be variable depending on airway resistance, respiratory system mechanics, and spontaneous efforts. Note in this schematic that the delivered tidal volume will be larger when patients are spontaneously breathing as the pressure delivery is additive to the patients' efforts, which results in higher flow and volumes. **C,** PRVC represents a hybrid mode. Each individual breath is a pressure-controlled type of breath. The level of pressure control, however, changes with each breath and is not set by the clinician. Instead, the clinician sets the target tidal volume, and the level of pressure control with each breath is adjusted incrementally to achieve the desired tidal volume. Note how the applied pressure will increase on the following breath when the tidal volumes do not achieve the target, and will decrease on a breath following one in which the tidal volume is greater than the target. The goal is that, on average, the patient will get the targeted tidal volume with more comfort for the patient. PRVC will easily achieve the target tidal volume when the patient is passive, but with variable effort, PRVC similarly will result in variable tidal volumes as the ventilator attempts to adjust unsuccessfully from breath to breath over time.

ventilator mode will target a specific tidal volume, PRVC is unique from true volume control, which delivers *flow-controlled breaths* with a fixed flow pattern to target a specific tidal volume. This mode is "advanced" in that it requires breath-to-breath analysis to determine how successful the prior level of support was at reaching the targeted volume; it then adjusts the support on each subsequent breath to get closer to the target volume. PRVC represents a simple form of partial closed-loop ventilation, which is further discussed in subsequent sections.

PRVC was initially created in an attempt to provide the benefits of both pressure-control mode and volume-control mode. By targeting a set volume, the benefits of volume control are maintained and allow for close control of the breath size. Tight control over delivered tidal volumes is critical for "lung-protective ventilation" (refer to Chapter 14), which includes limitation of overdistension and the resulting lung injury associated with large breaths. In addition, by targeting the tidal volume through a delivered pressure-regulated breath, the potential advantages associated with pressure control are demonstrated.

Pressure-control ventilation has been thought to provide more "comfortable" or "more physiologic" delivery of a breath. While volume control inherently is delivered via a fixed flow pattern, pressure-regulated breaths delivered in PRVC and pressure control have no fixed flow pattern; flow is based upon the applied pressure, the airway resistance, the underlying respiratory mechanics, and, most importantly for patient comfort, any additional patient effort. This has been thought to be particularly relevant to patients who are feeling what is known as "flow hunger" due to a high drive to breathe on the ventilator.

Flow hunger (which is further discussed in the consideration of flow asynchrony in Chapter 18) occurs when a patient desires either more flow or a different flow pattern than what is being controlled and delivered by the ventilator. PRVC has been thought to decrease flow hunger compared with volume control owing to the lack of fixed flow pattern; through this mechanism, the system provides more comfort for patients during mechanical ventilation. In addition, owing to the lack of fixed flow, the measured peak pressures on the ventilator may be lower in PRVC as compared with standard volume control (the plateau pressures should be identical because it is measured after the inspiration is completed; the patient's inspiratory efforts reduce pleural and airway pressure while gas is being pushed into the lungs, thereby reducing peak pressure). Lower peak pressures may be of benefit in patients with high airway resistance and in patients with frequent alarms for high pressure. Lastly, setting PRVC on the ventilator is very easy for clinicians and appears familiar compared with typical volume-control modes, with the primary difference being the absence of a set flow pattern in PRVC.

With these potential "benefits" from PRVC, a logical next question would be: Why it is not used as the default mode in all patients? At some sites, you will see this mode used as the standard of care, and for the most part, it can be considered an equivalent mode to volume control, albeit with differences in how individual breaths are delivered. It is also important to note as well that the proposed benefits from PRVC have not been proven in quality studies; there is minimal evidence that these proposed advantages lead to much difference in the care of or outcomes for patients. Furthermore, PRVC may have several disadvantages in some patient populations, which are important to understand. The first is that PRVC is not actually a *volume-control* mode. It only targets the set volume but can over- and under-shoot with each breath. This is particularly notable when patients are taking additional efforts with each breath, and it is easy for the delivery of larger-than-set volumes to occur. Consequently, in patients in whom very tight control is required, it is important to recognize this danger. As patients begin to breathe with more spontaneous efforts, the actual delivered volumes may be higher than otherwise desired. In addition, in situations in which breathing efforts are widely variable, the breath-to-breath adjustments may be inappropriate for any given breath because consistent efforts are needed for the system to know how much applied pressure is required for each breath to achieve the desired volume. Effort variability may be seen with neurogenic breathing patterns (ie, Cheyne-Stokes breathing), irregular spontaneous breathing, and in patients with intermittent agitation for whom the use of PRVC would need to be done with care.

PROPRIETARY CLOSED-LOOP VENTILATION MODES

Closed-loop mechanical ventilation refers to ventilator modes that continuously monitor patient respiratory output data and automate adjustment of the ventilator in response to perturbations in the data (**Figure 17-4**). The primary goal of these systems is to enhance patient comfort on the ventilator, which is hoped to enhance patient comfort and, consequently, patient-ventilator synchrony, thereby reducing the amount of sedation and analgesia required during the episode of acute respiratory failure. As discussed earlier, PRVC is one of the simplest forms of this type of closed-loop system; the resulting patient volumes are measured, and the ventilator automates the adjustment of pressure applied with each breath in response. While PRVC is a partially closed-loop system that is available on the majority of ventilators, more advanced and complex forms of closed-loop systems are often available as proprietary modes offered by specific manufacturers only on specific ventilator models.

Several proprietary closed-loop systems that are commercially available and have gained increased use over recent years include proportional assist ventilation (PAV), neurally adjusted

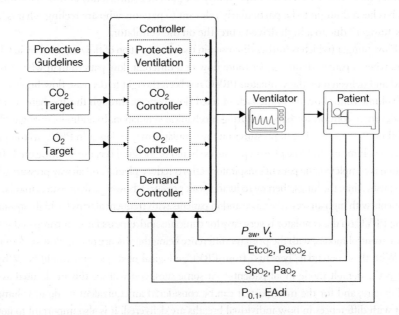

Figure 17-4: Closed-loop mechanical ventilation schematic. Closed-loop and partially closed-loop systems may have part or all of the abovementioned measurement signals and controllers listed. Clinicians typically dictate the specific targets that are desired for the patient, which can include specific oxygenation and CO_2 goals and/or specific "lung-protective" guidelines including pressure or volume goals. Multiple automated controllers within the ventilator work together to deliver the target settings. The ventilator then receives feedback from the patient, which can include numerous signals as illustrated; these are then read by the ventilator to determine how good a match there is between the feedback received and the clinical goals and target set by the provider; the control centers in the ventilator automatically make adjustments in the settings and the subsequent ventilation delivered to the patient. This dynamic approach occurs continually on a breath-to-breath basis to adjust incrementally the settings. (From Platen PV, Pomprapa A, Lachmann B, Leonhardt S. The dawn of physiological closed-loop ventilation-a review. *Crit Care*. 2020;24(1):121. Figure 4.)

ventilator assist (NAVA), adaptive support ventilation (ASV) and Intellivent-ASV, and SmartCare/PS weaning, which are discussed later. Although these advanced modes represent an exciting advancement in mechanical ventilation, the proprietary nature (and thus the often-hidden and patented underpinnings of the software and system), the more complex physiology, and the lack of high-quality data limit their generalizability. It is, however, likely that at least one of these types of advanced modes will be available within your ICU in the coming years and may even be one of the primary ventilator modes at your hospital, so we give a brief introduction to some of the more commonly used modes.

PROPORTIONAL ASSIST VENTILATION

This ventilator mode is a partially closed-loop form of mechanical ventilation designed to decrease patient work of breathing and improve patient-ventilator synchrony. The mode adjusts airway pressure in proportion to the patient's effort. Unlike other modes in which the physician presets a specific tidal volume or pressure, PAV lets the patient determine the inspired volume and the flow rate. This mode requires continuous measurements of resistance and compliance to determine the amount of pressure to give. The support given is a proportion of the patient's effort and is normally set at 80%. Therefore, this support is always changing according to patient's effort and lung dynamics on a breath-to-breath basis. If the patient's effort and/or demand are increased, the ventilator support is increased, and vice versa, to always give a set proportion of the breath (**Figure 17-5**). Unfortunately, setting the degree of inspiratory assist cannot be easily determined based upon the standard parameters, such as tidal volume or $Paco_2$ targets. Although 80% support is commonly used, it really is not clear what the right proportional support should be for patients, and this remains a limitation of the mode. Furthermore, the specific "safe" levels of inspiratory effort are still not well defined and may widely vary between patients depending on the type and severity of lung injury and/or diaphragm function.

Proportional assist ventilation

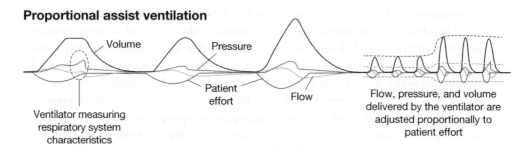

Volume   Pressure

Patient effort   Flow

Ventilator measuring respiratory system characteristics

Flow, pressure, and volume delivered by the ventilator are adjusted proportionally to patient effort

Figure 17-5: Proportional assist ventilation (PAV) schematic. With every spontaneous breath, the ventilator measures an estimate for the patients "effort" as well as the resistance and compliance of the patient's respiratory system. The mode estimates the total pressure that is needed to provide ventilation and then applies a certain proportion of that estimate via the ventilator (usually 60%-80%) with the remaining force generated by the patient. This means that in a patient with higher ventilator demands, the ventilator inherently is applying a larger total pressure to support each breath and, conversely, as ventilation requirements decrease, less support is applied. PAV has been demonstrated to improve patient-ventilator synchrony; however, there are few data to suggest that it is superior to traditional pressure support in terms of clinical outcomes. (From Mireles-Cabodevila E, Diaz-Guzman E, Heresi GA, Chatburn RL. Alternative modes of mechanical ventilation: a review for the hospitalist. *Cleve Clin J Med.* 2009;76(7):417-430. doi:10.3949/ccjm.76a.08043. Erratum in: *Cleve Clin J Med.* 2009;76(8):445. Figure 3.)

The data do not provide clear guidance on which patients might benefit from PAV. Several small studies have suggested that PAV may be superior to pressure support in terms of weaning to extubation, improved synchrony, and even improved sleep quality, but larger studies are needed to clarify the correct application. That being said, if this mode is available in your ICU, it appears generally safe to use interchangeably with pressure-support ventilation without any clear additional risks associated with the mode.

NEURALLY ADJUSTED VENTILATORY ASSIST

NAVA is a ventilator mode that shares similarity with PAV. Indeed, NAVA can be functionally thought of as a mode that replaces monitoring of airway pressure and flow signals with a measurement of neuronal effort generated from the patient. NAVA was initially designed with the goal to improve patient comfort and ventilator synchrony by improving the detection of a patient underlying effort with synchronization of the ventilator to these efforts.

In standard modes, conventional signals including flow, volume, and airway pressures are used to drive and control the ventilator operation; each of these parameters are mechanical manifestations of the patient's drive to breathe. In contrast, NAVA measures and monitors the electrical activity of the diaphragm (EAdi), as a more direct measure of respiratory drive, to rapidly detect inspiratory efforts. These signals are then used to trigger on and then cycle off the initiation and delivery of mechanical assistance from the ventilator while also regulating the level of support applied during the breath (**Figure 17-6**). Instead of utilizing pressure and flow changes measured at the airway (with the resulting delay in delivery of support), NAVA was designed to detect a patient' neuronal effort, with the idea that measuring this neuronal effort might reduce the delay in providing support and might achieve better titration of the level of support to the neuronal drive as opposed to surrogate measures of effort, which could be affected by muscle strength and other clinical factors.

NAVA measures EAdi via an esophageal probe similar to the probes discussed in Chapter 16. By determining the "effort" in this manner, the ventilator then delivers a level of pressure support that is proportional to the estimate of the patient's central respiratory drive (a concept of proportional assist that has some similarity with PAV). In addition to closely coordinated initiation of breath delivery and proportional levels of assistance relative to effort, the termination of an inspiratory effort is similarly determined based upon the EAdi value, which theoretically results in improved synchrony. Overall, there are limited data on NAVA to suggest that it is actually superior to traditional modes of ventilation. Nevertheless, several small studies suggest that NAVA is able to improve the inspiratory trigger delay, decrease the number of measured asynchrony events, and improve the ability to cycle off (ie, cease providing inspiratory support) during expiration. There are also several studies that suggest that NAVA may improve weaning specifically in difficult-to-wean patients; again, these are all small studies with unclear generalizability.

Importantly, the use of this mode is contingent upon the correct positioning of the esophageal probe to obtain quality EAdi signals from the diaphragm. Despite the potential and theoretical benefits compared with standard pressure support, the use of NAVA remains limited at this time. Barriers include the use of esophageal probes, the education required to master placement and use of the system, and the absence of large studies confirming the proposed benefits.

ADAPTIVE SUPPORT VENTILATION AND INTELLIVENT

ASV is a partially "closed-loop" ventilator mode in which the clinician targets a set desired total minute ventilation. The set minute ventilation is determined by the clinician based upon the anatomic dead space fraction and through empiric adjustment while monitoring CO_2 clearance, that

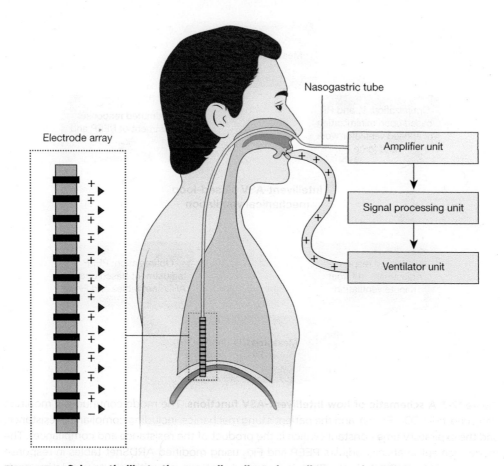

Figure 17-6: Schematic illustrating neurally adjusted ventilatory assist (NAVA). NAVA uses an esophageal probe, which is placed through the nose or mouth and extends from the thorax into the abdominal cavity through the diaphragm. The electrode array is positioned to allow for monitoring of diaphragm electrical activity (EAdi). A patient's inspiratory efforts can be monitored by the electrodes, and the amplitude of electrical activity is interpreted as a specific level of effort. The ventilator then provides assistance to the patient's inspiratory effort in an amount that is proportional to the level of neuronal effort. With more EAdi activity interpreted as a stronger inspiratory effort, a larger level of pressure support is applied from the ventilator. This is similar in some ways to proportional assist ventilation (PAV), which uses pressure and flow deviations to measure "effort." By measuring neuronal effort, however, NAVA allows for measurement of effort even in the presence of muscle weakness or auto-PEEP. PEEP, positive end-expiratory pressure.

is, achieving the desired $Paco_2$. The ventilator then uses breath-to-breath feedback from the airway resistance and lung compliance (stiffness) to determine the "best" combination of tidal volumes and respiratory rate for the patient to achieve the target minute ventilation. The algorithm uses established physiologic principles and formulas to determine the combination of rate and volume that minimizes both the applied mechanical work from the ventilator and the applied driving pressure. Furthermore, it allows a seamless transition between a fully controlled and fully spontaneous mode and can be used to automate weaning off the ventilator. In this mode, while volume and respiratory rate are automatically adjusted, applied PEEP and Fio_2 must be determined and set by the clinician, which is why this mode is considered only partially closed loop.

Intellivent-ASV furthers the concept of closed-loop ventilation to allow for full automation (**Figure 17-7**). Spo_2 measurements in real time provide the oxygenation feedback to the ventilator

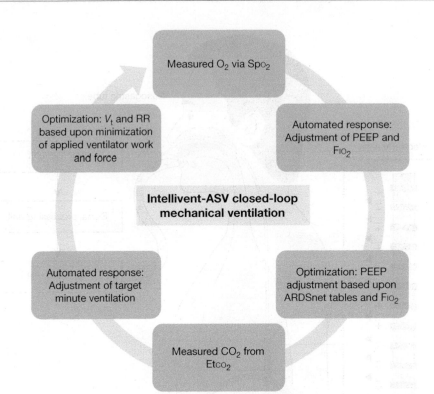

Figure 17-7: A schematic of how Intellivent-ASV functions. The mode continuously monitors Pao$_2$, end-tidal CO$_2$ (Etco$_2$), and the patient's lung mechanics, including compliance, resistance, and the expiratory time constant (which is the product of the resistance and compliance). The mode then automatically adjusts PEEP and Fio$_2$ using modified ARDSnet tables in response to changes in Spo$_2$. Similarly, the Etco$_2$ is measured continuously, with minute ventilation goals automatically adjusted to maintain the target CO$_2$ levels. Once a target minute ventilation has been determined by the ventilator, the respiratory rate (RR) and tidal volume (V_t) are then automatically adjusted based upon the patient's mechanics to minimize the applied power and driving pressures from the ventilator. In this mode, clinicians set the target Spo$_2$ and Etco$_2$ levels based upon the clinical condition of the patient. PEEP, positive end-expiratory pressure.

to adjust PEEP and Fio$_2$ based upon ARDSnet tables (see Chapter 13). End-tidal CO$_2$ (Etco$_2$) is measured in line with the ventilator, and the target minute ventilation is automatically adjusted as the Etco$_2$ increases and decreases. Minute ventilation is increased as the Etco$_2$ increases above the target levels and decreases when the Etco$_2$ drops below the target range. The ventilation controller then interacts with the ASV controller (above) to determine the best tidal volume and respiratory rate, given the required minute ventilation feedback from the Etco$_2$ monitor.

The small amount of existing data suggest that these modes are generally safe and function well in the majority of patients. These modes may speed up weaning and extubation in some patients and appear to target "safe" lung volume and pressure levels in passive patients with ARDS. There is, however, less control for the clinician over each specific variable as the management of the ventilator is increasingly automated. This lack of control may be suboptimal for some clinicians who prefer to have a greater role in determining the specific mix of variables inherent in mechanical ventilation. In other circumstances, when resources and personnel are limited, closed-loop automation could theoretically improve care with its ability to adjust as a patient's respiratory status waxes and wanes. At this time, high-quality evidence does not exist to determine the optimal application of these types of modes.

SMARTCARE/PS

SmartCare from Draeger represents an automated ventilator mode specifically dedicated to weaning. This ventilator mode continuously monitors respiratory rate, pressure-support level, tidal volumes, and other output variables and adjusts the level of support automatically to target the lowest possible ventilator support to maintain adequate ventilation. The hypothesis is this system will more rapidly demonstrate that a patient is ready for extubation and will challenge patients to wean at a faster rate. The mode then checks to ensure the patient is succeeding with weaning and subsequently transitions into an automated spontaneous breathing trial (SBT) when the predetermined thresholds have been met. There is some evidence in several small trials that such systems could be utilized to speed up extubation, but the optimal use and generalizability of this approach have yet to be fully demonstrated.

SUMMARY

While the vast majority of patients can be successfully ventilated using the traditional pressure and volume assist/control modes and pressure-support modes, the use of more advanced ventilator modes has increased in many ICUs internationally and within the United States. Some of these "advanced" modes—in particular PRVC—have become the standard of care at many hospitals because of the perceived advantages of applying a hybrid approach for ventilation, even though the data supporting these advantages remain limited at this time. Other advanced modes such as APRV may be beneficial in a small subset of patients, but if used improperly may be harmful; it also requires advanced levels of training and education. The use of partially or fully closed-loop mechanical ventilator systems will likely become more common as these systems advance technologically and are more widely available. Indeed, closed-loop system likely represents the future of mechanical ventilation and, in theory, could allow a more rapid response to changing patient conditions, tighter control and more consistent application of lung-protective settings, improved patient-ventilator interaction with decreased dyssynchrony, and faster weaning toward extubation.

KEY POINTS

- Standard modes used in most ICUs include pressure assist-control, volume assist-control, and pressure-support modes. Although labeled as "advanced modes," many of these are now used as the standard of care within ICUs instead of "standard modes."
- APRV applies an extreme version of inverse ratio ventilation in which the inspiratory time is longer than the expiratory time. APRV applies a high pressure (P_{high}) for a relatively long duration (T_{high}) with intermittent releases in pressure to a low pressure (P_{low}), which is held for a very short duration (T_{low}).
- APRV may in some cases help with lung recruitment and oxygenation, but if applied incorrectly, or in a patient who will not be able to recruit more lung with higher applied pressures, APRV can also be harmful.
- Closed-loop and partially closed-loop modes of mechanical ventilation utilize continuous feedback from the patient to adjust applied variables to the patient. These modes may vary from simple partial closed-loop adjusting target volume, to fully closed-loop systems that monitor oxygenation, carbon dioxide clearance, and lung mechanics.

- PRVC is a partially closed-loop mode that represents a hybrid between volume- and pressure-control modes. A given volume is targeted in PRVC, and the mode adjusts the applied pressure required to achieve this volume on a breath-by-breath basis.
- PAV is a partially closed-loop system that monitors markers of patient "effort" based upon flow and pressure changes and then applies support from the ventilator proportional to the patient's effort. If a patient is exhibiting a high respiratory drive, the ventilator will provide more support, and this support decreases as patient efforts decrease.
- NAVA is similar to PAV in that it applies a proportional level of assistance depending on patient effort, but instead of using airway pressure and flow as surrogates for effort, it measures actual diaphragmatic electrical activity to determine the level of neural effort.
- ASV is a partially closed-loop mode that monitors respiratory system mechanics and resistance to determine the optimal tidal volume and respiratory rate to minimize mechanical work and driving pressure with each breath.
- Intellivent-ASV utilizes the ASV mode but provides fully closed-loop support by automating minute ventilation to measured levels of end-tidal CO_2 and adjusts PEEP and FIO_2 based upon the measured oxygen saturation.
- SmartCare/PS is a partially closed-loop mode that purports to monitor the patient's readiness to wean from mechanical ventilation and automates the progressive decrease in support consistent with that readiness and transitions the patient to a SBT in an attempt to expedite extubation.

STUDY QUESTIONS AND ANSWERS

Questions

1. A 68-year-old woman with confirmed ARDS is undergoing mechanical ventilation with PRVC ventilation with tidal volume target set to 400 mL. The patient is starting to have intermittent irregular spontaneous efforts. Which of the following would you expect to see with this patient having irregular spontaneous efforts in PRVC?
   A. Consistent flow pattern during each inspiration
   B. Tidal volumes larger than what is set on the ventilator
   C. Consistent applied level of pressure with each breath
   D. Worsened flow asynchrony or "flow hunger"
   E. None of the above

2. There are five mechanically ventilated patients currently on your team with variable reasons for requiring intubation. Which of these patients might in theory benefit the most from being placed on APRV?
   A. A 45-year-old man with variceal bleed intubated for esophagogastroduodenoscopy (EGD) and ongoing bleeding who has been intubated for 2 days
   B. A 68-year-old woman with flair of existing chronic interstitial lung disease and fibrosis intubated and undergoing a pulse of steroids
   C. A 53-year-old morbidly obese man with acute pancreatitis, intubated overnight with ARDS, and persistent severe hypoxemia

D. A 36-year-old woman 3 weeks into her course of COVID pneumonia and ARDS

E. A 74-year-old man with chronic obstructive pulmonary disease (COPD) exacerbation secondary to pneumonia, intubated secondary to hypercarbia 2 days prior

3. A 67-year-old woman is recovering from a prolonged course of COVID pneumonia during which she required prolonged proning and paralysis. Her lungs have significantly recovered, but she has been noted to have profound weakness. She is noted to be awake and interactive with minimal oxygenation or ventilation issues on pressure support, but is having weak efforts that are often failing to trigger the ventilator despite lowering the trigger threshold. Which of the ventilator modes would be best for this patient?

A. Continue pressure support and tolerate the intermittently missed triggers.

B. Change to NAVA.

C. Change to PAV.

D. Change to control mode ventilation (either pressure or volume control).

E. None of the above.

Answers

1. **Answer B. Tidal volumes larger than what is set on the ventilator**

Rationale: Tidal volumes may be larger than the set target volume in patients who are ventilated with PRVC. This is because the tidal volume is not tightly controlled as would be seen in volume control. Instead, pressure supporting the inspiratory flow is minutely adjusted with each breath to achieve the target volume. In the setting of additional spontaneous breathing, especially if the efforts are irregular or with variable effort, the machine may be unable to accurately adjust the applied pressure to achieve precise tidal volume on each breath, and the delivered volumes may be both lower and higher than what is set. **A.** This is not correct because the flow in PRVC is not tightly regulated and a variable flow pattern will occur on a breath-to-breath basis depending on resistance, compliance, and degree of patient effort. A consistent flow pattern is a characteristic of volume assist/control ventilation. **C.** This is not correct as a consistent set pressure level applied with each breath is a characteristic of pressure assist/control ventilation. In PRVC, while each individual breath appears similar to a pressure-control breath, the level of pressure applied with each breath may be quite variable as the ventilator adjusts to achieve the volume goal. Particularly in this scenario, when the patient is having active spontaneous efforts, the pressure applied with each breath would likely be widely variable. **D.** This is not correct because PRVC typically improves the severity of flow asynchrony by not forcing the patient into a set flow pattern. As such, patients with spontaneous efforts can have what is thought to be more comfortable breathing with less evidence for the flow hunger associated with flow asynchrony.

2. **Answer C. A 53-year-old morbidly obese man with acute pancreatitis, intubated overnight with ARDS, and persistent severe hypoxemia**

Rationale: APRV is a mode that may have some benefit in patients with significant hypoxemia who are potentially recruitable. In this setting, recruitable means that significant regions of their lungs may be atelectatic and that the application of higher levels of pressure may help reopen the lungs and maintain recruitment, which helps improve lung mechanics and hypoxemia while potentially reducing lung injury. Of the scenarios given, this patient

(continued)

with early ARDS, with a high likelihood for collapse of the lungs due to his body habitus and pancreatitis, would be the most likely patient to benefit from APRV if applied correctly. **A.** A patient intubated for a procedure without significant other lung disease would be unlikely to derive any benefit from APRV. **B.** A patient with chronic lung injury and fibrosis would be unlikely to benefit from high-pressure application, and APRV would likely only be harmful in this patient. **D.** Although in theory this patient might have been considered a good candidate for APRV earlier in her course, the fact that she has had such a prolonged course suggests that she has likely developed some degree of lung fibrosis, which would make her a poor candidate for APRV; there would be little lung available for recruitment. **E.** Patients with COPD are poor candidates for APRV as they require more time for exhalation due to their underlying emphysema and obstruction. The short release times with APRV would not allow adequate exhalation and would worsen hyperinflation. As such, APRV should be avoided in patients with significant obstructive disease.

3. **Answer B. Change to NAVA**

   Rationale: In this case, the patient has a significant critical illness myopathy that has weakened her respiratory muscles to the point at which she is unable to generate sufficient flow and pressure change to trigger the ventilator. In this case, the use of NAVA, which measures the neuronal effort, would capture her attempts to breathe and rapidly coordinate assistance from the ventilator. **A.** Continuing pressure support may not be ideal if there are many missed efforts as the patient may be very uncomfortable or be unable to generate enough minute ventilation to breathe off her CO_2. **C.** Even though PAV has a similar function to NAVA in that it adjusts the level of support as patient effort changes, in this case, similar to pressure support, PAV still relies upon airway pressure and flow changes to sense triggering. As such, it would likely not be any better than pressure support in detecting and responding to patient efforts. **D.** Changing the patient to a fully controlled mode of ventilation might be necessary if NAVA is not available (which may be the case within your ICU). If the patient remains too weak to trigger the ventilator, then changing to a control mode may be needed for sufficient ventilation. If NAVA is available, however, then this may continue to encourage spontaneous breathing and allow for more patient comfort.

Suggested Readings

Jonkman AH, Rauseo M, Carteaux G, et al. Proportional modes of ventilation: technology to assist physiology. *Intensive Care Med*. 2020;46(12):2301-2313. doi:10.1007/s00134-020-06206-z.

Lellouche F, Brochard L. Advanced closed loops during mechanical ventilation (PAV, NAVA, ASV, SmartCare). *Best Pract Res Clin Anaesthesiol*. 2009;23(1):81-93. doi:10.1016/j.bpa.2008.08.001.

MacIntyre NR, Gropper C, Westfall T. Combining pressure-limiting and volume-cycling features in a patient-interactive mechanical breath. *Crit Care Med*. 1994;22(2):353-357. doi:10.1097/00003246-199402000-00030.

Platen PV, Pomprapa A, Lachmann B, Leonhardt S. The dawn of physiological closed-loop ventilation: a review. *Crit Care*. 2020;24(1):121. doi:10.1186/s13054-020-2810-1.

Zhou Y, Jin X, Lv Y, et al. Early application of airway pressure release ventilation may reduce the duration of mechanical ventilation in acute respiratory distress syndrome. *Intensive Care Med*. 2017;43(11):1648-1659. doi:10.1007/s00134-017-4912-z.

Ventilator Dyssynchrony

Elias Baedorf Kassis • Emmett A. Kistler

LEARNING OBJECTIVES

- Define ventilator dyssynchrony and summarize its clinical significance.
- Identify common types of ventilator dyssynchrony and their causes.
- Analyze common pathologic ventilator pressure/flow waveforms in different types of ventilator dyssynchrony.
- Identify management plans for both the patient and ventilator to mitigate ventilator dyssynchrony.

DEFINITION AND CLINICAL SIGNIFICANCE

When placing a patient with respiratory failure on mechanical ventilation, the goal is for the ventilator and any spontaneous breathing efforts made by the patient to work together synchronously. Ventilator dyssynchrony, when the machine and patient are not aligned, arises from an imbalance between a mechanically ventilated patient's respiratory efforts and the mechanical support provided by the ventilator.

Dyssynchrony is a common problem that affects most intubated patients but is often underappreciated and missed by clinicians. The frequency with which it occurs is not well documented; nevertheless, it is increasingly recognized as an important problem because the physiologic implications associated with ventilator dyssynchrony are numerous and potentially quite serious. Mismatched efforts between patient and ventilator can lead to increased work of breathing, derecruitment (ie, collapse of alveoli), and worsened gas exchange. Dyssynchrony can also cause variable tidal volumes, large and injurious pressure swings across the lungs, and lung overdistension, making it a likely contributor to the development of lung injury. Consequently, intensive care unit (ICU) providers try to minimize ventilator dyssynchrony by prescribing analgesics, sedation, and paralytics, which can contribute to prolonged ICU stay, increased duration of mechanical ventilation, and even worsened mortality.

There are multiple types of ventilator dyssynchrony, each of which has a different cause, impact, and solution(s) (**Table 18-1**). Of note, when we discuss the causes of each dyssynchrony, we will discuss the dominant patient and ventilator factors contributing to each subtype; it is important, however, to note that the patient and ventilator factors are often closely related and at times inseparable from each other. Ventilator dyssynchrony can be categorized based on how and when the mismatch in efforts take place during the typical breathing cycle: the initiation of the breath, when a breath is delivered, and during the breath. Although most often associated with inspiration, dyssynchrony can also occur during the patient's exhalation.

Despite how frequently these events occur and their negative implications for clinical care, recognition and management of ventilator dyssynchrony remain challenging for many ICU providers. We will take an in-depth look at the most common forms of dyssynchrony, discuss etiologies and identification of this phenomenon, and offer strategies for addressing mismatch between the patient and machine. As part of a practical approach to ventilator dyssynchrony, we address each type of dyssynchrony by examining etiologic factors pertaining to the patient and those attributable to the ventilator.

TRIGGER ASYNCHRONY

One of the key aspects of the patient-ventilator interaction is the ventilator's ability to detect when a patient is attempting to initiate a breath. When patients are fully passive without any spontaneous breathing efforts, the ventilator triggers the initiation of a delivered breath based upon the respiratory rate set by the clinician. However, when a patient is exhibiting spontaneous breathing (regardless of whether the ventilator is in fully spontaneous or assist-control mode), the patient initiates the breath, which is then delivered by the ventilator to align with the efforts made by the patient. The *trigger threshold* for activation of the ventilator, the time to detection by the ventilator of that patient effort, and the speed with which a breath can then be delivered by the ventilator determine the comfort experienced by the patient on the ventilator. In sum, the ventilator tries to mimic a "natural" breath.

TABLE 18-1 Overview of the Primary Types of Dyssynchrony

	Detection	Harm	Cause—Patient	Treatment—Patient	Cause—Ventilator	Treatment—Ventilator
Missed trigger	Pressure/flow deviations showing efforts not followed by a full breath	Inadequate ventilation Patient discomfort	Resp. muscle weakness Insufficient resp. drive Inability to overcome intrinsic PEEP	Lighten sedation Decrease airway resistance Decrease auto-PEEP	High sensitivity threshold Inadequate applied PEEP	Decrease trigger sensitivity Match auto-PEEP with set PEEP Improve auto-PEEP by decreasing RR Shorten I, lengthen E time
Auto-triggering	Small deviations in pressure/flow lead to ventilator-initiated breath without patient efforts	Increased tidal volume/ volutrauma Patient discomfort	Excess secretions Cardiac oscillations	Treat secretions Manage cardiac pathology	Low-sensitivity threshold Air leaks Fluid in the tubing	Increase trigger sensitivity Remove fluid in the tubing
Reverse triggering with or without breath stacking	Vent-initiated breath followed by buried patient effort May cause breath stacking, which is easy to detect Without breath stacking: scooping of pressure waveform and augmented volume during inspiration Flow/volume deviations during exhalation	Increased tidal volume/ volutrauma Transpulmonary pressure swings, Pendelluft Asymmetric stretch of dependent lung	Excess sedation, other causes such as hypocarbia, high masked drive possible, but unknown	Adjust and even decrease sedation Consider paralytics if associated with breath stacking or worsened hypoxemia	Unknown	Increase tidal volume Increase PEEP Trial alternative vent mode

(continued)

TABLE 18-1 Overview of the Primary Types of Dyssynchrony (continued)

	Detection	Harm	Cause—Patient	Treatment—Patient	Cause—Ventilator	Treatment—Ventilator
Premature cycling (aka Double triggering)	Prolonged patient effort prompts second vent-delivered breath Breath stacking Initial patient effort is distinct from reverse triggering	Increased tidal volume/ volutrauma Transpulmonary pressure swings	High respiratory drive Insufficient sedation	Increase sedation Consider paralytics Optimize respiratory drive	Inadequate ventilator support	Increase ventilation if safe with increased tidal volume and RR Increase inspiratory time
Flow asynchrony	Scooping of pressure waveform during inspiration	High WOB Self-induced lung Injury	High respiratory drive Patient discomfort	Increase sedation Optimize respiratory drive	Pattern of flow Volume-regulated modes	Increase flow Change flow ramp Change to pressure-regulated mode
Expiratory effort Dyssynchrony (aka Delayed cycling)	End-inspiratory spikes on pressure waveform	Derecruitment Auto-PEEP Missed triggers Hypoxemia	High airway resistance Auto-PEEP	Adjust sedation Reduce airway resistance	Prolonged inspiratory time	Increase V_e Decrease t / time

PEEP, positive end-expiratory pressure; RR, respiratory rate; WOB, work of breathing.

For the spontaneously breathing patient, the trigger threshold comprises a pressure or flow, generated by the patient. When the trigger threshold is met, the ventilator goes into action. *Pressure triggering* occurs when the ventilator detects a decrease in pressure in the airway secondary to a patient's inspiratory effort. Alternatively, with *flow triggering*, the ventilator measures the patient's inspiratory flow as the trigger to initiate a breath. Sensing this inspiratory "effort," the ventilator is activated and the breath is supported. Because a change in pressure determines flow for a given resistance, flow and pressure triggers are often used interchangeably.

Trigger asynchrony can occur with either pressure or flow triggering when the ventilator fails to recognize a patient's efforts to initiate a breath (missed triggers) or when the ventilator misinterprets an alternative stimulus (eg, vibration in the tubing or cardiac oscillations), as the patient's efforts to breathe and inappropriately delivers a breath (auto-triggers). Despite its name, double triggering and reverse triggering are distinctive types of dyssynchrony that fall into a separate category and will be addressed later in this chapter.

MISSED TRIGGERS

Missed triggers are among the most common types of ventilator dyssynchrony. A missed or ineffective trigger occurs when a mechanically ventilated patient attempts to breathe but the trigger threshold is not met and, consequently, initiation of a ventilator-delivered breath does not occur. Missed triggers can occur in any mode of ventilation and with both flow- and pressure-triggered breaths. Missed triggers occur for several reasons, which can be divided into two categories: those related to the patient and those related to ventilator settings.

With respect to clinical ramifications, attempts to breathe that are not mechanically supported can lead to significant distress for the patient and potentially injurious respiratory responses. More specifically, missed triggers are associated with dyspnea, increased respiratory muscle efforts, and ineffective breathing patterns such as rapid shallow breathing.

Causes of Missed Triggers

Patient Factors

A common cause for missed triggering is insufficient respiratory drive, which can limit the patient's ability to generate sufficient pressure or flow to meet or exceed the trigger threshold. Consider the excessively sedated patient newly transitioned to a pressure support mode who alarms for apnea because a lack of wakefulness hinders sufficient efforts to breathe. Although this patient may be making inspiratory efforts, the suppressed respiratory drive fails to generate sufficient pressure or flow to meet the trigger threshold. Respiratory drive may be decreased secondary to multiple causes including sedative agents, central nervous system injury, or encephalopathy because of toxin ingestion, severe sepsis, or other metabolic derangements, which decrease wakefulness.

Alternatively, a patient may be awake enough to breathe on their own, but respiratory muscle weakness prevents them from generating enough flow or pressure to prompt the ventilator to deliver a breath. Respiratory muscle weakness is common after prolonged mechanical ventilation (see Chapter 15) or may be attributable to primary neuromuscular pathologies such as Guillain-Barré, amyotrophic lateral sclerosis, or muscular dystrophy. It may also be secondary to severe restriction of the chest wall. Finally, auto–positive end-expiratory pressure (*auto-PEEP*; see Chapters 7, 11, and 12)—which can be seen in the patient in status asthmaticus or during an acute exacerbation of chronic obstructive pulmonary disease (COPD)—can prevent even the awake patient with normal respiratory muscle strength from meeting the trigger threshold. In these circumstances, patients have not completed a full exhalation by the time that the next breath is set to begin; pressure in the lungs is still greater than the pressure at the airway opening and gas is still moving out of the lungs. This residual expiratory pressure and flow need to be overcome by the inspiratory effort to reverse flow and create a negative deflection in pressure strong enough to trigger the ventilator.

Ventilator Factors

Missed triggering may result if the ventilator is set for a "low trigger sensitivity" (the ventilator is *relatively insensitive* to pressure or flow changes in the airway, ie, higher thresholds of effort required for triggering). The patient must generate a high amount of pressure or flow to initiate the mechanically delivered breath. Even patients with adequate respiratory drive and muscle strength may have difficulty creating enough flow or pressure if sensitivity is set too low or if the patient has auto-PEEP.

To counter the high trigger threshold associated with auto-PEEP as seen in the patient in status asthmaticus described earlier, one tries to set the machine PEEP just below (eg, a few cm H_2O pressure) close to the level of the total PEEP (**Figure 18-1**). When the patient initiates a breath and the airway pressure falls to a level slightly less than the applied PEEP, the ventilator is triggered to support the breath.

Inadequate *applied PEEP* (PEEP exerted by the ventilator) is a more specific circumstance leading to missed triggers that typically involves a patient with excess auto-PEEP.

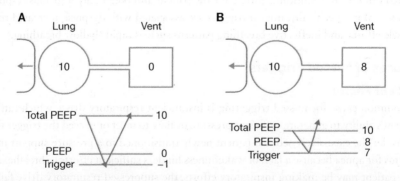

Figure 18-1: Schematic illustrating the effect of auto-PEEP in a patient with significant flow limitation. A, A patient with a significant auto-PEEP and zero PEEP applied by the ventilator, resulting in a total PEEP of 10 cm H_2O pressure. The patient initiates a breath and starts to reduce airway pressure, but the ventilator will not be triggered until the airway pressure overcomes the auto-PEEP and the trigger setting (-1 cm H_2O). The patient must generate a total of 11 cm H_2O pressure to trigger a breath. Failing to meet this threshold results in a missed trigger (the patient is trying to get a breath and the ventilator does not detect the inspiratory effort). **B,** By increasing the set PEEP, that is, the PEEP applied by the ventilator, closer to the level of the total PEEP, the patient only needs to generate a much smaller effort (to produce a change in pressure of 3 cm H_2O) to trigger the breath, decreasing the likelihood of causing a missed trigger event. PEEP, positive end-expiratory pressure.

Recognition of Missed Triggers

With the etiologies of missed triggers in mind, we can now discuss recognition of these events. On pressure and flow ventilator waveforms, missed triggers manifest as flow and/or pressure deviations that do not result in a triggered ventilator supported breath (**Figure 18-2**). These deviations can be subtle, and they can be more readily recognizable when an esophageal balloon is employed to monitor esophageal pressure (see Chapter 16), which provides an indication of pleural pressure changes secondary to inspiratory efforts. For a missed trigger, esophageal manometry will show a negative deflection in the esophageal pressure curve without a corresponding breath delivered by the ventilator.

Management of Missed Triggers

Management of missed triggers is directed at the underlying cause(s) and can be divided into interventions for the patient and interventions on the ventilator. Beginning with the patient, decreased respiratory drive because of excessive sedation requires optimization of the sedative regimen (holding sedation and/or employing agents with less profound effects on respiratory drive) and delaying the transition to patient-triggered modes such as pressure support until adequate wakefulness is present.

Some types of neuromuscular disease are reversible (such as critical illness myopathy or Guillain-Barré), whereas others are progressive (muscular dystrophy or amyotrophic lateral sclerosis). When applicable, treatment should be directed to the primary underlying cause of weakness. For the patient with advanced respiratory muscle weakness attributable to neurologic disease, therapeutic interventions are unfortunately lacking. Management instead necessitates discussion of long-term, ventilator-driven support for these patients if this intervention is within their goals of care. For patients with critical care myopathy, ensuring appropriate nutrition and normal electrolytes (particularly potassium and phosphate) may hasten recovery of muscle strength.

The patient with auto-PEEP should receive therapies aimed at reducing airway resistance/obstruction with drugs such as bronchodilators and steroids. Additionally, for the patient with dynamic hyperinflation because of obstructive lung disease, ICU providers must balance adequate management of the patient's secretion burden with minimizing airway stimulation (which can worsen secretions and provoke bronchospasm) through excessive suctioning.

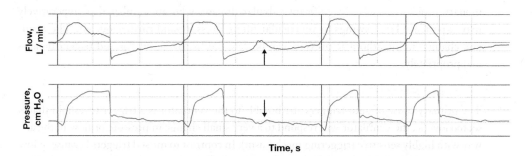

Time, s

Figure 18-2: **Recognition of missed triggering on waveforms.** Missed triggers typically can be seen both by bedside evaluation of patients, with observed inspiratory efforts not resulting in triggered breaths supported by the ventilator, and on waveforms where subtle pressure and flow deviations may suggest an effort that is not triggering the ventilator.

When considering missed triggers because of inappropriate ventilator settings, such as inadequate trigger sensitivity, missed triggers can be addressed by increasing the sensitivity. This equates to setting a lower pressure or flow threshold at which the ventilator will deliver a breath. As we will see in the next section, however, trigger threshold that is set too low can predispose a patient to auto-triggering.

With respect to the patient with high auto-PEEP, one must devise strategies to reduce missed triggers including lowering tidal volumes (larger tidal volumes can result in more auto-PEEP with longer required expiratory periods), decreasing the respiratory rate (allows for longer expiratory time), and PEEP matching, which requires measurement of the patient's total PEEP as illustrated in **Figure 18-2** and setting the applied PEEP just below that level, thereby reducing the total "effort" required by the patient to trigger a breath and decreasing the likelihood for a missed trigger event.

AUTO-TRIGGERS

Conceptually, auto-triggers represent the opposite of missed triggers (ie, the ventilator provides a breath despite the absence of an inspiratory effort in contrast to failing to respond to the patient's attempt to get a breath) and occur when trigger thresholds are fulfilled by stimuli *unrelated* to the patient's spontaneous breathing. Auto-triggers are due to deviations in airway pressure or flow related to secretions and/or intrathoracic swings in pressure independent of any inspiratory efforts from the patient. Excessive condensation in the ventilator tubing and leaks in the circuit can also be inciting factors.

Auto-triggers result in inappropriately delivered breaths, which can lead to patient discomfort and hyperventilation. Breath delivery out of phase with exhalation can, in some cases, lead to breath stacking, auto-PEEP, and injuriously large tidal volumes.

Causes of Auto-Triggers
Patient Factors
Patient-related causes of auto-triggers include excessive amounts of secretions or other fluids oscillating within the ventilator tubing or airways and cardiopulmonary pathology, which may produce significant intrathoracic pressure swings. Secretions and mucus can accumulate in the ventilator tubing, disrupting laminar airflow and provoking sufficient changes in pressure to trigger a mechanically delivered breath. Individuals with major cardiopulmonary problems, such as significant valvular disease, who are intubated perioperatively may experience large swings in ventricular filling pressure and cardiac output. The resultant changes in intrathoracic pressure can be detected by the ventilator and trigger breaths inappropriately.

Ventilator Factors
The primary cause of auto-triggers attributable to the ventilator is a trigger threshold that is set too low (ie, the ventilator will respond to a very small change in pressure or flow in the airway with highly sensitive triggering mechanism). In contrast to missed triggers because of low sensitivity, which can lead to failure to recognize patient efforts to breathe, excessively high sensitivity can result in delivery of a breath when there is no spontaneous inspiratory effort but there are other stimuli, for example, shivering or positional changes. An air leak or buildup of secretions or condensation fluid in the ventilator tubing can also cause auto-triggering;

pressure and flow changes from oscillation of the fluid in the tubing may be of sufficient amplitude to mimic an inspiratory effort.

Recognition of Auto-Triggers

On ventilator waveforms, indicators of auto-triggering include the association of ventilator-delivered breaths with heart rate or other cardiac stimuli as well as the lack of association of ventilator-delivered breaths with observed patient efforts to breathe. External tipoffs that the patient may be at risk for auto-triggers include increased fluid in ventilator tubing, physical exam signs of dynamic cardiac function (eg, strong apical impulse in the precordium), and data from invasive hemodynamic monitoring suggestive of high cardiac output and/or swings in intrathoracic pressure (**Figure 18-3**).

Management

Management of auto-triggering entails interventions to reduce risk factors by minimizing secretions and/or optimization of cardiac function (although aberrant cardiac status may be difficult to correct). On the ventilator, routine removal of fluid and secretions from the tubing is a simple but important approach to decrease auto-triggering. Additionally, trigger threshold can be increased (ie, reduced sensitivity of the ventilator), although the ICU provider must then monitor for missed triggers.

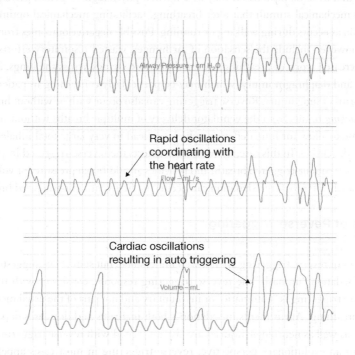

Figure 18-3: Recognition of auto-triggering on waveforms. Auto-triggering can be recognized when the ventilator is falsely reading pressure or flow changes that are independent of the patient's inspiratory effort. This can occur from fluid in the tubing or strong cardiac oscillations. Any time triggering is occurring in a fast, rhythmic fashion, and clinical exam reveals that breaths delivered by the ventilator are discordant with patient efforts, auto-triggering should be suspected.

REVERSE TRIGGERING

For patient-triggered breaths, the appropriate series of events is as follows: the patient exerts an effort to breath, enough pressure or flow is generated to meet a trigger threshold, and the ventilator is prompted to deliver a breath. *Reverse triggering*, another type of ventilator dyssynchrony, entails the opposite pattern in which a ventilator-initiated breath prompts an automatic patient inspiratory effort. It is termed "reverse triggering" as the trigger seems to occur in reverse of the typical trigger, with the ventilator conversely seeming to trigger the patient's inspiratory effort. For example, mechanical changes of the respiratory system resulting from a ventilator generated breath seem to precipitate a breath initiated by the patient. In other words, the respiratory mechanical activity prompted by the ventilator seems to provoke or couple with a neural discharge by the patient to produce another breath. These "neuromechanically coupled" inspiratory muscle contractions, which often appear with a regular and consistent timing and amplitude after the ventilator-initiated breath, which have previously been thought to be a reflexive response, are a form of respiratory entrainment, that is, an external stimulus triggers a physiologic response, as will be discussed later. Reverse triggering appears to be present in both healthy normal patients as well as critically ill patients with variable causes of severe lung injury, suggesting that a variety of stimuli are associated with reverse triggering.

The presence of reverse triggering noted during research studies of healthy volunteers suggests that in some instances it may be a normal physiologic response, perhaps as an adaptation to mechanical stimuli that alter breathing, facilitating mechanical optimization of the inspiration as occurs during walking or running. Possible negative outcomes from reverse triggering, however, include the sensation of air hunger, wasted respiratory efforts that contribute to increased work of breathing, elevated pressure swings across the lungs, and high tidal volumes and diaphragm injury, which may be particularly concerning in patients with more severe forms of lung injury. Reverse triggering can also occur with or without breath stacking. *Breath stacking* results from the ventilator delivery of multiple breaths without sufficient exhalation time to allow for lung deflation, which can lead to very large total inhaled volume and lung overdistension. In this case, the ventilator detects the reverse-triggered inspiratory effort, like a typical patient-triggered breath, and provides an additional pressure- or volume-targeted breath shortly after (before exhalation can occur) the first ventilator-triggered breath.

Causes of Reverse Triggering

Patient Factors

The causes of reverse triggering are not well understood, but some have suggested that deeper levels of sedation "unmask" the reverse triggering response, consistent with the notion that the reverse triggering is "automatic" or involuntary and not part of the usual mechanisms that control breathing. Adjustments in sedation—both increases and decreases depending on the patient—as well as neurologic injuries are also associated with reverse triggering.

From an evolutionary perspective, reverse triggering in most cases appears secondary to a type of neuromechanical coupling called respiratory entrainment. Respiratory entrainment occurs when the inspiratory muscles respond to an external physical stimulus rather than through the usual ventilatory control mechanisms. Respiratory entrainment is well described in mammalian bipedal and quadrupedal species, which link their breathing pattern during ambulation with their leg movements. Although this is often referred to as "reflexive," this interaction is more complex than the simple reflex and likely involves alternative neural pathways. In the case of patients who are mechanically ventilated with reverse triggering, the ventilator takes on a role analogous to ambulation in the example provided earlier, providing the "external" stimulus that triggers a respiratory response.

Ventilator Factors

On the ventilator, reverse triggering can occur in multiple different controlled modes of ventilation. The specific mechanism by which the ventilator provokes reverse triggering have not been fully defined, but low tidal volumes and low PEEP have been postulated to exacerbate reverse triggering, whereas higher minute ventilation (and hence lower Pco_2) has been postulated to decrease the occurrence of reverse triggering. Additionally, reverse triggering may disappear when patients are switched to a spontaneous support mode of ventilation when they have sufficient respiratory drive to not require a control mode.

Recognition of Reverse Triggering

When reverse triggering causes breath stacking (an inspiratory volume added to the prior tidal volume before exhalation has occurred), the events are easier to identify (**Figure 18-4**). Recognition of breath stacking should prompt an analysis of whether the initial breath was

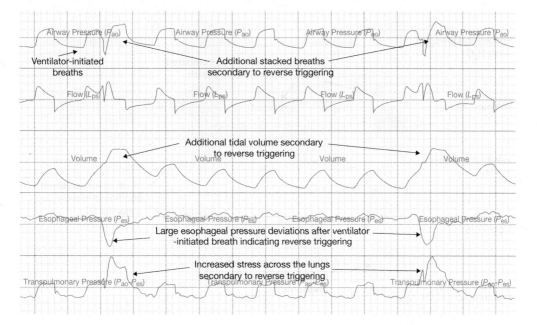

Figure 18-4: Waveform tracings from a patient exhibiting reverse triggering with breath stacking. Note how each breath is a ventilator-initiated breath not triggered by the patient. Most of the breaths are fully passive without any evidence of patient inspiratory effort. In the second and eight breaths, however, there are inspiratory efforts occurring (deflections in the flow and pressure tracings), which are buried within the initial ventilator-delivered breath suggestive of reverse triggering given the timing in the respiratory cycle and the absence of other patient-initiated breaths. These efforts occur toward the end of the ventilator inspiratory cycle extending into expiration and causing sufficient flow and pressure deviation to result in an additional triggered breath with stacking upon the prior breath. As can be seen, these stacked breaths result in large, delivered volumes and increased lung stress (as seen by the transpulmonary pressure tracing).

triggered by the patient or by the ventilator. If the initial breath was triggered by the ventilator, the resulting breath-stacking event is most likely secondary to reverse triggering. If the initial breath was triggered by the patient, the event is more likely to be premature cycling as will be discussed in the next section. In difficult or more subtle cases of reverse triggering, an esophageal balloon (see Chapter 16) may be needed to detect events. The esophageal balloon detects changes in pleural pressure secondary to inspiratory efforts and can more easily ascertain the initiation point of the patient effort relative to the ventilator-delivered breath.

Detection of reverse triggering without breath stacking may be more challenging, but can often be identified if waveforms are analyzed closely. The delayed active inspiratory efforts associated with reverse triggering often occur in a regular pattern after the ventilator-initiated breath. When reverse triggering occurs early during inspiration, it may manifest with "scooping" of the airway pressure waveform during inspiration similar in appearance to flow asynchrony (see Section "Flow Asynchrony"). This pressure scooping may be more obvious in patients on volume control ventilation, but it can be seen in patients on pressure-regulated modes as well. Flow waveforms may demonstrate increased inspiratory flow and tidal volumes may be magnified during reverse trigger breaths, particularly in pressure-regulated modes. In some cases, reverse triggering during inspiration may be strong enough to augment the delivered volume (**Figure 18-5**).

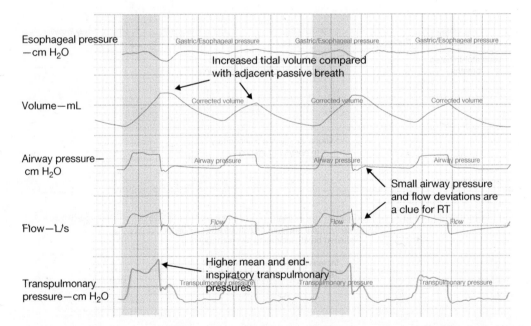

Figure 18-5: Waveform tracings from a patient exhibiting reverse triggering *without* breath stacking. This patient is showing frequent reverse triggering alternating with passive breaths in a typical pattern. Unlike in the prior example, the largest amount of inspiratory effort during reverse triggering is occurring during the ventilator inspiratory cycle leading to larger delivered volumes compared with the subsequent passive breaths, and higher transpulmonary pressure (the pressure or stress across the lungs). Note that the reverse trigger does extend somewhat into the expiratory phase, but there is not sufficient flow or pressure changes during expiration to trigger an additional stacked breath from the ventilator. Note that even though there are no stacked breaths, tidal volumes and lung stress are still higher than in similar passive breaths.

Reverse triggering during exhalation may be easier to detect as it appears the same regardless of ventilator mode. The inspiratory effort occurs during exhalation and may result in decreased expiratory flow, which can be seen on both the flow and volume tracings.

Management of Reverse Triggering

Why do we care about reverse triggering? As we described generally for ventilator asynchrony, these processes may lead to patient discomfort (dyspnea) and to large excursions in tidal volume and pressure that may lead to lung injury. Unfortunately, best practices in the management of reverse triggering are not well defined. Depending on the duration and amount of force exerted, reverse triggering may not always be harmful. Consequently, it is not always clear if reverse triggering needs to be addressed, but we suggest approaching reverse triggering as you might regular spontaneous breathing that does not meet guidelines for tidal volume and driving pressure in patients with variable susceptibility to ventilator-induced lung injury. Although it is likely acceptable to tolerate in patients with less severe illness, reverse triggering should be addressed in patients with more severe lung injury or at high risk for developing progressive lung injury (see the discussion on acute respiratory distress syndrome [ARDS] in Chapter 13); the larger volumes or pressure swings associated with reverse triggering events may lead to lung and diaphragm injury in these individuals.

If you decide to intervene and address the reverse triggering events, several treatment strategies may be considered sequentially. The initial step is to consider whether the reverse triggering is responsive to decreases or increases in sedation. Although initial descriptions of reverse triggering hypothesized that these events were secondary to "unmasking" of the coupling from deep sedation, in other patients it appears that lightening sedation may be the cause, and the clinician may not know for sure unless an empiric change in sedation is implemented. In less ill patients, the presence of reverse triggering may suggest that they are ready for transition to spontaneous breathing, which should be considered after balancing the risks of allowing the patient to spontaneously breathe (see the section on patient self-induced lung injury in Chapter 15).

ICU providers may trial higher PEEP and tidal volume settings to see if synchrony can be reestablished between patient and ventilator, again considering the potentially beneficial and harmful effects of making these adjustments on lung distension (see Chapters 13 and 15 for discussion on barotrauma). Additionally, in some cases in which patients have lighter sedation, reverse triggering may resolve by switching the patient to a pressure support mode allowing for decoupling of the patient's inspiratory efforts to the vent, and in some cases moving patients toward spontaneous breathing. If this is done, however, the risks and benefits from this switch must be considered carefully (eg, will the patient generate unacceptably high tidal volumes with pressure support?). Unfortunately, there is no clear algorithmic approach available for reverse triggering; we are often left with trial and error.

FLOW ASYNCHRONY

Flow asynchrony arises when the flow of air delivered by the ventilator does not match the patient's desired inspiratory flow. Flow asynchrony is common and underappreciated, particularly in patients with acute respiratory failure with high respiratory drive.

The consequences of flow asynchrony should not be underestimated. The patient's vigorous drive to breathe and the mismatch between desired and delivered flow may lead to significant patient discomfort and excessive inspiratory muscle work. The latter drives large swings in transpulmonary pressures and contributes to unsafe increases in tidal volume. Although perhaps more subtle than breath stacking and cycle length dyssynchrony, unrecognized persistent flow asynchrony could be a cause or marker of self-induced lung injury in patients who are sensitive to developing further lung injury.

Causes of Flow Asynchrony

Patient Factors

The primary driver of flow asynchrony appears to be a high patient respiratory drive, for example, because of stimuli from the lungs, chest wall, chemoreceptors along with behavioral factors (see Chapter 1). High respiratory drive can be attributable to primary respiratory pathology—severe pneumonia, asthma flare, ARDS, etc.—or from secondary causes such as agitation, pain, delirium, and acidemia. Younger, previously healthy patients in particular may exhibit robust respiratory drive leading to flow asynchrony.

Ventilator factors: Remember that when you set the ventilator, you have assumed control for the respiratory system and, if your settings are not congruent with the messages coming from the patient's ventilatory controller, problems may arise. Inspiratory flow may be set too low when in volume control mode. Certain flow ramp patterns can also contribute to the sensation of inadequate flow, particularly when the flow pattern is fixed (in volume control); the patient's desired flow pattern may be quite different from what the ventilator is providing. Factors other than flow, such as low minute ventilation, can exacerbate the sensation of inadequate flow. Finally, flow asynchrony is more prevalent in volume-based ventilation compared to pressure ventilation. In pressure-regulated and -controlled modes, there is no fixed flow pattern. Greater inspiratory efforts yield higher flow as the ventilator attempts to reach the set pressure. Flow asynchrony, however, may occur in any mode if the patient has a high respiratory drive accompanied by the muscle strength to generate large inspiratory efforts.

Recognition of Flow Asynchrony

Flow asynchrony manifests with scooping of the airway pressure tracing as the patient attempts to augment the flow delivered by the ventilator, which can be more clearly visualized in volume control settings (**Figure 18-6**). Flow enhancement may also be appreciated in different modes of ventilation, particularly pressure control, where higher tidal volumes generated by the patient can also be visualized. Esophageal manometry may facilitate recognition of flow asynchrony by demonstrating large swings in pleural pressure that correlate with scooping of the airway pressure tracing. At the bedside, the patient may demonstrate nasal flaring, accessory muscle use, and other signs of increased drive to breathe and associated excessive work of breathing.

Management of Flow Asynchrony

Focusing on patient-based strategies first, the approach of managing underlying risk factors applies to flow asynchrony as it did to trigger asynchrony. Although the first inclination may be to increase sedation—which may ultimately be the necessary management decision—ICU providers should thoroughly evaluate for and address alternative sources of high respiratory drive: is the patient in pain? Are they withdrawing from alcohol, or have they been made delirious by a medication? Could they have a new ventilator-associated pneumonia? Do they have a new metabolic acidosis? Given the well-documented adverse effects of excess sedation,

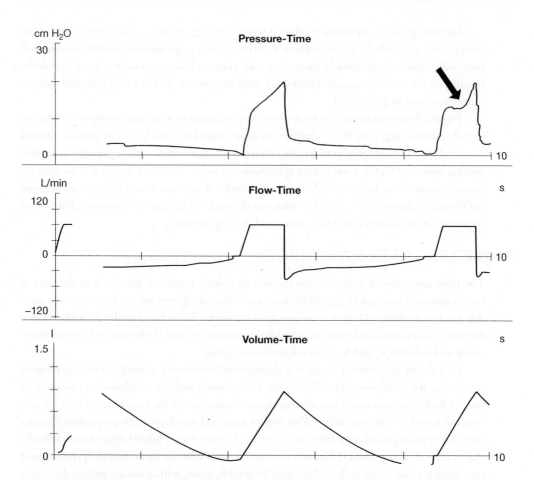

Figure 18-6: Waveform tracings showing the difference between a synchronous assisted breath (flow is appropriate for the patient's needs), and in the second breath, a demonstration of flow asynchrony (*arrow*; patient is trying to augment flow). Flow asynchrony occurs when the delivered flow is less than what the patient desires during inspiration. This desire for a higher flow is illustrated by a scooping of the pressure waveform and is usually seen when patients are triggering the initial breath and breathing spontaneously. Flow asynchrony may occur particularly when patients are in volume control mode during which flow is strictly controlled by the ventilator, and the set flow may be different from what the patient desires.

management of flow asynchrony warrants a comprehensive approach to the various factors that enhance respiratory drive prior to its suppression with sedating agents.

Several adjustments on the ventilator can alleviate the mismatch between delivered and desired flow. Unless the patient is in extremis, our strategy is to address one variable at a time, evaluate the efficacy of this change, and then adjust a second variable or the first variable again.

First, the flow and the pattern with which it is delivered can be optimized. Increasing flow may improve flow asynchrony, although increasing flow can result in higher peak pressures. Changing to a descending ramp flow can also be helpful (high flow at the beginning of the inspiration gradually decreasing as one gets to the end of the inspiration; this is what we do during spontaneous breathing), as this better matches the patient's initial flow demand as compared to other waveforms, particularly the square wave approach to flow regulation.

Increasing minute ventilation offers a second strategy, which can address a high respiratory drive, particularly if tidal volume is increased and respiratory acidosis is ameliorated. Increasing minute ventilation by increasing tidal volume, however, may not be an option depending on the underlying pathophysiology, such as in severe ARDS when low-tidal-volume ventilation must be prioritized.

Finally, flow asynchrony can be improved by changing to a separate mode of ventilation, namely transitioning from flow-restrictive volume control to a mode such as pressure control or one which allows the patient to largely determine their own flow such as pressure-regulated volume control (PRVC), a mode that is discussed in more detail in Chapter 17. As with increasing minute ventilation, switching to other modes of ventilation may alleviate asynchrony but ultimately impose a new risk depending on the underlying cause of respiratory failure and the impact of the changes on tidal volume and driving pressure.

CYCLE LENGTH DYSSYNCHRONY

The prior categories of dyssynchrony focused on patient-ventilator mismatch at the time of breath initiation between the patient's desires and the subsequent rate or flow at which air is delivered to the lung. We now turn our attention to the discordance in the patient's desired *duration* of inspiration and what the ventilator is permitting, and the transition between inspiration and exhalation, which is also referred to as *cycling*.

Cycle length dyssynchrony is due to a discrepancy between the patient's neural inspiratory time (what the ventilatory controller in the brain wants) and the ventilator's set inspiratory time. A healthy person at rest usually spends about one-third of the breathing cycle in inspiration and two-thirds in expiration. With higher rates and ventilation, the proportion changes such that inspiration and expiration are about equal in duration. This all happens automatically without you thinking about it. But when we set the ventilator, we determine the proportion of time in each phase of the cycle and we may be at odds, again, with what the patient desires. A mismatch in cycling time leads to a loss of coordination between the appropriate respiratory muscles and phase of breathing. For example, patient-driven inspiratory efforts exerted during ventilator-determined exhalation leads to wasted energy expenditure and patient discomfort. Furthermore, mismatched cycling can lead to breath stacking and large tidal volumes.

Cycle length dyssynchrony occurs in two distinctively different types of patterns, premature cycling and late cycling, based on when the discrepancy occurs. Premature cycling occurs when the set ventilator inspiratory time is less than the patient's desired neural inspiratory time, resulting in patient inspiratory efforts that extend into the ventilator's set expiration time. In contrast, delayed or late cycling entails the opposite scenario in which the ventilator inspiratory time exceeds the patient's inspiratory time and patients terminate the delivery of the breath and initiate expiration early through an expiratory effort. This section will focus on premature cycling, whereas delayed cycling will be described in the section discussing expiratory effort dyssynchrony.

PREMATURE CYCLING

Premature cycling occurs when the patient exerts inspiratory efforts that persist beyond the ventilator's delivered breath. When these inspiratory efforts extend into the ventilator's expiratory phase with sufficient intensity and duration, the ventilator can be triggered to deliver a second breath. The sum effect is the inappropriate early delivery of a second, "stacked" breath soon after the initial ventilator-delivered breath and before the patient's lungs have deflated.

Premature cycling leading to stacked breaths has also been named *double triggering or double cycling* in the literature. It is important to realize that premature cycling can result in more than two stacked breaths if the effort is very long and strong, which is why we prefer not to use the nomenclature "double triggering." The consequent breath stacking and volume accumulation from premature cycling can lead to overdistension and volutrauma.

Causes of Premature Cycling

Patient Factors

The primary patient-related cause of premature cycling is a high respiratory drive. In these patients, the high drive manifests as large and prolonged inspiratory efforts, or mistimed efforts generated by the patient and extending into the expiratory phase.

Ventilator Factors

The primary ventilator causes for premature cycling include a short set inspiratory time, insufficient flow, low tidal volumes, and/or low minute ventilation. With overlapping etiologies, premature cycling often coexists with other forms of ventilator dyssynchrony including flow asynchrony and expiratory effort dyssynchrony.

Recognition of Premature Cycling

Premature cycling is often easier to identify clinically than many of the previously described dyssynchrony categories. The classic pattern entails an initial patient-triggered breath with prolonged effort extending into the ventilator's exhalation phase, prompting a second stacked breath (**Figure 18-7**). Breath stacking caused by premature cycling may appear similar to that caused by reverse triggering. Premature cycling, however, is initiated by the patient, whereas breath stacking from reverse triggering entails a ventilator-initiated breath prompting an "automatic" inspiratory effort from the patient. Importantly, reverse triggering often occurs without breath stacking when the timing or the amplitude of effort does not result in an inappropriate early additional ventilator-delivered (stacked) breath.

On physical exam, double triggering manifests in multiple patterns and is often interspersed with other spontaneous efforts. The patient may be awake, agitated, and/or described as "overbreathing" or "bucking" the ventilator. In other instances, the clinical presentation is more subtle and requires a close observation of the ventilator waveform tracing.

Management of Premature Cycling

Management of premature cycling in many ways mirrors management of flow asynchrony. One should assess the patient for causes of high respiratory drive and intervene to reduce stimuli to the ventilatory control centers when possible (eg, correct metabolic acidosis). Increasing sedation—which has been demonstrated to reduce premature cycling—may be necessary to prevent breath stacking and lung injury, particularly for the patient who must remain on lung-protective settings.

Adjustments to the ventilator, such as lengthening the inspiratory time, can be made but doing so limits the max amount of flow that can be provided if one does not want to increase tidal volume (unless an inspiratory pause is instituted at the end of the inspiration to lengthen the portion of the cycle attributed to inspiration) and thus may aggravate flow asynchrony and further elevate respiratory drive. Similarly, lowering trigger sensitivity to increase the threshold at which a breath is initiated may improve the frequency of breath stacking, but lowering sensitivity may simultaneously worsen patient discomfort and respiratory efforts in some patients; consequently, this strategy is not universally recommended.

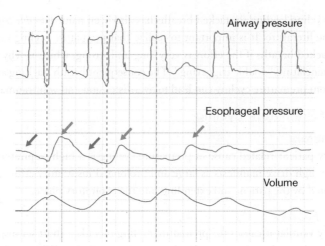

Figure 18-7: This is a patient with spontaneous efforts exhibiting premature cycling (also known as double triggering). Note that each initial breath, which is being triggered by the patient, can be seen by both the negative airway pressure and esophageal balloon pressure tracings. The inspiratory effort in this case (the *red arrow* indicates the initiation) causes esophageal pressure to fall and extends past the duration of the inspiratory time and into the expiratory phase resulting in a second triggered breath (shown by the vertical dotted line). Premature cycling resulting in double triggering may be confused with reverse triggering as both can result in similar appearing breath stacking. The two very different forms of dyssynchrony may be differentiated by looking at the initial breath of the breath-stacking couplet. If this initial breath is a ventilator-triggered breath (ie, it was not spontaneously triggered by the patient), then this breath stacking was most likely secondary to reverse triggering. If the initial breath was triggered by the patient, then the breath stacking was most likely secondary to premature cycling resulting in double triggering. Also note that this type of dyssynchrony is often found accompanied by other forms of dyssynchrony associated with high patient respiratory drive, including flow asynchrony and expiratory effort dyssynchrony, which you typically would not see with reverse triggering. Notably in this example, after the breath-stacking events, the patient has several expiratory efforts (as indicated on the figure by the *blue arrows*), which may be seen in patients with high respiratory drive attempting to augment expiratory flow.

If premature cycling is leading to dangerously high tidal volumes and escalating sedation requirements, the ICU provider must consider if the benefits of restrictive, lung-protective settings are outweighed by the cost of profound ventilator dyssynchrony. Rotating to less restrictive modes such as pressure support can alleviate premature cycling but may result in larger tidal volumes. Continuing with volume control but increasing the set tidal volume represents another option that has been demonstrated to decrease double triggering, but the ICU provider must be willing to tolerate higher tidal volumes and the potential risk for lung injury accompanying this.

EXPIRATORY DYSSYNCHRONY

After completion of the inspiratory phase (regardless of whether the breath was a spontaneous or vent-controlled breath), the expiratory phase is typically passive in most patients; exhalation is accomplished by the stored elastic energy of the respiratory system, which drives expiratory flow. Whereas typical expiration is passive, active expiratory efforts may be common in healthy patients during exertion, and may be common even at rest in patients with flow limitation and COPD. Similarly, during mechanical ventilation, expiratory efforts may be benign, but in some patients they may have the capacity to be harmful or even worsen other forms of dyssynchrony. In particular, this section focuses on two types of expiratory effort dyssynchrony: expiratory dyssynchrony, which occurs when the patient's expiratory efforts do not coincide with an open expiratory valve on the ventilator (a type of cycle length dyssynchrony called delayed cycling), or when the amplitude of the efforts to exhale are large enough to impact end-expiratory pressures and volumes.

In contrast to premature cycling in which the patient's inspiratory efforts extend beyond the ventilator's set inspiratory time, *delayed or late cycling* occurs when the patient transitions to exhalation while the ventilator continues in the inspiratory phase. The patient makes this transition by using their expiratory muscles to impair inspiratory flow and force the transition to expiration. Expiratory dyssynchrony also occurs when the patient exerts expiratory efforts late in the expiratory cycle, a phenomenon that is independent of delayed cycling.

Excessive expiratory efforts (with or without delayed cycling) may be evidence of attempts to augment expiratory flow and indicate respiratory distress. Alternatively, they may be minor and of little concern. This variability is in some ways similar to the varying degrees of flow asynchrony discussed earlier in this chapter; in those cases, the amplitude of the efforts and the severity of illness of the patient exhibiting these breathing patterns likely determine the potential for harm. Expiratory efforts may actually be quite common, particularly in patients with COPD, and can help augment inspiration in patients with a high respiratory drive by lowering the end-expiratory volume and making use of the outward recoil of the chest wall (now compressed by the expiratory muscles) to assist in the generation of flow. Conversely, expiratory efforts and delayed cycling can be evidence of respiratory distress and potentially cause low end-expiratory lung volumes leading to derecruitment, thereby negating the effect of PEEP. These effects have been postulated to worsen gas exchange and create high auto-PEEP. Additionally, the increased intrathoracic pressure with large expiratory efforts can, in some patients, cause hemodynamic instability with reduced venous return and impaired cardiac output.

Causes of Expiratory Efforts and Delayed Cycling

Patient Factors

The prototypical patient who develops delayed cycling is the patient with uncontrolled obstructive lung disease intubated for an acute asthma or COPD exacerbation. High airways resistance, bronchospasm, and abnormally high compliance necessitate a longer expiratory time, which, if not allowed by the ventilator, will lead to delayed cycling. Expiratory efforts may also occur in patients with ARDS and other pathology without flow limitation and high resistance. This latter group represents patients with high expiratory efforts that may be associated with other forms of dyssynchrony sharing a common underlying driver: excess drive to breathe.

Ventilator Factors

The most common ventilator reason for delayed cycling is a long set inspiratory time (and consequently, shorter expiratory time than desired by the patient) and/or insensitive expiratory trigger sensitivity. Additionally, although rare, leaks in the circuit can lead to prolonged ventilator inspiratory times that fall out of phase with the patient's inspiratory times.

Recognition of Delayed Cycling and Expiratory Efforts

Delayed cycling may manifest with subtle graphical changes (**Figure 18-8**) or profound dyssynchronous behavior (agitation of the patient). The pressure waveform will demonstrate an increase in airway pressure as the patient activates expiratory muscles while the ventilator's

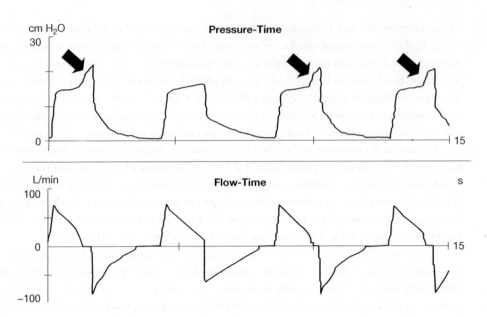

Figure 18-8: Waveforms of delayed cycling characterized by expiratory efforts (also known as delayed cycling; *arrows*) at the end of inspiration causing spikes in airway pressure. This occurs when the ventilator cycle time is "delayed" relative to the patient's desired inspiratory time, and the patient attempts to terminate the inspiratory effort by forcefully exhaling against the breath resulting in spikes in pressure. Note how this scooping might appear initially similar to flow asynchrony; however, an important difference is the flow asynchrony lowers the airway pressure during inspiration, whereas delayed cycling causes higher airway pressure.

inspiratory flow continues, albeit at a diminished level because of the patient's expiratory efforts. On the flow diagram, there will be a drop-off in flow when the patient cycles to exhalation but before flow drops to zero when the ventilator cycles to exhalation.

Recognition of high expiratory efforts independent of delayed cycling may often be more challenging based upon the waveforms unless an esophageal balloon is present (see Chapter 16). On physical exam, however, the expiratory efforts may be easier to detect. During these efforts the patient engages expiratory muscles during exhalation, causing a "rounding up" of the abdominal muscles, and discordant motion of the chest and abdomen.

Management of Delayed Cycling and Expiratory Dyssynchrony

Strategies to reduce delayed cycling and excess expiratory efforts begin with the patient, namely treating airway obstruction and reducing expiratory resistance (if present) with bronchodilators, steroids, and optimal pulmonary toilet techniques. Like other forms of dyssynchrony associated with high respiratory effort, addressing other etiologies of agitation and high respiratory drive is key. If these interventions are unsuccessful or not indicated, then increasing sedation temporarily may be necessary to shut down a high expiratory drive and prevent injurious swings in pressure.

With the ventilator, the main approach is to shorten the inspiratory time while prolonging the expiratory time. Some ventilators also allow for changing the sensitivity of the expiratory trigger. This changes the flow threshold at which the ventilator transitions from the inspiratory phase to the expiratory phase. Increasing the expiratory trigger sensitivity will functionally shorten the inspiratory time and perhaps allow for improved synchrony. This is particularly important for patients being managed with pressure support ventilation in whom patient distress is sometimes taken as a need for higher levels of pressure support ventilation rather than an adjustment in the expiratory trigger (see Chapter 6 for additional discussion of pressure support ventilation).

Other strategies on the ventilator include optimizing applied PEEP to account for auto-PEEP. This may reduce patient discomfort overall by lowering the threshold for triggering ventilator support and reduce respiratory drive by "satisfying" the stretch receptors of the lungs. Adjusting the level of pressure support provided by the ventilator is also a consideration with higher support providing larger tidal volumes, which could match the patient's high respiratory drive. Unfortunately, the larger tidal volumes that can result from higher support may prolong the required duration of expiration, result in worsened auto-PEEP, and conversely encourage more expiratory efforts. As with many forms of dyssynchrony, there is no perfect approach that can be applied to every patient, and treatment may require significant time at the bedside assessing empirically the individual patient's response to changes you make.

SUMMARY

Ventilator dyssynchrony results from a mismatch between patient and ventilator efforts, and comprehensive management necessitates optimization of both patient- and ventilator-related parameters. Dyssynchrony is associated with significant clinical implications such that prompt recognition and management is key. The multiple types of dyssynchrony span the respiratory cycle, from the trigger that initiates the breath, to the delivery of the breath itself, to termination of inspiration, and deflation during exhalation. Bedside analysis of pressure and flow waveforms is crucial to dyssynchrony identification, whereas esophageal manometry offers additional insight into the recognition of more subtle manifestations. Although adjusting sedation may ultimately be required to treat ventilator dyssynchrony, other management strategies, particularly adjustments in the parameters and settings of the mechanical ventilator, should be considered first given the well-documented deleterious effects of excess sedation.

See **Table 18-2** for a glossary of key terms from this chapter.

TABLE 18-2 Glossary of Key Terms	
Key Term(s)	Definition
Applied PEEP or extrinsic PEEP	Positive end-expiratory pressure exerted by the ventilator
Auto-PEEP or intrinsic PEEP	Positive end-expiratory pressure generated by high airways resistance, heterogeneous expiratory flow, and/or inadequate expiration time
Breath stacking	An injurious phenomenon in which consecutive inspiratory efforts occur without sufficient exhalation time to allow for lung deflation between inspirations. Breath stacking is associated with reverse triggering (ventilator-initiated breath stacking) and premature cycling (patient-initiated breath stacking).
Cycle length dyssynchrony	A type of ventilator dyssynchrony arising from a mismatch between the patient's inspiratory time and the inspiratory time set on the ventilator. The transition from inspiration to expiration is not synchronized, leading to uncoordinated and inefficient breathing efforts. There are two types: premature cycling (patient's inspiratory efforts extend beyond ventilator's inspiratory time) and delayed cycling (ventilator's inspiratory time extends beyond that of the patient).
Cycling	The transition from the inspiratory phase to the expiratory phase

(continued)

TABLE 18-2 Glossary of Key Terms (*continued*)	
Double triggering or double cycling	Another phrase for breath stacking that refers to two consecutive patient-triggered, ventilator-delivered breaths
Expiratory dyssynchrony	A type of ventilator dyssynchrony related to the timing and amplitude of the patient's expiratory efforts. Expiratory dyssynchrony occurs when the patient begins to exhale during the ventilator's inspiratory phase, or when the patient attempts to augment expiratory flow to the point of derecruitment and/or generation of auto-PEEP.
Flow asynchrony	A type of ventilator dyssynchrony in which the delivered flow does not match the patient's desired flow (desired flow usually exceeds delivered flow). Flow asynchrony can occur in any mode of mechanical ventilation, is associated with high respiratory drive, and can lead to patient discomfort, excessive work of breathing, and large swings in transpulmonary pressures.
Reverse triggering	A type of ventilator dyssynchrony in which a ventilator-initiated breath prompts an automated, often stereotyped (ie, outside the usual ventilatory control mechanisms) patient inspiratory effort. This inspiratory effort is out of phase with the ventilator and can be injurious in some circumstances.
Trigger sensitivity	Setting related to the trigger threshold that determines how much of a pressure or flow deviation is required to achieve the trigger threshold. Low-sensitivity settings require the patient to make larger changes in pressure or flow to achieve a trigger threshold and vice versa.
Trigger threshold	A ventilator setting that determines the quantity of flow or volume generated by the patient to then cause the ventilator to deliver a breath. When the trigger threshold is met, the ventilator is prompted to deliver a breath.
Trigger asynchrony	A type of ventilator dyssynchrony related to failed trigger recognition. There are two types: missed triggers in which the ventilator fails to recognize a patient's attempt to initiate a breath, and auto-triggers when the ventilator misinterprets an alternative stimulus as meeting the trigger threshold leading to an inappropriately delivered breath.

KEY POINTS

- Ventilator dyssynchrony comprises an imbalance between the patient's efforts to breathe and the support provided by the mechanical ventilator. It is common and underappreciated.
- Although consequences vary based on the type of dyssynchrony, general concerns include discomfort, injuriously large tidal volumes, unsafe swings in transpulmonary pressure, increased use of sedation and paralytics, prolonged duration of mechanical ventilation, and worsened mortality.
- Missed triggers arise from inadequate respiratory drive, insufficient respiratory muscle strength, or inability to overcome high trigger thresholds.
- Auto-trigger dyssynchrony may result from dynamic intrathoracic processes or excess fluid in the ventilator circuit/tubing, which prompts inappropriate delivery of a breath out of phase with the patient's efforts.

- Reverse triggering is poorly understood and, in some cases, may be an "automatic" physiologic adaptation that bypasses the normal central control mechanism governing our breathing. It is associated with deep sedation and changes in sedation.
- Flow asynchrony represents a mismatch between desired and delivered flow occurring in patients with high respiratory drive who are subject to restrictive ventilator settings. Management entails increasing flow, liberating tidal volumes (if possible), and changing to alternative ventilator modes.
- Cycle length dyssynchrony represents discrepancies in the transition from inspiration to exhalation between patient and ventilator.
- Premature cycling may lead to breath stacking and accompany high respiratory drive, whereas delayed cycling can lead to dynamic hyperinflation and requires management of high airways resistance.
- Expiratory dyssynchrony results from high expiratory resistance and flow limitation. Management strategies include treating uncontrolled obstructive lung disease while shortening inspiratory time and prolonging expiratory time.

STUDY QUESTIONS AND ANSWERS

Questions

1. You are called to the bedside to evaluate an intubated patient demonstrating a new breathing pattern. You notice the following waveforms (as shown in **QFigure 18-1**) on the ventilator:

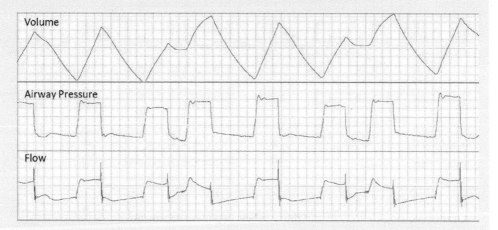

Which of the following is the least likely to be the cause of this pattern?
A. Neurologic injury
B. Depth and duration of sedation
C. Recent changes in sedation
D. Insufficient flow
E. None of the above

2. A 45-year-old man develops a viral respiratory infection and is intubated for hypoxemic respiratory failure with a P:F ratio of 150. He is placed on low-tidal-volume ventilation and develops an irregular breathing pattern. You are called to the bedside and notice that the patient is having breath-stacking events with the patient triggering the ventilator frequently with spontaneous breathing efforts.

(continued)

Of the following options, what is the next best step in management?
A. Liberate tidal volumes.
B. Obtain a stat computed tomography (CT) head.
C. Bolus and increase propofol infusion.
D. Increase PEEP.
E. Decrease inspiratory time.

3. A patient with unknown past medical history is found in an unresponsive state and does not rouse to sternal rub. He is intubated for airway protection and placed on pressure support ventilation. A CT scan of the head is unremarkable, and toxicology studies are pending. An alarm begins sounding in his room. As you examine the patient at the bedside, you note the below pattern on the ventilator:

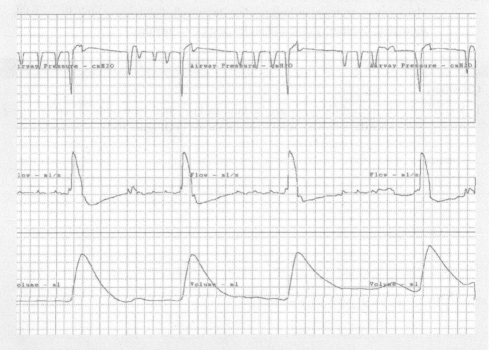

Of the following choices, what is the next best step in management?
A. Increase sedation to diminish injurious efforts.
B. Place the patient on volume control.
C. Goals of care conversation regarding tracheostomy
D. Decrease PEEP.
E. Decrease trigger sensitivity.

4. A 72-year-old patient with COPD is admitted to the ICU after being intubated for respiratory distress with profound work of breathing. She is placed on volume control with V_t 6 mL/kg, respiratory rate 15 breaths/min, applied PEEP of 5 mm H_2O, F_{IO_2} 0.5, and the standard I:E ratio. An expiratory hold demonstrates a total PEEP of 10 mm H_2O. She is hemodynamically stable. You note the following pressure waveform (as shown in **QFigure 18-2**) on the ventilator:

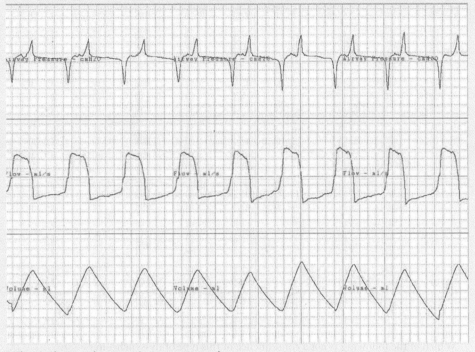

What is the next best step in management?
   A. Decrease PEEP.
   B. Disconnect the endotracheal tube from the ventilator.
   C. Increase the inspiratory time, decrease the expiratory time.
   D. Decrease inspiratory time, increase expiratory time.
   E. Paralyze the patient.

5. A 55-year-old woman is diagnosed with methicillin-resistant *Staphylococcus aureus* (MRSA) pneumonia that causes hypoxemic respiratory failure and leads to intubation. She is placed on a volume-based mode with lung-protective settings. She is tachycardic, hypertensive, and febrile and on exam she easily rouses from a sedated state when staff walk into the room. Her blood gases show that she is acidemic. Analyzing her ventilator, you note the following waveform (as shown in **QFigure 18-3**):

(continued)

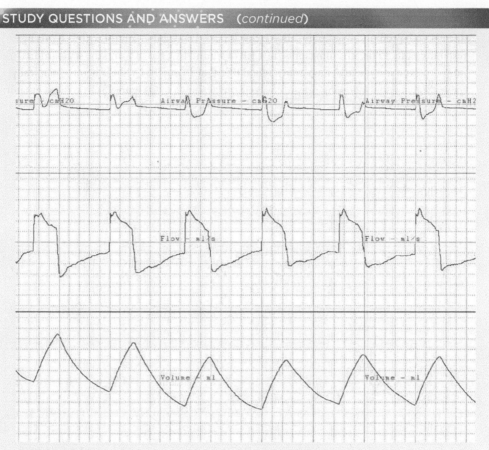

Which of the following is not a consequence of this type of dyssynchrony?

A. Auto-PEEP

B. Large swings in transpulmonary pressures

C. Patient discomfort

D. Increased tidal volume

E. None of the above

Answers

1. Answer D. Insufficient flow

Rationale: This is an example of reverse triggering with breath stacking initiated by the ventilator. Although the exact pathophysiology is not fully understood, reverse triggering is implicated in neurologic injuries, in patients with prolonged sedation exposure, and in patients with recent changes in sedation who may be rousing from a deeply sedated state (Options **A, B,** and **C**).

The first breath is initiated by the patient; subsequent breath stacking is not attributable to reverse triggering but rather other causes such as premature cycling. This scenario warrants evaluation for causes of high respiratory drive out of proportion to the delivered support such as in the case of insufficient flow (Option **D**).

2. **Answer C. Bolus and increase propofol infusion**

   Rationale: This patient is demonstrating premature cycling with double triggering and breath stacking. Clinically, this pattern is the result of a young patient with a high respiratory drive being placed on restrictive ventilator settings as part of ARDS management. The double triggering comprises the patient's attempt to increase his minute ventilation, but the result is injuriously large tidal volumes that could propagate the patient's lung injury and lead to worsened outcomes if left unchecked.

   The next best step in management is to increase sedation to ensure synchrony with the low-tidal-volume approach during this vulnerable time in the course of the patient's disease. Liberating tidal volumes (Option **A**) would reduce dyssynchrony by helping to match the patient's respiratory demand, but this change is not indicated during early ARDS when higher tidal volumes are known to correlate with worsened outcomes. Double triggering is not typically associated with acute neurologic pathophysiology such that urgent head imaging is not indicated (Option **B**). Increasing PEEP and decreasing the inspiratory time (Options **D** and **E**) may be necessary over time, but the first priority is to adequately sedate the patient to limit additional lung injury.

3. **Answer B. Place the patient on volume control**

   Rationale: This patient is demonstrating missed triggers, which are likely the result of a depressed mental status leading to insufficient respiratory drive and difficulty achieving the ventilator's trigger threshold. Because the patient is alarming for apneic events, the next best step in management is to place the patient on a mode that offers a set respiratory rate to reduce apneic events while the patient is allowed to awaken.

   The patient was intubated for airway protection and had no evidence for lung injury. As such, increasing sedation (Option **A**) on a patient already having apneic events will result in more harm than benefit. Although goals of care conversations in general should be pursued, discussion of a tracheostomy this early in the patient's course (Option **C**) is not yet indicated, particularly because the patient has not yet had an opportunity to recover from a theoretical acute insult, which is more likely than irrecoverable respiratory muscle weakness. The presence of auto-PEEP and inability to meet the trigger threshold can produce missed triggers, but no other evidence of auto-PEEP is provided and even if it were present, increasing applied PEEP rather than decreasing it (Option **D**) would be the correct intervention. Finally, decreasing trigger sensitivity (Option **E**) would make this patient more prone to missed triggers and apneic events as the threshold at which a breath is triggered would be increased.

4. **Answer D. Decrease inspiratory time, increase expiratory time**

   Rationale: This patient with uncontrolled obstructive lung disease with evidence of auto-PEEP is demonstrating evidence of expiratory dyssynchrony. The next best step is to allow the patient with presumably high expiratory resistance additional time to exhale by increasing the expiratory time. Other viable adjustments on the ventilator include decreasing the respiratory rate and increasing the tidal volumes.

   Increasing the inspiratory time (Option **C**) would have the opposite effect and propagate expiratory dyssynchrony. An increase in PEEP rather than decrease in PEEP (Option **A**) should be considered to allow for better PEEP matching to improve recruitment and gas exchange. Disconnecting the patient from the ventilator (Option **B**) to allow complete exhalation may be necessary if her auto-PEEP worsens to the point of causing hemodynamic

(continued)

collapse but based on her stable hemodynamics other interventions should be attempted first. Although a paralytic (Option **E**) would abolish expiratory muscle tone, data supporting its use in expiratory dyssynchrony are lacking such that other strategies should be employed first.

5. **Answer A. Auto-PEEP**

   Rationale: This is an example of flow asynchrony. The patient is in volume control ventilation with descending ramp flow, but this does not match the high-flow needs of the patient that extend longer than the initial delivered flow. This results in the "scooping" seen in the pressure tracing as patients attempt to augment the inspiratory flow, with the flow being set and not able to further increase. Flow asynchrony is a common, underappreciated form of ventilator dyssynchrony with numerous clinical implications including large tidal volumes, shifts in transpulmonary pressures, and patient discomfort (Choices **B**, **C**, and **D**). Auto-PEEP is not a common consequence of flow asynchrony.

Suggested Readings

Akoumianaki E, Lyazidi A, Rey N, et al. Mechanical ventilation-induced reverse-triggered breaths: a frequently unrecognized form of neuromechanical coupling. *Chest*. 2013;143(4):927-938.

Baedorf-Kassis E, Su HK, Graham AR, Novack V, Loring SH, Talmor DS. Reverse trigger phenotypes in acute respiratory distress syndrome. *Am J Respir Crit Care Med*. 2021;203:67-77.

Blanch L, Villagra A, Sales B, et al. Asynchronies during mechanical ventilation are associated with mortality. *Intensive Care Med*. 2015;41(4):633-641.

Chanques G, Kress JP, Pohlman A, et al. Impact of ventilator adjustment and sedation-analgesia practices on severe asynchrony in patients ventilated in assist-control mode. *Crit Care Med*. 2013;41(9):2177-2187.

de Wit M, Miller KB, Green DA, Ostman HE, Gennings C, Epstein SK. Ineffective triggering predicts increased duration of mechanical ventilation. *Crit Care Med*. 2009; 37(10):2740-2745.

Gentile MA. Cycling of the mechanical ventilator breath. *Respir Care*. 2011;56(1):52-60.

Gilstrap D, MacIntyre N. Patient-ventilator interactions: implications for clinical management. *Am J Respir Crit Care Med*. 2013;188(9):1058-1068.

Kondili E, Xirouchaki N, Georgopoulos D. Modulation and treatment of patient-ventilator dyssynchrony. *Curr Opin Crit Care*. 2007;13:84-89.

Sottille PD, Albers D, Smith BJ, Moss MM. Ventilator dyssynchrony—detection, pathophysiology, and clinical relevance: a narrative review. *Ann Thorac Med*. 2020;15(4):190-198.

Thille AW, Rodriguez P, Cabello B, Lellouche F, Brochard L. Patient-ventilator asynchrony during assisted mechanical ventilation. *Intensive Care Med*. 2006;32(10):1515-1522.

Dyspnea and Mechanical Ventilation

Jeremy B. Richards • Richard M. Schwartzstein

LEARNING OBJECTIVES

- Describe the mechanisms of dyspnea in mechanically ventilated patients.
- Delineate specific diagnostic approaches to identifying and characterizing dyspnea in critically ill, mechanically ventilated patients.
- Define the concept of "dyssynchrony" with mechanical ventilation.
- Discuss the adverse symptomatic, physical, and psychological outcomes of mechanical ventilation for critically ill patients.
- Identify therapeutic interventions to address dyspnea and discomfort in mechanically ventilated patients.

INTRODUCTION

The decision to place a patient on mechanical ventilation is complex and depends upon a variety of factors, such as laboratory information (abnormal blood gases), or clinical features of the case, such as dyspnea, increased work of breathing, markedly altered mental status, and/or extreme fatigue. Dyspnea refers to the sensation of breathlessness or discomfort of breathing, often experienced by individuals with severe respiratory conditions. When a patient's dyspnea reaches a level that they cannot manage on their own, the decision to intubate and support them on mechanical ventilation may be made. Sedation is almost always administered prior to intubating a patient and placing them on mechanical ventilation in order to minimize discomfort and ensure that the patient does not struggle with the process of intubation or breathe in ways that conflict with the ventilator. Ultimately, mechanical ventilation, although associated with a range of potential complications, provides life-saving support for patients who have difficulty breathing because of respiratory disease, and it is important to weigh these various factors carefully before making the decision to treat a patient with mechanical ventilation.

Many clinicians predict that by having the ventilator assume the "work" of breathing, the patient will experience less dyspnea. However, this notion is based on an overly simplistic view of the origins of dyspnea. In fact, many and perhaps most individuals with acute respiratory failure experience dyspnea with mechanical ventilation such that sedation is required to relieve anxiety and analgesics are employed to decrease the sense of breathlessness associated with their disease and mechanical ventilation; ultimately, these medications facilitate patient-ventilator interactions and patient synchrony with the ventilator.

Unfortunately, approximately 25% of individuals with respiratory failure and mechanical ventilation will experience mental health problems, including posttraumatic stress disorder (PTSD), following their illness, which may be due to both the lack of control of their breathing and the experience of dyspnea with mechanical ventilation. Given these considerations, it is important to ensure optimal sedation and analgesia for patients treated with mechanical ventilation, particularly immediately after intubation. Titrating sedation, which largely is directed at anxiety, and analgesia, to reduce the discomfort of the endotracheal tube and the dyspnea arising from the underlying respiratory problem, can help to achieve synchrony with mechanical ventilation as well as decrease the risk of adverse psychological outcomes. Furthermore, by understanding the underlying causes of the patient's respiratory failure and providing proper care and support, we can achieve optimized, patient-centered clinical outcomes. Mechanical ventilation is an important tool that can improve a patient's chances of survival from acute critical illness and respiratory failure, but it is essential to be aware of both the risks and benefits when making decisions regarding its use.

Dyssynchrony can be a significant issue with mechanical ventilation, and it is important to note that discomfort manifest as "fighting" the ventilator, by which we mean the patient appears to be struggling (eg, use of accessory muscles, facial expressions suggesting discomfort, pulling against restraints in bed) to achieve a different breathing pattern, for example, at a higher breathing rate or inspiratory flow or tidal volume, may be an indication of dyssynchrony. Dyssynchrony is a complicated issue that goes beyond discomfort (as is discussed in Chapter 18), but patient discomfort is a contributing factor to the observation, "the patient is 'fighting the ventilator.'" Dyssynchrony needs to be addressed for mechanical ventilation to be effective, and analgesia is the primary therapeutic intervention to achieve patient comfort and improve adherence to and synchrony with mechanical ventilation. Dyssynchrony can be complex to manage, but with the combination of sedation, analgesia and titration of mechanical ventilation settings, both patient comfort and quality of care can be improved.

This chapter reviews strategies for identifying dyspnea in mechanically ventilated patients, the mechanisms by which dyspnea is produced, how ventilator settings can exacerbate this problem, and therapeutic options for addressing dyspnea and discomfort in mechanically ventilated patients. Dyspnea can be identified and quantified in patients treated with mechanical ventilation in multiple ways: clinical observation, direct questions to the patient, and facial scales. Mechanisms of dyspnea include discordance between a patient's respiratory drive and the desired flow or volume as compared to what is provided by the ventilator. Treatment of dyspnea can include titration of ventilator settings as well as nonpharmacologic and pharmacologic approaches to help make patients more comfortable during mechanical ventilation. Mechanical ventilation can be a life-saving tool, but it is important to understand its risks and benefits in order to provide the best outcomes for patients. When healthcare professionals provide physiologically informed, patient-centered compassionate care and support, individuals on mechanical ventilation can experience optimized symptom management and clinical outcomes.

IDENTIFYING DYSPNEA

Identifying and assessing dyspnea is a complex process that requires a comprehensive evaluation of the patient's clinical status. Dyspnea can be affected by multiple factors, including physiologic and psychological stimuli (**Figure 19-1**) as well as environmental factors; clinician awareness of and vigilance for the possibility of dyspnea in mechanically ventilated patients is critical for identifying it. Clinical observations may include increased work of breathing in mechanically ventilated patients—a respiratory rate and/or tidal volume elevated above the rate and volume set by the ventilation, the use of accessory muscles of respiration, and/or diaphoresis, or other signs of increased work of breathing, are all signs of dyspnea.

Once identified, dyspnea should be assessed using both patient-reported and observed measures. Patient-reported symptom intensity scales can be used to assess the severity of dyspnea and identify associated psychological issues such as anxiety, agitation, frustration, fear, and/or anger. Observed measures, such as inspiratory and expiratory flow characteristics, can be used to determine the underlying physiologic causes of dyspnea. Incomplete exhalation, for example, characterized by ongoing expiratory flow prior to transitioning from exhalation to inhalation, can be a sign of increased airways resistance, increased work of breathing, and dyspnea. Large drops in airway pressure during triggering of the ventilator may be an indication of a high drive to breathe, and reduction in peak inspiratory pressure with volume ventilation

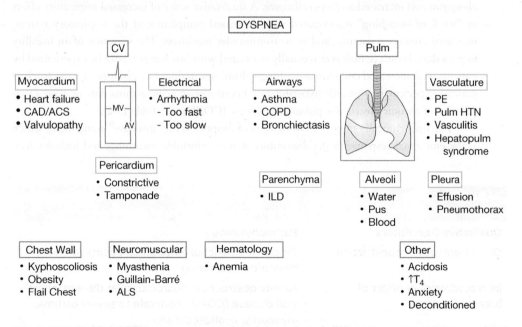

Figure 19-1: Multiple different processes involving several different organ systems can lead to the sensation of dyspnea. Note that most of the cardiovascular processes cause dyspnea by leading to increased pulmonary vascular pressures. ACS, acute coronary syndrome; ALS, amyotrophic lateral sclerosis; CAD, coronary artery disease; COPD, chronic obstructive pulmonary disease; HTN, hypertension; ILD, interstitial lung disease.

may indicate the patient is using inspiratory muscles in an effort to achieve a greater inspiratory flow or volume than is being provided by the ventilator. Overall, a multifaceted assessment of dyspnea is necessary for the provider to gain as complete a sense of a patient's circumstances as possible, which will guide the interventions (discussed later) chosen as most appropriate to address dyspnea.

MECHANISMS OF DYSPNEA

Although generally characterized as an "uncomfortable sensation of breathing," dyspnea is not a single symptom or process. Rather, dyspnea is a multidimensional experience that can be characterized by the intensity of discomfort, the quality of the symptoms of breathlessness, and the affective components, which reflect the individual's emotional response and the circumstances in which dyspnea is occurring.

The concept of "intensity" of discomfort can be characterized as the severity of the sense of breathlessness. Although there is no universally agreed upon scale for quantifying the intensity or severity of dyspnea, subjectively describing dyspnea as mild, moderate, or severe, or asking patients to rate intensity on a scale from 0 to 10 (by pointing with a finger), as they often do for pain, are among the approaches used to assess and describe this component of breathlessness in mechanically ventilated patients.

The "quality" of dyspnea is informed by the multiple underlying pathophysiologic mechanisms of dyspnea, and the words used can provide hints to the underlying process responsible for the dyspnea (**Table 19-1**). Specifically, a sensation of "air hunger" can be associated with an increased drive to breathe, whereas "chest tightness" is frequently associated with bronchospasm and increased airways resistance. A qualitative sense of increased respiratory effort or "work of breathing" is associated with decreased compliance of the respiratory system, increased airways resistance, and/or neuromuscular weakness. The sensation of an inability to get a deep breath (which is also usually associated with "air hunger") can be experienced by patients with increased end-expiratory lung volume and reduced inspiratory capacity (such as patients experiencing dynamic hyperinflation because of an acute asthma flare or acute exacerbation of chronic obstructive pulmonary disease [COPD], see **Table 19-2**).

The final clinically important dimension of dyspnea is the "affective" component, which is the emotional response to the discomfort of uncomfortable breathing, and includes fear,

TABLE 19-1	The Language of Dyspnea: Association of Qualitative Descriptors and Physiologic Mechanisms of Shortness of Breath
Qualitative Descriptors	**Pathophysiology**
Chest tightness or constriction	Bronchoconstriction, interstitial edema (asthma, myocardial ischemia)
Increased work or effort of breathing	Airway obstruction, neuromuscular disease, chest wall disease (COPD, moderate to severe asthma, myopathy, kyphoscoliosis)
Inability to get a deep breath	Hyperinflation (COPD, asthma)
Air hunger, need to breathe, urge to breathe	Increased drive to breathe (CHF, pulmonary embolism, moderate to severe airway obstruction)
Heavy breathing, rapid breathing, breathing more	Deconditioning

CHF, congestive heart failure; COPD, chronic obstructive pulmonary disease.

TABLE 19-2	Clinical Examples
Language of dyspnea	• A patient with COPD develops respiratory failure because of an acute exacerbation from a viral respiratory illness. She is very dyspneic and describes her discomfort by saying "I can't get enough air" and that she is doing increased "work" to breathe. The decision is made to intubate her and initiate mechanical ventilation. After intubation, the patient is very comfortable on mechanical ventilation—her sense of "air hunger" and increased work of breathing has been ameliorated. • In contrast, a patient with status asthmaticus experiences the sensations of "chest tightness" and increased work of breathing. He is intubated by his clinical team, which relieves the sense of increased work but not the "chest tightness," which appears to originate from stimulation of lung/airway receptors and is unaffected by mechanical ventilation. He remains uncomfortable despite intubation and initiation of mechanical ventilation.

COPD, chronic obstructive pulmonary disease.

anxiety, frustration, and depression. This psychological aspect of dyspnea is important for both symptom management and longer-term patient outcomes. As mentioned earlier, a substantive proportion of patients who survive respiratory failure and mechanical ventilation experience long-term psychological sequelae, and the affective experience of dyspnea during mechanical ventilation likely contributes to these adverse psychological and cognitive outcomes.

Drive to Breathe and Mechanical Response

The interaction between the patient's drive to breathe and consequent outgoing or efferent neural output to the inspiratory muscles and the resulting mechanical response of the system leading to incoming or afferent information from receptors in the airways, lungs, muscles, and chest wall may significantly affect the intensity of breathing discomfort. This phenomenon is called "efferent-reafferent dissociation" or "neuromechanical dissociation."

The drive to breathe is a complex physiologic process that involves peripheral and central nervous system input and coordination. Chemoreceptors, which detect and monitor the levels of carbon dioxide, oxygen, and pH within the bloodstream, irritant receptors, and mechanoreceptors that monitor mechanical processes such as "stretch" and movement, all provide information to the central nervous system about the status of the respiratory system. If chemoreceptors detect increased levels of carbon dioxide in the bloodstream, a potent signal is generated, prompting increased respiratory effort to endeavor to increase ventilation and normalize carbon dioxide levels. If irritant receptors in the airways are activated from inhaled particles, a signal is generated, creating increased output from the central controller (and possibly a cough) and a sense of uncomfortable breathing.

The "mechanical response" to dyspnea is informed by the interaction between the respiratory control center in the central nervous system and the neuromuscular activity of the respiratory system (**Figure 19-2**). Specifically, as ventilation occurs, neural outgoing (efferent) signals are sent to the respiratory muscles and simultaneously outgoing signals are sent in parallel to the sensory cortex (corollary discharge), which appears to be important in the creation of the "sense of effort" to breathe. As ventilation occurs, a variety of peripheral mechanoreceptors are stimulated that send neural (afferent) information *back* to the brain. These signals, which are sent to the sensory cortex in the brain, appear to be a way for the body to monitor the response to the efferent signals—flow receptors in the upper airway, stretch receptors in the lung, muscle and joint receptors in the chest wall all provide information on the movement generated by the respiratory system in response to the outgoing signals driving ventilation. If there is discordance between what the brain "wants" (as characterized by the outgoing, efferent messages

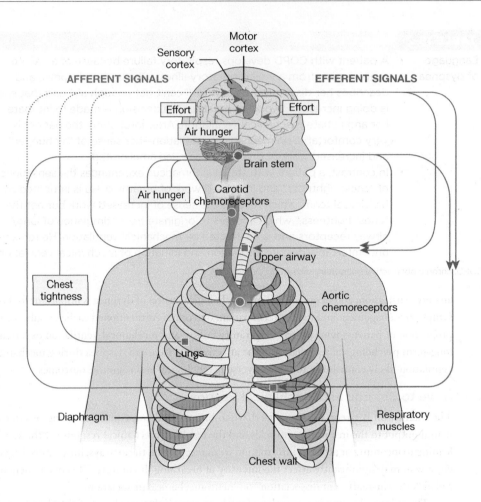

Figure 19-2: The afferent and efferent signals that contribute to dyspnea. (Redrawn from Efferent and afferent signals that contribute to the sensation of dyspnea. In: Schwartzstein RM. Approach to the patient with dyspnea. Post TW, ed. UpToDate. April 12, 2022. Topic 1436 Version 33.0.)

and processed as the corollary discharge to the sensory cortex as noted earlier) and what is "achieved" (the degree of flow and stretch generated by the respiratory system that is codified in the afferent messages), the intensity of dyspnea is increased. This phenomenon, when outgoing signals from the brain are not matched by the incoming signals from the respiratory system, this efferent-reafferent mismatch, contributes to the severity of breathing discomfort (**Table 19-3**).

TABLE 19-3	Clinical Examples
Efferent-reafferent mismatch	• If you run up 10 flights of stairs and you are told to breathe as fast as you want but to only take shallow breaths, you will be very uncomfortable because your brain wants you to take deeper breaths. Similarly, if you are told to inhale slowly (low inspiratory flow), you will also be uncomfortable because your brain wants you to take faster breaths (with higher inspiratory flow). All of these sensations may occur even with normal arterial blood gas measurements.

DYSPNEA AND MECHANICAL VENTILATION

The relationship between mechanical ventilation and dyspnea is not straightforward, and the notion that mechanical ventilation will always reduce a patient's work of breathing and sensations of dyspnea is an oversimplification. For some patients, to the extent that positive pressure ventilation removes the work of breathing, those individuals whose respiratory failure is primarily related to problems with the ventilatory pump (see Chapter 1) will have reduced dyspnea with mechanical ventilation.

Furthermore, to the extent that gas exchange and stimulation of peripheral and central chemoreceptors leads to increased drive to breathe and dyspnea, initiation of mechanical ventilation with supplemental oxygen, and appropriate alveolar ventilation to achieve acceptable partial pressure of arterial carbon dioxide ($Paco_2$), dyspnea will be lessened or even fully relieved. However, acute hypoxemia is a relatively weak stimulus for dyspnea, and in most cases, acceptable Pao_2 can be achieved with a variety of delivery modes for supplemental oxygen without needing to initiate mechanical ventilation.

Dyspnea can be exacerbated by mechanical ventilation when the ventilator settings (eg, rate, tidal volume, inspiratory flow, duty cycle [T_i/T_{tot}]) are not matching what the patient "wants" from a physiologic perspective. As a specific example, low tidal volume ventilation is a critical component of evidence-based care of patients with acute hypoxic respiratory failure (particularly those with acute respiratory distress syndrome [ARDS]); however, because of profound dyspnea resulting from a high drive to breathe, patients with ARDS want to take large volume breaths to attempt to alleviate the sensation of breathlessness associated with increased lung water, decreased lung compliance, and hypoxemia. This disconnect or mismatch between what a patient "wants" and what the ventilator is providing for tidal volumes, in particular, can exacerbate a patient's dyspnea (efferent-reafferent mismatch). Furthermore, as noted earlier, dyspnea originating from stimulation of pulmonary receptors is generally not alleviated by the initiation of mechanical ventilation.

One approach to addressing dyspnea associated with mechanical ventilation is to allow the patient to have more control of their respiratory cycle and patterns. Specifically, for patients who are experiencing significant dyssynchrony with mechanical ventilation, transitioning from a "controlled" mode of ventilation (see Chapter 5) to a "support" mode of ventilation (Chapter 6) allows a patient to set their own respiratory rate and inspiratory flow and tidal volume. This allows a patient to match their respiratory efforts and ventilatory output to their intrinsic drive to breathe, thereby reducing or eliminating efferent-reafferent mismatch and the associated dyspnea.

For many patients, however, it may not be clinically appropriate to transition from a "controlled" mode of ventilation to a "support" mode. Patients with moderate or severe ARDS, for example, should be treated with a low tidal volume, low "stretch" mode of ventilation to reduce volutrauma and barotrauma, which decreases mortality and optimizes clinical outcomes. Other strategies may be employed, however, in an effort to "satisfy" the high drive to breathe. Increasing inspiratory flow, for example, may increase comfort even if tidal volume is constrained. In addition, an end-inspiratory pause, that is, keeping the patient at their highest lung volume during the respiratory cycle for a second or two, may stimulate mechanoreceptors in the lung, which may also reduce dyspnea. If these strategies fail, adequate sedation and analgesia is required to achieve ventilator synchrony and to reduce the sensation of dyspnea and breathlessness that occurs with efferent-reafferent mismatch. Close clinical monitoring is critical in these circumstances to identify when sedation can be safely decreased or discontinued, given that oversedation can prolong the duration of mechanical ventilation, prolong hospital length of stay, increase the risk and severity of delirium, and increase long-term psychological and cognitive adverse outcomes for critically ill patients.

In addition to optimizing the judicious use of sedation, increasing positive end-expiratory pressure (PEEP) may alleviate dyspnea for mechanically ventilated patients who cannot be transitioned from a "controlled" to "support" mode of ventilation; patients with decreased compliance of the respiratory system develop a low functional residual capacity (FRC). Low FRC predisposes the patient to develop atelectasis, which stimulates mechanoreceptors in the lung that lead to increased respiratory drive and dyspnea. Application of higher levels of PEEP with the ventilator may open atelectatic regions of lung and reduce dyspnea in addition to enhancing oxygenation. Alternatively, patients with elevated end-expiratory lung volumes from dynamic hyperinflation (such as in the setting of an acute asthma flare or acute COPD exacerbation) may also benefit from increased PEEP. Patients with severe airflow obstruction may experience incomplete exhalation because of increased expiratory airways resistance, resulting in a phenomenon referred to as "auto-PEEP" or "intrinsic PEEP," which describes increased end-expiratory pressures because of trapped air from incomplete exhalation (see Chapters 7 and 11). By increasing the PEEP delivered by the ventilator to match the patient's intrinsic PEEP, one can reduce the inspiratory effort needed to trigger the ventilator.

MEDICATIONS FOR DYSPNEA

As mentioned earlier, sedation may be necessary for some mechanically ventilated patients to optimize ventilator synchrony and to decrease their sensation of dyspnea. Sedative medications can reduce awareness, promote amnesia, and/or decrease anxiety or agitation. In addition to sedatives, other medications (specifically, opiates, an analgesic medication) can be used to directly address the sensation of dyspnea without directly causing amnesia and reduced awareness. One must be cautious about using sedation alone because these agents do not alter dyspnea; small neuroimaging studies suggest that the brain may still process noxious stimuli, such as pain, even while the patient is sedated with propofol to the point that they appear "comfortable."

Opiates are the only class of medications that has been clinically demonstrated to directly reduce the sensation of dyspnea and uncomfortable breathing. Opiates can also decrease the discomfort associated with intubation, reducing the intensity of oropharyngeal and laryngeal signaling attributable to the endotracheal tube. Opiates can be provided as intermittent boluses on an "as needed" basis, and/or as a continuous infusion. In the intensive care unit (ICU) setting, fentanyl is the opiate of choice given its short half-life and rapid time to onset of action. Hydromorphone is also frequently used to address dyspnea and discomfort in the ICU setting; morphine is generally avoided because of the potential adverse effects of its metabolites (including neurotoxic effects such as hyperalgesia, allodynia, myoclonus, and seizures).

Sedation, with the goal of decreasing awareness and promoting amnesia, can be achieved with propofol and/or benzodiazepines. Propofol is very effective at promoting somnolence and amnesia, thereby reducing the patient's drive to breathe. However, some studies (as noted earlier) have demonstrated that even with deep sedation from propofol, the amygdala may be activated, indicative of persistent and significant discomfort; this observation may help explain why the incidence of postrespiratory failure mental health issues is so high. Benzodiazepines are no longer first-line agents for sedation in critically ill patients because of their strong association with increased delirium and its associated adverse psychological and cognitive outcomes, but they may still be used in certain clinical circumstances. Benzodiazepines are effective at achieving anxiolysis and can relieve the fear, anxiety, and sense of loss of control associated with dyspnea; however, benzodiazepines do not directly or effectively address other qualitative aspects of dyspnea such as "air hunger," "chest tightness," or "increased work of breathing." Similarly, dexmedetomidine, an alpha-2 agonist, effectively decreases anxiety and agitation, but does not directly address qualitative manifestations of dyspnea.

SUMMARY

Dyspnea is a complex physiologic, neurologic, and affective process that is very common in critically ill patients, including those with acute respiratory failure requiring mechanical ventilation. Although dyspnea can be assessed in a variety of ways, clinician awareness of this debilitating symptom is critical to identify and treat dyspnea in mechanically ventilated patients. Understanding the mechanistic pathophysiology of dyspnea is necessary to inform optimal treatment of dyspnea and to specifically determine whether and how mechanical ventilation will alleviate or worsen dyspnea. Although necessary for many patients with acute hypoxic respiratory failure, low tidal volume ventilation will almost invariably worsen dyspnea if a patient's drive to breathe is high, necessitating the use of opiates and/or sedative medications to address dyspnea and its sequelae.

KEY POINTS

Dyspnea is a common symptom in patients with acute respiratory failure. An understanding of the physiologic mechanisms underlying dyspnea enables you to manage ventilator dyssynchrony and provide appropriate medications to avoid or relieve breathing discomfort.

- A significant portion of patients with acute respiratory failure treated with mechanical ventilation will suffer from mental health issues if they survive the acute illness.
- Identifying dyspnea in the intubated, sedated patient may be difficult. In awake patients, always inquire about dyspnea. Facial expressions and ventilator dyssynchrony may also be indicators of dyspnea.
- Dyspnea is associated with high respiratory drive, often because of gas exchange abnormalities, or stimulation of pulmonary or cardiovascular receptors from a variety of diseases. Elevated respiratory drive leads to sensations such as air hunger and/or inability to get enough air.
- Bronchospasm commonly produces a sensation of chest tightness that is not relieved by the institution of mechanical ventilation.
- Mismatch between what the patient desires with respect to the output of the respiratory system (tidal volume, inspiratory flow, respiratory rate) and what is provided by the ventilator increases the intensity of dyspnea, particularly "air hunger."
- If a patient has a high respiratory drive but must be managed with low tidal volume ventilation, consider increasing inspiratory flow and/or instituting an inspiratory pause to reduce dyspnea.
- In patients with increased airway resistance and dyspnea on the ventilator, assess for the presence of intrinsic PEEP, which may be contributing to an increased work of breathing.
- For patients with dyspnea who are managed with mechanical ventilation, analgesics directed to address dyspnea should be used in treatment along with sedation.

STUDY QUESTIONS AND ANSWERS

Questions

1. A 63-year-old man is admitted with acute hypoxic respiratory failure because of COVID-19 pneumonia. Chest x-ray demonstrates diffuse airspace opacities consistent with ARDS. He is intubated and mechanical ventilation is initiated with volume assist control and the following settings: tidal volume 400 mL (7 L/kg of predicted body weight), respiratory rate 22 breaths/min, PEEP of 8 cm H_2O, and a FIO_2 of 60%. An arterial blood gas obtained on these settings demonstrates a pH of 7.34, $PaCO_2$ of 48 mm Hg, and PaO_2 of 82 mm Hg. The peak inspiratory pressure on the ventilator is 28 cm H_2O with a plateau pressure of 26 cm H_2O. He is receiving propofol and fentanyl via continuous infusions. He is noted to be dys-synchronous with mechanical ventilation, with tidal volumes ranging from 300 to 700 mL and a respiratory rate of 30 to 34 breaths/min. Which of the following is the most appropriate intervention?
   A. Decrease the PEEP to 5 cm H_2O.
   B. Increase the FIO_2 to 100%.
   C. Decrease the tidal volume to 350 mL (6 mL/kg of ideal body weight).
   D. Increase the dose of propofol.
   E. Decrease the dose of fentanyl.

2. A 26-year-old woman presented with status asthmaticus and because of markedly increased work of breathing she was intubated and initiated on mechanical ventilation. Approximately an hour after intubation, you are called to the bedside because of significant patient discomfort and dyssynchrony with the ventilator. The patient is on a volume assist control mode of ventilation with a set tidal volume of 360 mL (6.5 mL/kg of predicted body weight), set respiratory rate of 24 breaths/min, PEEP of 5 cm H_2O, and a FIO_2 of 70%. Her peak inspiratory pressure is vacillating between 12 and 40 cm H_2O and her plateau pressure is unmeasurable because of her high respiratory rate and spontaneous respiratory efforts. She is taking tidal volumes of 300 to 1000 mL, her actual respiratory rate is 30 to 36 breaths/min, and her oxygen saturation is 91%. She is receiving propofol and fentanyl via continuous infusion. The respiratory therapist reports that the patient's measured PEEP is 12 cm H_2O. An arterial blood gas has been obtained, but the results are pending. In addition to increasing sedation, which of the following is the most appropriate next step in her care?
   A. Initiate a continuous benzodiazepine infusion.
   B. Increase the patient's PEEP to 10 cm H_2O.
   C. Increase the patient's set respiratory rate from 24 to 28 breaths/min.
   D. Decrease the patient's tidal volume from 360 to 320 mL (6 mL/kg of predicted body weight).
   E. Decrease the patient's FIO_2 to 50%.

3. A patient experiencing an acute exacerbation of COPD would be expected to describe their sensation of breathlessness with which of the following phrases?
   A. "Increased effort to breathe"
   B. "Air hunger"
   C. "Unable to get a deep breath"
   D. All of the above
   E. None of the above

Answers

1. **Answer D. Increase the dose of propofol**

   Rationale: Given that this patient has ARDS with a low Pao_2/Fio_2 ratio (137), it is not appropriate to transition from a controlled mode of ventilation to pressure support ventilation. Rather, continuing low tidal volume ventilation and addressing ventilator dyssynchrony with optimized sedation is the most appropriate clinical intervention. Increasing the dose of propofol (along with opiates) to decrease his drive to breathe (and decrease efferent-reafferent mismatch) will also address his sense of dyspnea, thereby helping to achieve synchrony. Decreasing fentanyl at this point would be counterproductive for managing the patient's dyspnea and dyssynchrony. Given the severity of the patient's respiratory failure and hypoxemia, decreasing the delivered PEEP is not clinically indicated (and, regardless, would not address dyssynchrony and dyspnea in this patient who likely already has a low FRC) and although increasing the delivered PEEP could help with the patient's "comfort" with mechanical ventilation, the more important first intervention is to address dyssynchrony with increased sedation. Increasing the Fio_2 is also not necessary, as although his Pao_2/Fio_2 ratio is low, his Pao_2 is acceptable (and increasing the Fio_2 would not address or improve dyspnea). Decreasing his tidal volume is not indicated, as his plateau pressure is within acceptable ranges, and decreasing the tidal volume would likely worsen (rather than improve) dyspnea and dyssynchrony.

2. **Answer B. Increase the patient's PEEP to 10 cm H_2O**

   Rationale: This patient is experiencing increased intrinsic PEEP (or "auto-PEEP"), because of incomplete exhalation and air trapping resulting in elevated expiratory pressure. With the measured PEEP greater than the applied PEEP, the patient must do excessive inspiratory work to drop airway pressure to the level of the PEEP applied by the ventilator in order to trigger the next breath; this increases the work of breathing and the patient's dyspnea. By increasing the PEEP applied by the ventilator to just below the measured PEEP, the patient must drop the airway pressure only slightly to reach the applied PEEP and trigger next ventilator-delivered breath. This can help to reduce the patient's perceived work of breathing and decrease her sensation of dyspnea. Initiating a benzodiazepine infusion is premature without first endeavoring to rectify the underlying cause of the dyspnea and to achieve adequate sedation with propofol and fentanyl—the adverse effects of benzodiazepines are not inconsequential, and avoiding benzodiazepines, if possible, is desirable. The patient's respiratory rate is already higher than the set rate, such that increasing the set rate from 24 to 28 breaths/min will have no effect on the patient's work of breathing or clinical circumstances. Similarly, decreasing the tidal volume is both not clinically indicated (her tidal volume is already within the target range of 6 to 8 mL/kg of ideal body weight) and decreasing her tidal volume will not address dyssynchrony or increased work of breathing. Finally, with an oxygen saturation of 91%, decreasing the patient's Fio_2 is not clinically appropriate (and will likely worsen, rather than help, her dyspnea and ventilator dyssynchrony).

3. **Answer D. All of the above**

   Rationale: An acute exacerbation of COPD is characterized by increased airways resistance and incomplete exhalation, which results in increased end-expiratory lung volumes from air trapping; breathing at high lung volumes shortens inspiratory muscles, which make them

(continued)

less effective. This factor, along with the decreased compliance of the respiratory system at high volumes, increases the work and effort to breathe. The sensation of "air hunger" is associated with an increased drive to breathe, which is common in an acute COPD exacerbation because of stimulation of and signaling from airway irritant receptors. The sensation of an inability to get a deep breath (which is also usually associated with air hunger) can be experienced by patients with increased end-expiratory lung volume and reduced inspiratory capacity, which frequently occurs in patients with severe or very severe COPD during an acute exacerbation.

Suggested Readings

Brunelli A, Charloux A, Bolliger CT, et al. Dyspnea in the ICU: an evidence-based review. *Chest*. 2009;136(5):1337-1348.

Demoule A, Hajage D, Messika J, et al. Prevalence, intensity, and clinical impact of dyspnea in critically ill patients receiving invasive ventilation. *Am J Respir Crit Care Med*. 2022;205(8):917-926.

Gentzler ER, Derry H, Ouyang D, et al. Underdetection and undertreatment of dyspnea in critically ill patients. *Am J Resp Crit Care Med*. 2019;199(11):1377-1384.

Hofbauer RK, Fiset P, Plourde G, Backman SB, Bushnell MC. Dose-dependent effects of propofol on the central processing of thermal pain. *Anesthesiol*. 2004;100(2):386-394.

Lee K, Burry LD, Bannon L, et al. Non-pharmacological interventions for sedation in critically ill adults: a systematic review. *BMC Critical Care*. 2016;15(1):216.

Parshall MB, Schwartzstein RM, Adams L, et al. An official American Thoracic Society statement: update on the mechanisms, assessment, and management of dyspnea. *Am J Respir Crit Care Med*. 2012;185(4):435-452.

Reade MC, Finfer S. Sedation and delirium in the Intensive Care Unit. *N Eng J Med*. 2014;370:444-454.

Schmidt M, Banzett RB, Morelot-Panzini C, Dangers L, Similowski T, Demoule A. Unrecognized suffering in the ICU: addressing dyspnea in mechanically ventilated patients. *Intensive Care Med*. 2014;40(1):1-10.

Schmidt M, Demoule A, Polito A, et al. Dyspnea in mechanically ventilated critically ill patients. *Crit Care Med*. 2011;39(9):2059-2065.

Schwartzstein RM, Campbell ML. Dyspnea and mechanical ventilation: the emperor has no clothes. *Am J Respir Crit Care Med*. 2022;205(8):864-865.

Worsham CM, Banzett RB, Schwartzstein RM. Dyspnea, acute respiratory failure, psychological trauma, and post-ICU mental health: a caution and a call for research. *Chest*. 2021 Feb;159(2):749-756.

Index

Note: *Pages followed by an "f" denote figures; those followed by a "t" denote tables.*